Musculoskeletal Infection

American Academy of
Orthopaedic Surgeons
Symposium

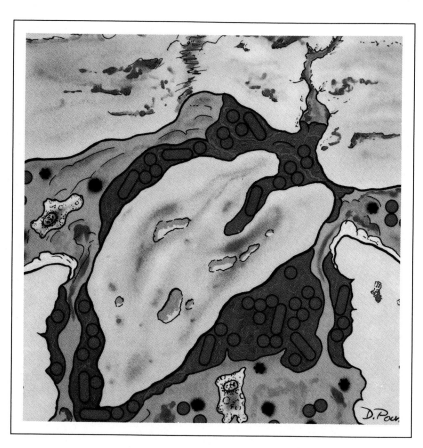

A sinus tract, the result of progressive inflammation and abscess formation, develops as the focus of a resistant infection.

Musculoskeletal Infection

Edited by
John L. Esterhai, Jr., MD
Associate Professor
Department of Orthopaedics
Hospital of the University of Pennsylvania
University of Pennsylvania School of Medicine
Philadelphia, Pennsylvania

Anthony G. Gristina, MD
President and Senior Scientist
The Musculoskeletal Sciences Research Institute
Herndon, Virginia

Robert Poss, MD
Professor of Orthopaedic Surgery
Harvard Medical School
The Brigham & Women's Hospital
Boston, Massachusetts

with 98 illustrations

Workshop
Dallas, Texas
Nov. 8–10, 1990

Supported by the
American Academy of Orthopaedic Surgeons

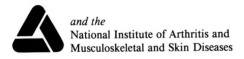

and the
National Institute of Arthritis and
Musculoskeletal and Skin Diseases

American Academy of Orthopaedic Surgeons
222 South Prospect Avenue
Park Ridge, IL 60068

American Academy of Orthopaedic Surgeons

Musculoskeletal Infection

Library of Congress Cataloging-in-Publication Data

Musculoskeletal infection/edited by John L. Esterhai, Jr., Anthony
   G. Gristina, Robert Poss; supported by the American Academy of
   Orthopaedic Surgeons and the National Institute of Arthritis and
   Musculoskeletal and Skin Diseases.
      "Workshop. Hyatt Regency, Dallas Texas, Nov. 8–10, 1990."
      Includes bibliographical references and index.
      ISBN 0-89203-053-4
      1. Musculoskeletal system—Infections—Congresses.   2. Orthopedic
   implants—Complications and sequelae—Congresses.   I. Esterhai,
   John L.   II. Gristina, Anthony G.   III. Poss, Robert.   IV. American
   Academy of Orthopaedic Surgeons.   V. National Institute of Arthritis
   and Musculoskeletal and Skin Diseases (U.S.)
      [DNLM: 1. Infection—congresses.   2. Musculoskeletal Diseases—
   microbiology—congresses.   3. Musculoskeletal Diseases—therapy—
   congresses.   4. Orthopedics—congresses.   WE 251 M985 1990]
   RC925.5M8788   1992
   616.7—dc20
   DNLM/DLC
   for Library of Congress   91-58690
                                                                     CIP

Printed in Mexico.

Contributors and Workshop Participants

David Amir, MD†
Senior Orthopedic Surgeon
Orthopedic Department, Hadassah
  Hospital
Hebrew University
Jerusalem, Israel

James M. Anderson, MD, PhD*†
Professor of Pathology
Macromolecular Science and Biomedical
  Engineering
Institute of Pathology
Case Western Reserve University
Cleveland, Ohio

Robert E. Baier, PhD†
Associate Professor
Department of Biomaterials
University of Buffalo
Buffalo, New York

Joel B. Baseman, PhD*†
Professor and Chairman
Department of Microbiology
The University of Texas Health Science
  Center
San Antonio, Texas

Bernard S. Bloom, PhD*†
Research Professor
University of Pennsylvania
Philadelphia, Pennsylvania

Tracey Bonfield, PhD†
Postdoctoral Fellow
Institute of Pathology
Case Western Reserve University
Cleveland, Ohio

Barbara D. Boyan, PhD*†
Professor and Director of Orthopaedic
  Research
Department of Orthopaedics
The University of Texas Health Science
  Center
San Antonio, Texas

Barry D. Brause, MD*†
Clinical Associate Professor of Medicine
Cornell University Medical College
New York, New York

Jason H. Calhoun, MD†
Associate Professor
Division of Orthopedic Surgery
The University of Texas Medical Branch
Galveston, Texas

Gordon D. Christensen, MD*†
Associate Chief of Staff for Research and
  Development
Harry S. Truman Memorial Veterans
  Hospital
Columbia, Missouri

Jose Cobos, MD†
Orthopaedic Surgery Resident
Division of Orthopaedic Surgery
The University of Texas Medical Branch
Galveston, Texas

Thomas A. Einhorn, MD*†
Associate Professor of Orthopaedics
The Mt. Sinai School of Medicine
New York, New York

John L. Esterhai, Jr., MD*†
Associate Professor
Department of Orthopaedics
Hospital of the University of Pennsylvania
University of Pennsylvania School of
  Medicine
Philadelphia, Pennsylvania

David Eyre, PhD†
Burgess Professor of Orthopaedics &
  Biochemistry
University of Washington
Seattle, Washington

Robert H. Fitzgerald, Jr., MD*†
Professor and Chairman
Department of Orthopaedic Surgery
Wayne State University School of
  Medicine
Detroit, Michigan

Jeffrey S. Gelb, BS†
Medical Student
University of Pennsylvania School of
    Medicine
Philadelphia, Pennsylvania

Layne O. Gentry, MD*†
Clinical Professor of Medicine,
    Microbiology, and Immunology
Baylor College of Medicine
Houston, Texas

Ronald J. Gibbons, PhD*†
Director
Forsythe Dental Center
Boston, Massachusetts

Moses Goddard, MD*†
Assistant Professor, Surgery
Section of Artificial Organs, Biomaterials,
    and Cellular Technology
Brown University
Providence, Rhode Island

Stephen L. Gordon, PhD*
Director, Musculoskeletal Diseases
    Program
National Institute of Arthritis and
    Musculoskeletal and Skin Diseases
Bethesda, Maryland

Anthony G. Gristina, MD*†
President and Senior Scientist
The Musculoskeletal Sciences Research
    Institute
Herndon, Virginia

Ulrich Gross, MD†
Professor
Institute of Pathology
Klinikum Steglitz
Free University of Berlin
Berlin, Germany

Hans Hager, MD†
Instructor
Department of Internal Medicine
Division of Infectious Diseases
The University of Texas Medical Branch
Galveston, Texas

Magnus Hook, PhD*
Professor of Biochemistry
University of Alabama at Birmingham
Birmingham, Alabama

Harriet Williams Hopf, MD*†
Fellow, Department of Anesthesia
University of California, San Francisco
San Francisco, California

Mark C. Horowitz, PhD*†
Associate Professor
Department of Orthopaedics and
    Rehabilitation
Yale University School of Medicine
New Haven, Connecticut

Thomas K. Hunt, MD†
Professor of Surgery
University of California, San Francisco
San Francisco, California

Robert L. Jilka, PhD†
Department of Medicine
Section of Endocrinology and Metabolism
Indianapolis Veterans Administration
    Medical Center
Indianapolis, Indiana

Aruna Khare, PhD†
Senior Research Scientist
Department of Orthopaedics
The University of Texas Health Science
    Center
San Antonio, Texas

Jack E. Lemons, PhD*†
Director of Orthopaedic Surgical Research
University of Alabama at Birmingham
Birmingham, Alabama

Craig L. Levitz, BA†
Medical Student
University of Pennsylvania School of
    Medicine
Philadelphia, Pennsylvania

Rob Roy MacGregor, MD*†
Professor of Medicine
University of Pennsylvania School of
    Medicine
Philadelphia, Pennsylvania

Jon T. Mader, MD*†
Acting Chief
Division of Infectious Diseases
The Marine Biomedical Institute
Galveston, Texas

Tom Marshall, DDS†
Wilfred Hall Medical Center
University of Texas
School of Health Care Sciences
San Antonio, Texas

Stephen J. Mathes, MD†
Professor and Head
Division of Plastic and Reconstructive
    Surgery
University of California
San Francisco, California

Katharine Merritt, PhD*†
Associate Professor
Department of Biomedical Engineering
Case Western Reserve University
Cleveland, Ohio

Anne E. Meyer, PhD*†
Principal Research Scientist
Industry/University Center for Biosurfaces
University of Buffalo
Buffalo, New York

Brent R. W. Moelleken, MD*†
Chief Resident in Surgery
Department of Surgery
University of California
San Francisco, California

C. Müller-Mai, MD†
Institute of Pathology, Klinikum Steglitz
Freie Universität Berlin
Berlin, Germany

Quentin N. Myrvik†
Vice-President and Senior Scientist
The Musculoskeletal Sciences Research
    Institute
Herndon, Virginia

Paul T. Naylor, MD, PhD*†
West Knoxville Orthopedic & Sports
    Medicine Clinic
Knoxville, Tennessee

Carl L. Nelson, MD*†
Professor and Chairman
Department of Orthopaedic Surgery
University of Arkansas for Medical
    Sciences
Little Rock, Arkansas

Carl W. Norden, MD*†
Executive Director
Anti-Infectives
Lederle Laboratories
Medical Research Division
Pearl River, New York

Michael J. Patzakis, MD*†
Professor and Interim Chairman
Department of Orthopaedic Surgery
University of Southern California
School of Medicine
Los Angeles, California

Steve A. Petersen, MD†
Assistant Professor
Department of Orthopaedic Surgery
Wayne State University School of
    Medicine
Detroit, Michigan

William Petty, MD*†
Professor and Chairman
Department of Orthopaedics
University of Florida College of Medicine
Gainesville, Florida

Robert Poss, MD*
Professor of Orthopaedic Surgery
Harvard Medical School
The Brigham & Women's Hospital
Boston, Massachusetts

Cheryl L. Puskarich, PhD†
Adjunct Assistant Professor
Department of Orthopaedic Surgery
University of Arkansas for Medical
    Sciences
Little Rock, Arkansas

Lawrence C. Rosenberg, MD*†
Professor of Orthopaedic Surgery
Albert Einstein College of Medicine
Bronx, New York

Vincent Ruggiero, BS†
Medical Student
University of Pennsylvania
School of Medicine
Philadelphia, Pennsylvania

David J. Schurman, MD*†
Professor and Acting Head, Division of
    Orthopaedic Surgery
Stanford University School of Medicine
Stanford, California

Zvi Schwartz, DMD, PhD†
Senior Lecturer
Department of Periodontics
Hebrew University-Hadassah
Faculty of Dental Medicine
Jerusalem, Israel

Jona Sela, DMD†
Professor of Oral Pathology
Hebrew University-Hadassah
School of Dental Medicine
Jerusalem, Israel

W. Andrew Simpson, PhD†
Associate Career Scientist
Department of Veterans Affairs
University of Missouri
Columbia, Missouri

R. Lane Smith, PhD*†
Associate Professor of Research
Division of Orthopaedic Surgery
Stanford University School of Medicine
Stanford, California

Larry D. Swain, DDS, MS†
Assistant Professor
Department of Orthopaedics
The University of Texas Health Science
    Center
San Antonio, Texas

Victor V. Tryon, PhD†
Assistant Professor in Microbiology
Department of Microbiology
The University of Texas Health Science
    Center
San Antonio, Texas

Andreas F. von Recum, DVM, PhD*†
Professor and Head
Department of Bioengineering
Clemson University
Clemson, South Carolina

Joseph L. Whalen, MD, PhD†
Illinois Southwest Orthopedics
St. Elizabeth's Hospital
Granite City, Illinois

Alfred S. Windeler, DDS, PhD†
Clinical Professor
Division of Biomaterials
The University of Texas Health Science
    Center
San Antonio, Texas

Kazuhiro Yamaguchi, MD†
Research Associate
Institute of Pathology
Case Western Reserve University
Cleveland, Ohio

Nicholas P. Ziats, PhD†
Assistant Professor of Pathology
Institute of Pathology
Case Western Reserve University
Cleveland, Ohio

---

* Workshop Participant
† Contributor to this volume

Contents

Contents

Section Four   **Host Defenses**

Section Five   **Therapeutics**

Preface

Despite moderate success, there remain not infrequent, and all too often serious, complications associated with orthopaedic trauma care and reconstruction secondary to musculoskeletal sepsis. No topic is of more current interest than infection. The complexity of bone, cartilage, soft tissue, and biomaterial interaction in the face of infection provides a significant number of unresolved issues.

Despite the advent of new antibiotics; trauma, osteomyelitis, and arthroplasty grading systems; and improved knowledge concerning microbial adhesion and biomaterial-centered infections, there is an ongoing need for focused, interdisciplinary research and maximum interaction between scientists and clinicians if patient care is to be improved.

The recent publication of texts devoted to orthopaedic infection and the space allotted to the topic in the Academy's *Orthopaedic Knowledge Update, Instructional Course Lectures,* and review courses are indicative of the impact of musculoskeletal infection on society. And yet, much of the relevant basic science work is being performed and presented outside the orthopaedic community. Only one of the 48 sessions at the Orthopaedic Research Society meeting in March 1991 was devoted to infection. By comparison, 37 papers presented at the recent Interscience Conference on Antimicrobial Agents and Chemotherapy (ICAAC) involved musculoskeletal sepsis and related antibiotic development.

The closed workshop from which this book was derived was held in Dallas, Texas, from November 8 through 10, 1990. The specific goals were: (1) to achieve a state-of-the-art understanding of the mechanisms involved in the pathogenesis of musculoskeletal sepsis; (2) to address chemotherapeutic and surgical treatment regimens; (3) to identify the most appropriate directions and questions for ongoing research; (4) to provide a forum for the interchange of ideas among physicians and scientists from various disciplines; (5) to develop collaborative relationships for future research; and (6) to provide a reference book, in a timely fashion, that would compile the information discussed at the workshop and make it available both for the participants and for the scientific community.

The participants at this workshop attempted to integrate current basic science knowledge concerning musculoskeletal infection with the persistent problems faced by clinicians and to identify points of confusion and incomplete understanding. The presentations were outstanding and the discussions were sophisticated, spirited, and intellectually stimulating. Because of enthusiastic participation and diligent work by all concerned, future directions for research based on these data and conclusions have been suggested and should result in new strategies and tactics for improving both our knowledge and clinical outcomes.

The format included didactic lectures and Gordon conference-type discussions during the day. In the evening, small group workshop discussions focused on the directions for future research. Meals were shared together on site, which allowed additional time for interchange. The final session of the conference was devoted to presentations by the rapporteurs and group leaders and to discussion of the research suggestions that had been developed and refined throughout the lectures, earlier discussions, and small group workshops.

The invited participants included basic scientists and clinicians, each of whom had agreed to provide abstracts of their presentations prior to the meeting. Many were able to provide initial drafts of their chapters at that time. The chapters of this book represent the information discussed during their presentations, the exchange of ideas during the discussions that followed each presentation, and the recommendations of the breakout sessions designed to define future questions for directed research activity.

Obviously, the scope of musculoskeletal infection cannot be covered in an encyclopedic fashion during a three-day workshop designed in part to define future research goals. With that understanding, we divided the subject into five broad topic areas, each with multiple subsections. The chapters of this book are grouped into sections that deal with these topic areas.

The first section was designed to help scientists from multiple disciplines understand the problem of musculoskeletal sepsis from what for them would be new points of view. The section leader was Barry Brause. Bernard Bloom presented the topic of the economics of health care and the impact, morbidity, and cost to society, medicine, and government of musculoskeletal infection. Anthony Gristina introduced the concept of the molecular mechanisms of sepsis. Michael Patzakis and Brause helped the basic scientists appreciate the surgeon's and infectious disease physician's perspective of the problem.

The second section, led by Joel Baseman, focused on the microorganisms responsible for the problem. Gram-positive organisms and the pathogenesis of staphylococcal infection were presented by Gordon Christensen. Gram-negative and polymicrobial infections were discussed by Katharine Merritt. Microbial adhesion in the arthritides, emphasizing mycoplasma and the spirochetes causing Lyme disease and syphilis, was covered by Baseman. Ronald Gibbons detailed the work from the dental field on bacterial adhesion. David Schurman and Lane Smith discussed bacterial biofilm and infected biomaterials, prostheses, and artificial organs.

Section three, led by Andreas von Recum, involved interface and matrix interactions—the biochemistry of adhesion to biomaterials and tissue. Jack Lemons presented the requirements and rationale for choosing metals, polymers, and ceramics for surgical implants. Barbara Boyan detailed the response of bone-forming cells to ceramic surfaces in vitro and in vivo. Anne Meyer discussed the effect of surface properties on biologic adhesion and the macromolecular films that are formed on biomaterial surfaces after implantation. The importance of surface microtexture to a favorable tissue response was highlighted by von Recum. Lawrence Rosenberg explained the relevance of proteoglycans and collagens of the extracellular matrix of articular cartilage to the pathogenesis of septic arthritis. Moses Goddard closed this section with a report on his research to bypass the host immune system working with bioartificial neural prostheses.

Section four focused on host defense mechanisms and was led by William Petty. In the first presentation of this section he reviewed the humoral and cellular mechanisms of immune defense. James Anderson then discussed the biocompatibility of biomedical polymers. The third discussion, by Mark Horowitz and Thomas Einhorn, focused on the effect of endotoxin on bone cell function, allograft incorporation and fracture repair. In the last chapter of this section, Rob Roy MacGregor discussed the immunocompromised host, identifying diseases and therapies that impair normal host defense mechanisms.

Section five, chaired by Layne Gentry, addressed therapeutic issues. Brent Moelleken presented information on the effect of growth factors on wound healing and the adverse effects of poor wound vascularity on neutrophil function. Harriet Hopf discussed the role of oxygen supply and nutrition in wound repair and infection. Gentry discussed antibiotic therapy. Jon Mader defined the issues surrounding the use of antiseptics. Carl Norden explained the clinical applications of the lessons learned from animal models of musculoskeletal sepsis. John Esterhai offered thoughts on the treatment of intra-articular sepsis. Robert Fitzgerald explained the pharmacokinetics of antibiotics in normal and osteomyelitic bone. Carl Nelson discussed the effect of patient nutritional status on clinical treatment outcome.

The individual chapters in this volume address specific issues. There is the promise of great future success. We stand on the verge of understanding cartilage and chondrocyte metabolism and articular cartilage repair. The day will come when we will not have to lament that the reparative, regenerative capacity of articular cartilage is limited. We will comprehend the mechanism by which infection adversely affects fracture healing. Biomaterial integration with human tissue will have been accomplished. We will be able to target and spend our health care resources wisely.

The workshop accomplished the desired objectives. There was valuable communication between clinicians and basic scientists. The participants learned a great deal from each other, actively made plans to collaborate on new work, and left the meeting with renewed vigor. No attempt was made to prioritize questions for future research. The workshop did call attention to the myths and shortcomings of current therapeutic methods.

The workshop and the preparation of this text took a great deal of time from normal duties and family. The reward was the opportunity to learn from outstanding physicians and scientists. I hope that this text will provide not only a review but also a stimulus to basic science and clinical research programs. I pray that a similar meeting just a decade hence will demonstrate exciting progress in our understanding of and our ability to prevent and defeat musculoskeletal sepsis.

This volume is dedicated to the Creator, who gives life and wisdom, and to mentors at home and at work.

JOHN L. ESTERHAI, JR., MD

Acknowledgments

The intellectual stimulus and the funding for this workshop and publication were provided by the National Institute of Arthritis and Musculoskeletal and Skin Diseases (NIAMS) of the National Institutes of Health and the Advisory Committee on Research of the American Academy of Orthopaedic Surgeons. We would like to thank the participants from NIH and the Academy who contributed unselfishly to the completion of the project.

Special thanks must be made to Stephen L. Gordon, PhD, the Director of the Musculoskeletal Diseases Program at NIH, for his commitment to and encouragement of the project.

Both the workshop and this publication are visible proof of the priority that the Board of Directors and membership of the Academy place on excellence in research, education, and patient care. Marilyn L. Fox, PhD, assistant director, publications, helped to organize the workshop and ensure timely publication. Bruce Davis, senior medical editor, managed the publications project and edited the manuscripts. Loraine Edwalds and Monica Trocker handled book production, and Geraldine Dubberke did the word processing. Karen Schneider, the workshop coordinator, helped to organize and plan the workshop.

Everyone associated with this workshop was saddened by the loss of Wendy Schmidt, the Academy's senior editor from 1987–1991, who died in May 1991. Wendy had initiated the editing of the manuscripts for this book as she had for prior symposia published by the Academy. She was a tireless, superbly skilled editor, who could make the roughest of manuscripts a polished work.

Lastly, we express our deep appreciation to the physicians and scientists who generously contributed their expertise and time. Their enthusiasm for their work, willingness to accept additional assignments, and openness to share not only their work but also their ideas and theories at the workshop and here in print made the symposium a scientific success. Their friendship and good humor made it a pleasure.

JOHN L. ESTERHAI, JR., MD
ANTHONY G. GRISTINA, MD
ROBERT POSS, MD

Section One

Microorganisms

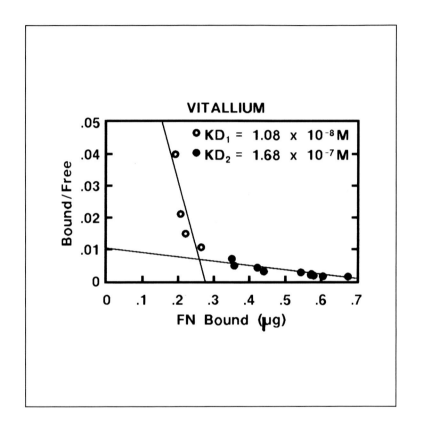

Introduction

John L. Esterhai Jr, MD

The first chapter in Section I deals with the economic impact of musculoskeletal infection on society, medicine, and government. Economics is the study of the apportionment of scarce resources among alternative ends. After a brief discussion of the laws of economics and the effectiveness of the marketplace, Bloom and I emphasize that the criteria necessary for a market to operate effectively have been lacking in the health industry.

In an attempt to determine the financial impact of musculoskeletal infection, we searched for information concerning the deleterious effects of infection complicating total hip arthroplasty, open reduction and internal fixation of long bone fractures, and arthritis. When compared with the data available on the anatomy, biochemistry, bioengineering, microbiology, pharmacology, physiology, and surgical techniques related to these orthopaedic problems, there is little information on the financial impact of infection. An extensive search of the literature failed to turn up the kinds of well-designed, controlled studies that are the basis of scientific advances in other aspects of medicine.

The cost of health care in the United States has risen to $1.23 billion dollars per day, and yet little money is allocated to study epidemiology, economics, outcomes, and quality-of-life issues for patients. Outcome studies will help patients and their physicians validate what we do and how we do it. The authors support initiatives to evaluate health care cost issues, emphasize prevention, and renew our dedication to research and innovation. If leaders of the orthopaedic community do not define and address the questions, others will.

In the second chapter, Gristina, Naylor, and Myrvik present a thorough introduction to the concept of molecular mechanisms of biomaterial-centered sepsis. The fundamental mechanism is microbial colonization of synthetic implants and damaged tissues. The authors introduce the concept of the biophysics of adhesion, explaining that the process is modulated by the host environment and the chemical composition of the implant. The successful integration of the implant requires molecular bonding of the host's cells to the implant surface. Conditioning films and matrix proteins direct subsequent events, both qualitatively and quantitatively. Because gram-positive and gram-negative bacteria have multiple adherence proteins and attachment mechanisms, a single strategy to block bacterial adherence is not possible.

Once bacteria have become adherent, they change phenotypically and become much harder to eradicate. Biofilm produced by the bacteria and the chemical composition of the biomaterial itself affect the organism's sensitivity to antimicrobial drugs. Thus, there is a race between eukaryotic host cells and bacteria to colonize and adhere to the implanted surface. The challenge presented to the physician and scientist is to identify and develop those matrix proteins that will specifically direct host cell adherence, while not serving as ligands for the receptors on the surfaces of bacterial cells.

The primary objectives of the orthopaedic surgeon are to restore function and to prevent infection. Chapter three, written from a surgical perspective, discusses the classification of open fractures and the care of patients with open traumatic wounds. Patzakis raises the controversial issues of primary wound closure, timing of soft-tissue transfer, and problems with secondary contamination. Infections complicating the internal fixation of fractures and the surgeon's dilemma of whether to retain or remove the hardware are discussed. Adequate debridement of traumatic injuries and a thorough, thoughtful approach to postoperative infections are emphasized. Stability has a positive effect on the treatment of infection in the presence of an ununited fracture. Appropriate fixation and dead space management are called for if the surgeon is to be successful.

In the final chapter of section I, Brause introduces the important issues surrounding antibiotic therapy. He provides an overview of the infectious disease approach to the diagnosis, prevention, and treatment of musculoskeletal infection. Antibiotic selection, at first empiric, is refined on the basis of initial laboratory findings of organism type and antibiotic sensitivity. After the definitive regimen is designated, its effectiveness must be confirmed. Antibiotics penetrate living bone, hematoma, and vascularized soft tissue. There is no indication that they penetrate large bony sequestra or fibrotic scar. Implantable delivery systems have been developed to provide a high local concentration of antibiotics with a minimum of systemic side effects. The timing and duration of antibiotic therapy are addressed, as is the effectiveness of newer oral agents. Lastly, the author presents the provocative issue of the use of prophylactic antibiotics in patients with prosthetic devices who must undergo subsequent procedures that will produce bacteremia. The rationale for attempting to protect such patients includes: the significant morbidity associated with a prosthetic joint infection; the fact that patient population, bacteria, and procedures associated with bacteremias are identifiable; and the belief that such procedures can cause prosthetic joint infections. The author supports the development of appropriate regimens.

Chapter 1

Musculoskeletal Infection: Impact, Morbidity, and Cost to Society, Medicine, and Government

Bernard S. Bloom, PhD
John L. Esterhai, Jr, MD

Introduction

Economics is the study of the apportionment of scarce resources among alternative ends. Generally, money is used to allocate means among objectives. Those who have money get the resources; those who do not, do without. Anyone who understands this relationship has captured the essentials of economics. Everything else is elaboration on this central theme.

Like all intellectual endeavors, economics has its own maxims. To ignore these ultimately places the enterprise in peril. The first law of economics is that all resources are limited: nothing is infinite or free. This is most especially and poignantly being driven home to us as we grapple with environmental issues of clean air and water. We have presumed that by not paying for or affixing a monetary value for air, that it is free. We are paying a high price for allowing air pollution to continue. It is not only noxious but unhealthy. The estimated financial burden to improve air quality causes consternation. The amount of money required to reduce the current levels of pollution by even a small amount seems disproportionately great.

The second law of economics is that all resources have alternative uses. Different products can be produced with the same raw materials. For example, the basic inputs of land, labor, capital, and management skill can be used to produce many different products and services. However, if these resources are used to produce one product, such as military hardware, the same resources cannot be used to produce surgical instruments.

The third law states that people have different wants. If a population decides that they want more medical care services, they cannot use those same resources for public transportation, police protection, or vacation spending. If they decide to allocate more money for the medical care of the indigent, they cannot use the same resources to further basic science research. Their wants and desires are collectively expressed in the goods and services that are purchased. If resources were without limit and free of charge, we would not have to make choices, but, by definition, resources are limited. We must choose. We have had little to guide us in making strategic health care choices. In most other economic markets, money determines who gets the resources or the product of the combination of resources. The medical market has not been thought to work like markets for other goods and services. Money has not been the major key that allowed entry to the medical marketplace as it has for other markets.

Certainly one can ask, "What does the economic market really do?" First, the market allocates resources in the most efficient manner possible. Second, it uses money as the medium of exchange by which resources are allocated and the outputs of goods and services are purchased. Third, it helps provide a way to determine value. Assessing value is simply relating the costs, usually defined in terms of money, to the outcomes, which can be defined, at least in health care, as lives saved, hospitalization prevented, physical, social, and psychological function improved, or patient satisfaction increased.

At the same time, there are economic criteria for defining the competitiveness and efficiency of a market. It is only in the competitive market that the forces of supply and demand play out so that the greatest value is obtained for the money or resources spent. The more economic criteria that are met within a market, and the more competitive it is, the more likely it is that the greatest value will be achieved by the largest number of people. Five basic criteria define an economically competitive market. (1) There must be many suppliers, e.g., physicians. (2) No supplier can affect the price. (Is this true in medical care? Can any physician charge, to a great extent, what he or she wants?) (3) There must be substitutability of products. This criterion is not met in medical care. It is difficult to substitute an antibiotic for a cast in the treatment of a fracture of the ulna. (4) There must be easy access to and exit from the market. It takes at least twelve years after completion of high school for a physician to be ready for independent practice. The specific training required to become a physician or nurse makes it extremely difficult to transfer those skills to another field. (5) Perfect information has to be available to both the purchaser and the seller. In medical care the physician has a near monopoly on information. The patient has limited information, often culled from the popular press. The patient often comes to a physician at a time of great physical or emotional stress, reducing the likelihood of making a rational decision.

The economic criteria needed for the market to operate effectively have been lacking in the health industry. This has reduced the impact of the laws of economics on medical care. To a large extent this explains the reasons for the uncontrolled rise in health care costs in all Western countries. Whether these costs are too high or not high enough is another issue. The economists would always ask, "Too high relative to what alternative or to what outcome?"

Frequency and Costs of Musculoskeletal Infection

What do we know about the economics and outcomes of the treatment of musculoskeletal infection? We will use three examples; total hip replacement; open reduction and internal fixation of a long bone fracture; and treatment of septic arthritis. We will examine these conditions with special reference to epidemiology, economics, and quality-of-life issues.

Data were obtained from three sources. First, an extensive review of existing literature was undertaken to obtain information pertinent to our objectives. Second, data on hospital and physician payment and length of stay for each entity were obtained from a study of inpatient Medicare recipients at the Hospital of the University of Pennsylvania. Third, a separate analysis of increased costs and increased length of hospital stay caused by infection in patients with the above medical problems was done by MediQual Systems, Inc., Applied Research Division, Worcester, MA.

Hip replacement

In 1987 approximately 135,000 total hip replacements were performed in the United States. Nearly 70% involved patients 65 years of age and older (fewer than 7% were younger than 45; fewer than 24% were between 45 and 64). Nearly two thirds were provided to women.[1]

Overall mortality for hip replacement is approximately eight per 1,000.[2] Therefore, we can calculate that, of the 135,000 patients who received replacement hips in 1987, approximately 1,080 died. From a study of Medicare patients at the Hospital of the University of Pennsylvania, we know that the mean length of stay is 9.5 days for hip replacement. Payments by Medicare, including hospital, surgeon, anesthesiology, and other payments, averaged nearly $15,000 per patient admission. Among patients younger than 65 years of age, mean length of stay was 9.8 days, and payment by their insurers averaged $11,806 per hospitalization.

Wound infection occurred at the rate of nine per 1,000 in primary procedures and 30 per 1,000 for secondary procedures.[3] Unfortunately, because we do not know the ratio between primary and subsequent procedures, we cannot determine the number of people with deep wound infection following total hip replacement. Standard treatment for deep wound infection following total hip replacement involves hospitalization for removal of the infected device followed by six weeks of intravenous antibiotic therapy, which is provided at home, if possible. Eisenberg and Kitz[4] estimated the direct medical cost for the antibiotics to be $1,972 in 1986. Medical care inflation between 1986 and 1990 would have increased this to a minimum of $2,537. A subsequent readmission for reimplantation of a new total hip is required, followed by extended rehabilitation.

A study by Cushner and Friedman[5] estimated the indirect costs of hip replacement in 1988. A total of $121 million was attributed to work loss by the patient and $147 million to work loss of the significant other. The bulk of these costs occurred during the period of recuperation, those months following the actual surgical procedure and hospitalization. This was particularly noteworthy for the losses sustained by the homemaker; 94.8% of the loss occurred during the recuperative

Table 1 Open reduction of fractures of the long bones with internal fixation*

	No. of Patients	Male (%)	Female (%)	Age (%)		
				<45	45–64	65+
Humerus	32,000	46.9	53.1	56.3	21.9	21.8
Radius and ulna	38,000	55.3	44.7	65.8	18.4	15.8
Femur	163,000	36.2	63.8	15.3	10.5	74.2
Tibia and fibula	117,000	55.6	44.4	58.1	25.6	16.3

*No. of patients = 350,000; year of study, 1987.

period. Total work loss was relatively small because more than two thirds of the patients requiring hip replacement are over the age of 65 years. Most of these patients do not work for remuneration outside of the home.

Open reduction of long bone fractures with internal fixation

Approximately 350,000 long bone fractures occur annually in the United States (Table 1).[1] Except for fractures of the proximal femur at the hip, most occur nearly equally in males and females.

We cannot estimate with any certainty how many people sustain fractures annually. We do not know how many of the 350,000 fractures occur as multiple fractures in the same patient. Mortality, though, is 18 per 1,000 per annum in these cases.[6] The rate of infection differs with the type of fracture, varying from 10 per 1,000 population for Gustilo type 1 fractures to over 25% of all patients with type 3 fractures.[7]

On average, patients stay 5.8 days in the hospital. The average cost of the hospital stay for a Medicare patient undergoing internal fixation for long bone fractures is $8,240. Most people with long bone fracture with internal fixation are under 65 years of age, and the cost of their medical care is $6,164 per admission, with each stay lasting a mean of 5.9 days. However, infection increases the cost of care by 20.5% per patient and increases the hospital stay by a mean of 2.1 days (36.2%) per hospitalization.

Recent work at the University of Arkansas has helped to define the cost of complications in patients with long bone fractures. Puskarich and Nelson have documented a 16% increase in cost when complications develop. The average length of hospital stay was 12 ± 6 days for patients without an infection and 26.5 ± 13 days for patients who developed a wound infection. Their calculations suggest that the national yearly cost secondary to infection in the treatment of long bone fractures is $271 million.

Septic arthritis

Septic arthritis is a classic example of a low frequency, high consequence event. It strikes approximately 19,000 patients each year, of whom nearly two thirds are male, and more than 60% are younger than 45 years of age.[1] More than one patient out of four with septic arthritis is less than 15 years of age. Septic arthritis has a high rate of untoward consequences with an annual mortality of 90 per thousand. More than 1,710 people died in 1987 from complications associated with this diagnosis.[8] There is an overall rate of complication related to septic arthritis of 190 per 1,000 or a total of 3,610 in 1987.[8] Among those over 60 years of age, 52% have a serious complication (2,470 people in 1987).[9] Thus, although the young are disproportionately affected by septic arthritis, it is mainly those over the age of 60 who suffer the high rates of complications, as shown by the fact that the average hospital stay for Medicare patients with septic arthritis at the Hospital of the University of Pennsylvania is 5.8 days, at an average cost to Medicare of $9,799.00. The average stay for patients younger than 65 years is 3.8 days, and their insurers pay $5,588 per hospitalization.

Discussion

This study sought to determine how much is known about the epidemiology, economics, and outcomes of musculoskeletal infection complicating the care of patients with total hip arthroplasty, open reduction with internal fixation of long bone fractures, and septic arthritis. The answer, unfortunately, is that rather little is known, especially when compared with the principles of microbiology, anatomy, bioengineering, physiology, biochemistry, pharmacology, and the surgical techniques used in their care. We found very few data on outcomes: physical, social, psychologic, and cost. Additionally, we have essentially no information on value, which relates the inputs of treatment to the outcomes of care. For example, there is little information on the exact ratio of primary to secondary or tertiary hip replacement other than information culled from the personal experience of clinicians. The indirect effects of infection on hip replacement, open reduction of long bone fracture, and arthritis in terms of work loss and the need for early disability retirement for patients and significant others are unknown. These costs—work loss and disability—are generally many times the costs of diagnosis and treatment for these entities. We could find no quantitative studies of disease treatment and its effects on pain, depression, or anxiety. We could find no information on the duration of and expenditures for rehabilitation and nursing home care following acute treatment or the long-term effects of rehabilitation on physical, social, and psychological activities of daily living. This does not mean that these data do not exist. Rather, our extensive search of the literature and discussions with other knowledgeable people in the field did not turn up the kinds of well-designed, controlled studies that are the basis of any scientific studies in medicine.

The Honorable Mark Hatfield, the presidential guest speaker at the 58th Annual Meeting of the American Academy of Orthopaedic Surgeons, held in March 1991, stated that between 1980 and 1988 health care costs in the United States increased 117%, which represents 11.5% of the gross national product.[10] In 1950 health care cost $1 billion per month. In 1990 the sum was $1.23 billion per day.

Probably less than 5% and more likely less than 2% of research funds in orthopaedics are devoted to epidemiology, economics, and quality of life of patients with musculoskeletal disease. It would be easy to call for more research funds to increase the number of investigators who deal with these important deficits, but we all know that large increases in funding will not be available over the next few years at the least. The economists would then ask, "Where are we to get the money to answer these questions? What are we willing to substitute in order to broaden the research agenda in orthopaedics? To which areas will new funds be devoted?" Ultimately, the question becomes, "What array of answers do we need now?"

Outcome studies will help patients and physicians decide together about care by validating what we do and how we do it. Each of us will need to work to improve quality of care and to help assess quality assurance. Provider quality means that our credentials are measured against objective criteria. Institutional quality measures the quality of hospitals against standards such as clinical outcomes. Service quality measures whether access to care and timeliness meet standards. Clinical quality measures whether care is appropriate and produces the desired outcome. Perceived quality measures how those who receive care view their care. We need to begin to place emphasis on outcomes rather than processes of care. The outcomes measured should be those important to patients.

The needs of the patient, profession, and payer do not necessarily conflict. Rather, they can be complementary. However, leaving the decisions to the payers, whether government or private insurers, will tend to lead to a skewed view in which the emphasis will be on keeping costs as low as possible, perhaps ignoring issues of value, access, quality, and equitability for patients and providers. Health care is a limited resource. Money, technology, and manpower are limited resources. Senator Hatfield suggested (1) elevating health care and health care cost issues to a strategic and national focus equivalent to that given to Defense; (2) emphasizing prevention; and (3) renewing the emphasis on research and innovation.

References

1. *National Hospital Discharge Survey 1987, Detailed Diagnoses and Procedures.* U.S. Public Health Service, Series No. 13 DHHS Pub. No. (PHS) 89–1761. Washington, DC, US Government Printing Office, 1989.
2. Mok DM, Bryant, KM: Ring uncemented plastic on metal hip replacements: Results from an independent unit. *J Royal Soc Med* 1989;82:142–144.
3. Harris WH, Sledge CG: Total hip and total knee replacements: First of two parts. *N Engl J Med* 1990;323:725–731.
4. Eisenberg JM, Kitz DS: Savings from outpatient antibiotic therapy for osteomyelitis. *JAMA* 1986;255:1584–1588.

 5. Cushner F, Friedman RJ: Economic impact of total hip arthroplasty. *South Med J* 1988;81:1379–1381.
 6. Broos PLO, Strappaerts KH, Luiten EJT, et al: The importance of early internal fixation in multiply injured patients to prevent late death due to sepsis. *Injury* 1987;18:235–237.
 7. Gustilo RB, Merkon RL, Templeman D: The management of open fractures. *J Bone Joint Surg* 1990;72A:299–304.
 8. Epstein JH, Zimmerman B III, Ho G Jr: Polyarticular septic arthritis. *J Rheumatol* 1986;13:1105–1107.
 9. Vincet GM, Amirault JD: Septic arthritis in the elderly. *Clin Orthop* 1990;251:241–245.
10. Hatfield M: The health care delivery problems as seen from Washington, DC. Presented at the 57th Annual Meeting of the American Academy of Orthopaedic Surgeons, Anaheim, CA, Mar 9, 1991.

Chapter 2

Molecular Mechanisms of Musculoskeletal Sepsis

Anthony G. Gristina, MD
Paul T. Naylor, MD, PhD
Quentin N. Myrvik, PhD

Introduction

Quite by chance, the extensive use of biomaterials and antibiotics in orthopaedic surgery has resulted in an understanding of molecular mechanisms in musculoskeletal sepsis that is providing insights for all disciplines in medicine.

Advances in medical and biomaterial sciences have led to the development of many implantable biomaterial devices, including orthopaedic plates and rods; total joints; intravenous, arterial, and peritoneal catheters; contact lenses and ocular implants; and pacemakers and artificial hearts. The design rationale for these implants is that they are constructed from biologically "compatible" or "inert" materials (metals, alloys, and polymers) of appropriate strength, corrosion resistance, and design function. Clinical experience with these implants has demonstrated not only strength and design problems, which are reasonably correctable, but also the formidable obstacles of biomaterial-centered infection and failure of implant integration into host tissues.

Biomaterial-centered infection leads to increased morbidity, cost, and possible mortality. This scenario is most dramatic in the case of the artificial heart, for which infection rates approach 100% for devices implanted for longer than 90 days. Massive infection and septic emboli are the usual cause of death.[1,2] In orthopaedic patients, an infected total joint is usually destined for a staged revision or a Girdlestone procedure to eradicate the infection, subjecting the patient to significant morbidity.[3–5]

The fundamental pathogenic mechanism in biomaterial-centered sepsis is microbial colonization of biomaterials and adjacent damaged tissues. Colonization occurs because bacteria have developed a unique and preferential ability to adhere to inanimate substrata. Microbial adhesion is basically a chemical bonding of bacterial extracapsular structures to the surface of an implant.

Failure of implant integration is indicated by tissue necrosis and inflammation at the interface between biomaterial and soft tissue or bone. This inflammatory layer is more extensive in the presence of polymers such as polymethylmethacrylate than it is in metal alloys.[6] This inflammatory interface ultimately leads to failure of soft-tissue coaptation and stability and results in pain and prosthetic failure. True integration (molecular or atomic bonding to surrounding bone or other tissues) is believed to represent homeostasis, prolonging implant life under useful loads or expected stress and decreasing the likelihood of infection.[7,8]

Failure of integration apparently allows the biomaterial's surface to serve as a substratum for bacterial colonization.[1,2] A biomaterial surface not integrated by tissue cells presents an available glycoprotein-conditioned substratum for which bacteria have specific receptors.[1,9,10]

Bacterial adhesion is as difficult to prevent as integration is to obtain because bacteria are more environmentally adaptable than eukaryotic cells. Bacteria have been shown to possess specific receptors for a number of host serum proteins and carbohydrates that coat implants and are apparently able to adhere nonspecifically to biomaterial surfaces as well.[11-14] Importantly, musculoskeletal sepsis in bone or cartilage involves the same mechanisms found in biomaterial infection.

Adherent bacteria manifest behavior that is phenotypically different from that of free-floating forms, as demonstrated by decreased susceptibility to antimicrobials.[15-17]

Thus, the challenge to biomedical engineering is to program biomaterial surfaces for host colonization or integration rather than microbial adhesion. This will be no small task.

The Biophysics of Adhesion

The in situ behavior of a biocompatible prosthesis is directed by its structure, composition, and atomic scale characteristics and by the specifics of the host environment. Implanted biomaterials are placed in a fluid environment that contains serum proteins, ions, cellular debris, matrix proteins, and, possibly, bacteria. The interaction of biomaterials with these constituents is subject to the principles of colloidal chemistry and theoretical physics.

Derjaguin and Landau[18] and Verwey and Overbeck[19] developed the so-called DLVO theory, which states that immersed objects have a tendency to draw objects to their surfaces. This theory further elaborates on the forces that draw these objects together and how this affects adhesion. The DLVO theory proposes that there are two positions of thermodynamic stability near a submerged surface in a colloidal solution. One at long range (1 to 10 mm from the surface) is composed of a variety of weak forces that attract particles, including gravitation, electrostatic attraction, chemotaxis, London-Van der Waals attraction, and surface tension. A second thermodynamic position occurs at short range (less than 1 mm from the surface) at which both attractive and repulsive forces predominate. At this point, London-Van der Waals forces and steric configurations repel particles, and hydrophobic, co-valent, hydrogen, and ionic bonding forces attract particles.

As a consequence of the counterbalancing forces present, a particle is positioned first at long range or the "secondary minimum." The positioning of particles at the "secondary minimum" is defined as adsorption and is theoretically a reversible process. Once repulsion is overcome by stronger attractive forces and the particle moves to within 1 mm of the surface, it enters the "primary minimum" and short-range attractive forces predominate. At this level, adherence is effected and the particle is essentially irreversibly bound.[1,18,20]

This entire process is modulated by the host environment and the implant's chemical composition. The native biomaterial surface be-comes coated with serum and matrix proteins on contact with the environment, changing the surface free energy of the implant.[9,10] Also, mechanical forces such as coughing, peristalsis, ciliary action, mucus entrapment, and fluid flow shear may disrupt long-range forces. The biomaterial's chemical composition dictates surface free energy and surface tension, initially influencing protein absorption. The oxide lay-ers of the biomaterial's surfaces with grain boundaries, pinhole defects, and segregation also direct binding because binding energy may be greater at these surface perturbations.[8]

Williams and Williams[21] demonstrated that the biomaterial's com-position can affect protein binding to metals with regard to spatial resolution of protein absorption on biomaterial surfaces and absorp-tion per unit area. They reported that albumin binds to pure silver, titanium, and tantalum foils at 4.34 $\mu g/cm^2$ for silver and only 0.05 $\mu g/cm^2$ for tantalum and titanium. They also demonstrated that there was heterogenicity of absorption of albumin to silver scintered with 10% titanium and tantalum. These data show albumin adhering to the silver particles preferentially. Williams and Williams also noted via contact angles that silver is less hydrophilic than titanium, which may help explain albumin binding.

Naylor and associates[22] demonstrated that fibronectin binds differ-ently to a variety of common orthopaedic biomaterials depending on the biomaterial's composition (Fig. 1). Our analysis revealed that fi-bronectin bound to the hydrocarbon polymers polymethylmethacry-late and ultra-high-molecular-weight (UHMW) polyethylene in greater quantities per unit area than to the three metals tested, although the binding constants were the same for both metals and polymers (Fig. 2).[22]

Thus, as we select materials to serve as biologic implants, we should test them for their ability to bind serum and matrix proteins that will enhance cellular integration.

Eukaryotic Cell Adhesion

The successful integration of a biomaterial implant into a host en-vironment requires molecular bonding of host cells to the biomaterial's

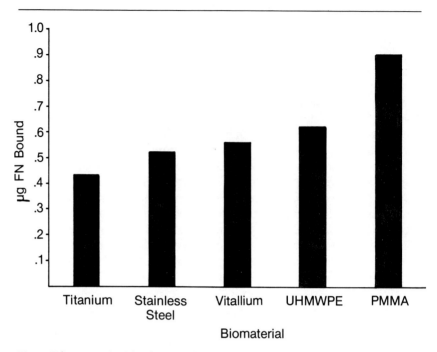

Fig. 1 *Fibronectin (FN) binding to different biomaterials (30 mg offered). UHMWPE, ultra-high-molecular-weight polyethylene; PMMA, polymethylmethacrylate.*

surface. Eukaryotic cells mediate this process through cell membrane receptors (integrins) that specifically bind to surface-adherent proteins in a typical receptor-ligand fashion.[23] This process is used daily in cell culture techniques in which plastic tissue-culture plates are coated with fibronectin or extracellular matrix proteins to establish optional growth of adherent cells. The specific coating protein used (laminin, fibronectin, collagen, or extracellular matrix material) depends on the tissue cell type to be grown, because different cell types require different matrixes for optimal growth.

The typical tissue-culture plate is made of a plastic polymer with a relatively low surface energy (20 to 30 dynes/cm), which is believed to be less adherent for cells than surfaces with greater free energies (plastics coated with proteins or some metals exhibiting surface energies of more than 40 dynes/cm).

Klein-Soyer and associates[24] have shown that plastic tissue-culture plates do not provide good adhesion and growth surfaces for human endothelial cells unless they are coated with fibronectin or chemically modified by covalently introducing nitrogen radicals to produce a positively charged surface with a surface energy comparable to extracellular matrix. Therefore, a biomaterial's chemical composition may play a central role in getting host cells to adhere to the biomaterial before bacteria do.

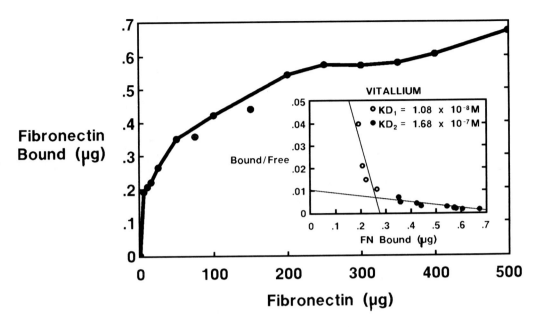

Fig. 2 *Fibronectin binding to Vitallium.*

Grinnell and Geiger[25] examined fibroblast adhesion to fibronectin-coated beads and planar glass coverslips to determine the effects of topography and hydrophobicity on eukaryotic cell adhesion. Previous reports stated that cell substratum adhesion occurs in a series of steps, beginning with cell membrane integrins binding with substratum ligands accompanied by cytoskeletal and cytoplasmic reorganization. There are two types of cellular adhesion in this process—close adhesions and focal adhesions.

Close adhesions generally occur before focal adhesions and are sufficient for cell spreading and cell motility. Close adhesions are characterized by local microfilament and α-actinin accumulation on the ventral surface of adhering cells.[25] Focal adhesions are located primarily on the margins of spreading cells and reveal microfilament bundles, vinculin plaques, tropomyosin, and α-actinin clusters. Focal adhesions increase the strength of cell attachment and limit cell mobility.

Grinnell and Geiger[25] demonstrated that focal adhesions are formed more readily on planar surfaces than on beads 16 mm in diameter. They also demonstrated that focal adhesions are more numerous and larger on planar hydrophilic surfaces than on planar hydrophobic surfaces. They suggested that the biomaterial's composition and topography can play a role in forming stable substratum complexes (that is, integration).

17

Although focal and close adhesions are necessary to keep cells bound to surfaces, their formation is preceded by specific receptor-ligand interactions mediated by membrane-bound molecules, integrins, and their corresponding substratum ligands (fibronectin, laminin, vitronectin, osteoponsatin, collagens, fibrinogen, Von Willebrand factor, and thrombospondin).

Ruoslahti and Pierschbacher[14] reviewed this specific binding process and reported that all these adhesive proteins share a common peptide sequenced arginine-glycine-aspartic acid (RGD) in their cell recognition site. These cellular receptors or integrins are a structurally similar family of transmembrane heterodimeric proteins. These authors also reported that surfaces coated with RGD peptides, like fibronectin, could promote cellular adhesion and, conversely, that RGD sequences could prevent cellular attachment to fibronectin control surfaces.

Although many extracellular matrix proteins have RGD sequences, they only react with specific integrins, possibly secondary to steric interference, as suggested by the effect of the RGD sequence containing the protein laminin on neurons. Neurons grown on laminin-coated surfaces begin to form neurites, whereas other RGD sequences containing matrix proteins cannot elicit such a response.[14]

Further evidence for RGD protein-integrin specificity is demonstrated by the genetic defect in Glanzmann's thrombasthenia in which 6pIIb/IIIA are missing from the patient's platelets. These platelets fail to aggregate, creating bleeding problems.[14]

Unfortunately, this binding mechanism is also subject to use by parasites and bacteria secondary to their environmental adaptations. The syphilis spirochete and trypanosomes have been reported to recognize fibronectin in a RGD-dependent fashion.[12,14] Thus, simple precoating of a biomaterial with extracellular matrix proteins to enhance integration may also invite opportunistic pathogens. Unfortunately, the more we learn about cellular adhesion mechanisms, the more we find that bacteria are using these same processes.

The Bacteria

Bacteria are a diversified group divided into two large classifications, gram-positive and gram-negative organisms. Within each of these major categories, there are a number of different genera and species. All have short reproduction times, allowing significant changes in genetic and phenotypic expressions. Thus, when studying bacterial adhesion mechanisms, one should expect multiple mechanisms and great variability in their expression.

Generally, well-known pathogens such as *Staphylococcus aureus*, *Pseudomonas aeruginosa.* and *Escherichia coli* are commonly involved in biomaterial- and musculoskeletal-centered sepsis. However, when bacteria adhere to surfaces, phenotypic changes occur that appear to affect virulence. These changes may help explain a unique aspect of biomaterial-centered infection, the transformation of normally com-

Table 1 Adherence of coagulase-negative staphylococci to biomaterial disks

Biomaterial	Organisms (Log 10 CFU/Disk)*		
	S epidermidis	*S hyicus*	*S hominis*
Stainless steel	6.33	5.95	5.33
UHMW polyethylene	6.70	6.34	5.28
PMMA	7.60	6.60	5.92

*Organisms were allowed to adhere to the biomaterials for 24 hours. CFU, colony-forming units; UHMW polyethylene, ultra-high-molecular weight polyethylene; PMMA, polymethylmethacrylate.

mensal, autochthonous bacteria to apparently virulent pathogens.[1,26] For example, although *Staphylococcus epidermidis* is normally a common nonpathogenic saprophyte of human skin, it has emerged as a serious causative organism in biomaterial-related and nosocomial infections, especially in immunosuppressed patients.[27] Several strains of *S epidermidis* produce the extracellular polysaccharide slime that is believed to be associated with virulence.[1,13,26] *P aeruginosa* is the most frequently identified cause of corneal keratitis associated with extended-wear contact lenses.[28]

The literature on bacterial adherence to biomaterials shows binding to be very species specific. Ludwicka and associates[29] reported that staphylococcal strains bind to various polymeric surfaces in a strain-specific fashion with regard to surface hydrophobicity and ionic and hydrogen bonding. Hogt and associates[30] presented data indicating that *S epidermidis* species bind more readily to hydrophobic surfaces than to hydrophilic surfaces (polytetrafluoroethylene-co-hexafluoropropylene versus cellulose acetate), again noting a species specificity.

Data from our laboratory reveal that binding of *S epidermidis* strains to stainless steel, UHMW polyethylene, and polymethylmethacrylate is influenced by the biomaterial's composition and the organism's ability to elaborate an extracellular polysaccharide. Three species of *S epidermidis* adhered more to polymethylmethacrylate than to the other biomaterials (Table 1).[17] The production of an exopolysaccharide slime by the organism also increased adherence to the biomaterials by one order of magnitude. Knox and associates[31] demonstrated that when the culture environment for a single species of *Streptococcus* was altered by changing the culture nutrients, pH, and surface hydrophobity, adherence varied so much that no correlation could be made between surface hydrophobity and adherence. The differences seen with different growth conditions in their study were attributed to the organism's ability to change phenotypically with local environmental conditions. This same process is relevant to treating biomaterial-adherent organisms with antibiotics, because the environment on a biomaterial surface is different from the environment a bacterium encounters when floating free in a liquid medium, thereby causing phenotypic changes between free and adherent organisms in otherwise similar nutrient conditions.[15-17]

Conditioning Film and Matrix Proteins

The above-mentioned studies were of bacteria adhering to biomaterials in vitro under very defined conditions and are not directly applicable to in vivo settings in which an implanted biomaterial is almost immediately coated by host serum and matrix proteins, ions, cellular debris, and carbohydrates. This initial coating or conditioning film also directs subsequent events in cellular adhesion both qualitatively and quantitatively. As a consequence, much attention has been directed toward bacterial adherence to serum and matrix proteins. Fibronectin-bacteria interactions have been extensively studied as have collagen-, fibrinogen-, and laminin-bacteria interactions.[13,32-35]

Fibronectin is a ubiquitous 440–kd serum and matrix protein that has many functions, including cell-to-cell attachment, cell adherence to surfaces, and clot stabilization.[36] It enhances chemotaxis and is important in directing embryogenesis and nerve regeneration. Fibronectin enhances macrophage and neutrophil activity.[36] Kuusela[37] was the first to report that fibronectin binds S $aureus$ when the bacterium has developed mechanisms for adhering to serum and matrix proteins. Since then, many investigators have reported fibronectin binding to a variety of bacterial species and surfaces, exhibiting saturation kinetics and apparent association constants in the range of 10^8 to 10^9 M (Fig. 2).[22] Recent reports have shown that bacterial binding to fibronectin occurs at RGD sequences in the fibronectin molecule. Proctor[36] reported a correlation between bacterial invasiveness of clinical isolates of S $aureus$ and fibronectin receptors per bacterium, further implicating fibronectin as a ligand for bacterial adherence.

Vaudaux and associates[33] reported that polymethylmethacrylate coverslips implanted subcutaneously in guinea pigs for four weeks specifically bound S $aureus$ and that this binding could be inhibited by antibodies to fibronectin and by trypsin treatment, indicating fibronectin's role in the in vivo coating of biomaterials and subsequent bacterial adherence. Oga and associates (unpublished data/personal communication, August, 1990) showed that biomaterials implanted into the peritoneal cavities of mice that receive S $epidermidis$ inoculations several days later develop adherent organisms. Noteworthy in this study is the effect biomaterials have on the number of bacteria adherent per unit (Table 2). Their data show that polymethylmethacrylate binds significantly more bacteria than titanium, ceramics, or hydroxyapatite, indicating a biomaterial-specific quantitative adherence. This may be related, in part, to polymethylmethacrylate's ability to bind more fibronectin than the other biomaterials.

Reports also indicate specific staphylococcal adherence to fibrinogen, laminin, collagen, and fibrin. Vercellotti and associates[23] presented data indicating that gram-positive organisms can bind fibronectin, laminin, and type IV collagen, whereas gram-negative organisms cannot, indicating different binding mechanisms or protein receptors for the gram-negative organisms. This contrasts with a report by Speziale and associates[38] that provided evidence that E $coli$ adheres to laminin.

Table 2 Adherence of *S. epidermidis* (SE-46) to biomaterials in a mouse peritoneal cavity

No. ($\times$ 10⁴) of Bacteria*	Biomaterials			
	Ceramic†	Hydroxyapatite	Polymethylmethacrylate	Titanium
Experiment 1				
No. on biomaterial	81	275	10,510	16
No. in cavity	136	1,390	760	219
Adhesion ratio	0.496	0.173	13.8	0.74
Experiment 2				
No. on biomaterial	173	229	2,920	195
No. in cavity	802	1,861	608	1,640
Adhesion ratio	0.216	0.123	4.8	0.19
Experiment 3				
No. on biomaterial	1,049	192	28,068	515
No. in cavity	6,280	329	861	2,510
Adhesion ratio	0.167	0.584	32.6	0.205
Experiment 4				
No. on biomaterial	301	809	9,839	759
No. in cavity	1,099	5,120	460	2,582
Adhesion ratio	0.274	0.158	21.4	0.294
Experiment 5				
No. on biomaterial	588	97	14,048	230
No. in cavity	2,013	110	1,006	630
Adhesion ratio	0.292	0.882	14.0	0.365
Experiment 6				
No. on biomaterial	242	3,421	20,937	243
No. in cavity	510	5,175	691	3,001
Adhesion ratio	0.470	0.061	30.3	0.081
Experiment 7				
No. on biomaterial	1,195	1,619	6,037	25
No. in cavity	1,376	7,612	78	191
Adhesion ratio	0.867	0.213	77.4	0.131
Average				
No. on biomaterial	519	949	13,204	283
No. in cavity	1,745	3,085	638	1,539
Adhesion ratio	0.397	0.401	27.75	0.156

*Adhesion ratio = the number of bacteria bound to biomaterial divided by the number in the peritoneal cavity. All experiments were done in triplicate.
†Aluminum oxide.

There is a great deal of species diversity, however, which may explain the different results obtained by these laboratories. Simpson and associates[32] have shown that the gram-positive *Streptococcus pyogenes* they studied bound fibronectin via lipoteichoic acid, which uses a different receptor site on the fibronectin molecules than does *S aureus*. This indicates that the fibronectin molecule has multiple binding sites for different bacterial receptors.

Gram-negative and gram-positive bacteria are structurally different, which accounts for their different adherence mechanisms. Gram-negative bacteria have an outer lipopolysaccharide layer that gram-positive organisms lack, and they display proteinaceous structures called pili and fimbriae that extend from the organism. Pili and fimbriae specifically bind the cellular proteins, matrix proteins, and glycolipids.

The different binding domains for gram-positive and gram-negative organisms can be beneficial for humans, as demonstrated by Abraham and associates.[13] These authors presented data on bacterial colonization of the oropharyngeal cavity by *S pyogenes*, a gram-positive component of the normal flora, via fibronectin on the epithelial cell surface. When the buccal epithelial cells become devoid of fibronectin, they allow adherence of pathogenic gram-negative organisms, indicating that fibronectin may play a protective role in modulating oropharyngeal ecology.

It appears that gram-positive and gram-negative organisms have multiple adherence proteins and many mechanisms for use with a variety of serum, cellular, and human matrix proteins. These mechanisms are species and environment specific and are easily modulated so that a single strategy to prevent bacterial adherence to biomaterials is not possible.

Bone as Substratum

Bone is a composite structure composed of calcium hydroxyapatite crystals and a collagen matrix. Calcium phosphate crystals (45 $\times$ 29.9 $\times$ 3 nm) are formed in plates between collagen fibrils. The collagen organic matrix is arranged as three noncoaxial helical polypeptides composed principally of proline, hydroxyproline, glycine, and alanine. Proline-rich proteins seem to act as ligands for bacterial adhesion.[39] Traumatized bone is devoid of normal periosteum and blood supply, exposing collagen protein matrix and acellular crystal faces to which bacteria may bind. Bone sialoprotein may also act as a ligand for bacterial receptors in osteomyelitis.[40]

Cartilage and Intra-Articular Surfaces

Recent studies indicate that the pathogenesis of intra-articular sepsis is based on the ability of certain strains of staphylococci to bind preferentially to a cartilage matrix.[41,42]

Microscopic examination of infected joints in humans and in a rabbit model indicated that bacteria predominantly colonized cartilaginous and not synovial surfaces.[42] These findings support the biochemical identification of collagen receptors on the surfaces of strains of *S aureus*. The acellular articular cartilage surface (lamina obscurans) offers no resistance to colonization by *S aureus*. Several strains of *S aureus* produce collagenase, which, along with host-originated inflammatory products, is probably the main cause of progressive cartilage destruction. The mechanisms involved in bacterial adhesion to collagen epitopes in articular sepsis and to collagen in osteomyelitis may also be relevant to allograft infections or to the addition of collagen and hydroxyapatite to the surface of a biomaterial. Binding by collagen receptors is inhibited by a synthetic peptide (proline-glycine-proline) similar to the collagen epitope.[42,43]

Biofilm-Bacterial Survival and Antibiotic Resistance

Bacteria adhere to surfaces as a survival mechanism. In their adherent state they can form microcolonies that become enshrouded in an extracellular matrix of polysaccharides, ions, nutrients, and other environmental constituents. Quantitative studies of natural ecosystems have established that 99% of bacteria exist in adherent biofilm microcolonies.[1] Previous reports have also shown that both human and other natural biofilm microcolonies are usually populated by more than one species of bacteria. In natural environments, bacteria in biofilms have been shown to be resistant to antagonists, predator organisms, antibiotics, and biocides.

Biofilm has been postulated to protect the bacteria and to act as a virulence factor.[44,45] The extracellular polysaccharide matrix can function like an ion exchange resin, concentrating valuable metabolic nutrients and ions within the microcolony. It has also been reported to inhibit macrophage activity.[46] Some bacteria use capsular polysaccharides as adhesion molecules. The biofilm may also aid in intercellular communication and transfer of genetic material.

Although bacterial adherence and the subsequent development of an extracellular biofilm may function to protect the organisms, this is not the only factor involved in the increased virulence of bacteria adherent to biomaterials. Adherent organisms are routinely more resistant to antibiotics than their planktonic forms when assayed in identical culture mediums. This is not a reflection of the antibiotic's ability to reach the organism, because bacteria that produce and those that do not produce exopolysaccharide both display this phenomenon. Initially, it was proposed that the biofilm impeded antibiotic penetration into the microcolony; however, studies suggest that resistance is based on phenotypic changes in surface-adherent colonies.[47,48] Nichols and associates[47,48] have shown that antibiotics penetrate the exopolysaccharide matrix and that a diffusion barrier does not exist.

Recent reports also suggest that resistance to antibiotics may also be explained by increased levels of betalactamase within the biofilm when certain bacterial species are present.[49]

Data from our laboratory indicate that the biomaterial also affects the organism's sensitivity to antimicrobial drugs (Table 3).[15] Three species of coagulase-negative staphylococci were analyzed for the minimum inhibitory concentrations and minimum bactericidal concentrations of several antibiotics while growing free in suspension or adhering to three different biomaterials, stainless steel, UHMW polyethylene, and polymethylmethacrylate. Several significant trends were noted. First, all three organisms were more resistant to antimicrobials when adhering to polymethylmethacrylate than when adhering to stainless steel.[16] This effect was not related to exopolysaccharide production because all three organisms displayed this phenomenon whereas only *S epidermidis* (RP-12) is a significant exopolysaccharide producer. *Staphylococcus hominis* (SP-2) is a nonproducer and *Staphylococcus hyicus* (SE-360) produces only minimal quantities of slime. Thus, the elaboration of slime did not correlate with increased antibiotic resistance.

We also studied the effect that exposure time to antibiotics at concentrations well above minimum inhibitory concentration levels had

Table 3 Antibiotic sensitivities

Organisms	Antibiotic (MBC in μg/ml)			
	Nafcillin	Daptomycin	Vancomycin	Gentamicin
S hominis				
Suspension	0.5	1	8	16
Stainless steel	8.0	1	16	32
UHMW polyethylene	0.5	16	8	32
PMMA	128.0	16	64	128
S. hyicus				
Suspension	0.5	2	16	2
Stainless steel	8.0	16	16	32
UHMW polyethylene	8.0	16	32	32
PMMA	>256.0	32	128	64
S. epidermidis				
Suspension	0.5	2	8	256
Stainless steel	128.0	2	32	256
UHMW polyethylene	>256.0	32	32	>256
PMMA	>256.0	16	32	>256

*Organisms were allowed to adhere to the biomaterials for 24 hours before exposure to antibiotics for 24 hours. MBC, minimum bactericidal concentration, UHMW polyethylene, ultra-high-molecular-weight polyethylene; PMMA, polymethylmethacrylate.

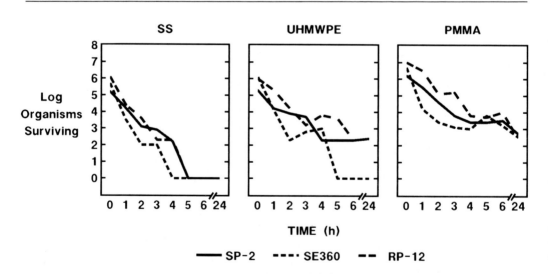

Fig. 3 *Killing kinetics of Daptomycin (16 μg/ml) against coagulase-negative staphylococcal species. Organisms were allowed to adhere to the biomaterials for one hour before exposure to antibiotics for various times. Surviving adherent organisms are shown for each exposure time. SS, stainless steel; UHMWPE, ultra-high-molecular-weight polyethylene; PMMA, polymethylmethacrylate. (Reproduced with permission from Naylor PT, Myrvik QN, Gristina A: Antibiotic resistance of biomaterial-adherent coagulase-negative and coagulase-positive staphylococci. Clin Orthop 1990;261:126–133.)*

Table 4 Adherence of *Staphylococcus epidermidis*

Experiment	No. of Bacteria (CFU/Disk)*		
	Polymethylmethacrylate	Polymethylmethacrylate With Tobramycin	Adherence Ratio
1	5.0×10^5	3.5×10^4	14.3
2	3.5×10^5	1.0×10^5	3.2
3	3.8×10^5	1.9×10^4	20.0
4	1.0×10^5	2.4×10^4	4.2
5	0.8×10^5	2.3×10^4	3.5
Average	2.8×10^5	4.2×10^4	6.9

*CFU, colony-forming units. Adherence ratio = the number of CFU adherent to polymethylmethacrylate divided by the number adherent to polymethylmethacrylate with tobramycin. (Reproduced with permission from Oga M, Arizono T, Sugioka Y, et al: The inhibition of bacterial adhesion to a tobramycin-impregnated polymethylmethacrylate substratum. *J Orthop Res*, in press.)

on the survival of biomaterial-adherent organisms (Fig. 3).[15] When all three coagulase-negative species were challenged in this fashion with Daptomycin, a cycle lipopeptide antibiotic, a definite effect was noted. None of the bacteria could be eradicated from the polymethylmethacrylate surface in 24 hours of exposure whereas all organisms succumbed to Daptomycin within several hours when adherent to stainless steel. Those data indicate that the biomaterial in some way modulates the microclimate about the biomaterial surface so that bacteria respond in a phenotypically different manner.

The experiments suggest that bacteria undergo phenotypic change when planktonic suspension organisms adhere to biomaterials and that changes are species specific and biomaterial dependent. This process is probably also modified by environmental pressures, such as nutrients, temperature, pH, and the like. Therefore, analyzing bacterial sensitivity to antibiotics in biomaterial-centered infections requires more than simple extrapolation of in vitro suspension assays.

Oga and associates[50] showed that a species of *S epidermidis* (SE-46) that is sensitive to tobramycin by standard bacterial tube dilution assay techniques readily adheres to polymethylmethacrylate disks impregnated with high concentrations of tobramycin (Table 4). In their study, adherence occurred even while the tobramycin-laden disks eluted 73.2 and 20.3 µg/ml of tobramycin during the first 24 and 48 hours, respectively, into the culture medium. This finding is relevant to the present treatment of infected prosthetics and wounds with antibiotic-laden polymethylmethacrylate beads and blocks that act as reservoirs or depots for antibiotics.

References

1. Gristina AG: Biomaterial-centered infections: Microbial adhesion versus tissue integration. *Science* 1987;237:1588–1595.
2. Gristina AG, Dobbins JJ, Giammara B, et al: Biomaterial-centered sepsis and the total artificial heart: Microbial adhesion vs tissue integration. *JAMA* 1988;259:870–874.
3. Buchholz HW, Elson RA, Engelbrecht E, et al: Management of deep infection of total hip replacement. *J Bone Joint Surg* 1981;63B:342–353.

4. Eftekhar NS: Long-term results of cemented total hip arthroplasty. *Clin Orthop* 1987;225:207–217.

5. Eftekhar NS, Nercessian O: Incidence and mechanism of failure of cemented acetabular component in total hip arthroplasty. *Orthop Clin North Am* 1988;19:557–566.

6. Kozinn SC, Johanson NA, Bullough PG: The biologic interface between bone and cementless femoral endoprostheses. *J Arthrop* 1986;1:249–259.

7. Albrektsson A: The response of bone to titanium implants. *CRC Crit Rev Biocompat* 1985;1:53–84.

8. Kasemo B, Lausmaa J: Surface science aspects on inorganic biomaterials. *CRC Crit Rev Biocompat* 1986;2:335–380.

9. Baier RE, Meyer AE, Natiella JR, et al: Surface properties determine bioadhesive outcomes: Methods and results. *J Biomed Mater Res* 1984;18:327–355.

10. Baier RE: Conditioning surfaces to suit the biomedical environment: Recent progress. *J Biomech Eng* 1982;104:257–271.

11. Proctor RA: The staphylococcal fibronectin receptor: Evidence for its importance in invasive infections. *Rev Infect Dis* 1987;9(suppl 4):S335–S340.

12. Thomas DD, Baseman JB, Alderete JF: Enhanced levels of attachment of fibronectin-primed *Treponema pallidum* to extracellular matrix. *Infect Immun* 1986;52:736–741.

13. Abraham SN, Beachey EH, Simpson WA: Adherence of *Streptococcus pyogenes*, *Escherichia coli*, and *Pseudomanas aeruginosa* to fibronectin-coated and uncoated epithelial cells. *Infect Immun* 1983;41:1261–1268.

14. Ruoslahti E, Pierschbacher MD: New perspectives in cell adhesion: RGD and integrins. *Science* 1987;238:491–497.

15. Naylor PT, Myrvik QN, Gristina A: Antibiotic resistance of biomaterial-adherent coagulase-negative and coagulase-positive staphylococci. *Clin Orthop* 1990;261:126–133.

16. Gristina AG, Hobgood CD, Webb LX, et al: Adhesive colonization of biomaterials and antibiotic resistance. *Biomaterials* 1987;8:423–426.

17. Gristina AG, Jennings RA, Naylor, PT, et al: Comparative in vitro antibiotic resistance of surface-colonizing coagulase negative staphylococci. *Antimicrob Agents Chemother* 1989;33:813–816.

18. Derjaguin BV, Landau L: Theory of the stability of strongly charged lyophobic sols and of the adhesion of strongly charged particles in solutions of electrolytes. *Acta Physiochem URSS* 1941;14:633–656.

19. Verwey EJW, Overbeck JTG: *Theory of Stability of Lyophobic Colloids.* London, Elsevier, 1948.

20. Gristina AG, Naylor P, Myrvik Q: Infections from biomaterials and implants: A race for the surface. *Med Prog Technol* 1988;14:205–224.

21. Williams RL, Williams DF: The spatial resolution of protein adsorption on surfaces of heterogeneous metallic biomaterials. *J Biomed Mater Res* 1989;23:339–350.

22. Naylor PT, Ruch D, Brownlow C, et al: Fibronectin binding to orthopedic biomaterials and its subsequent role in bacterial adherence. *Trans Orthop Res Soc* 1989;14:561.

23. Vercellotti GM, McCarthy JB, Lindholm P, et al: Extracellular matrix proteins (fibronectin, laminin, and type IV collagen) bind and aggregate bacteria. *Am J Pathol* 1985;120:13–21.

24. Klein-Soyer C, Hemmendinger S, Cazenave JP: Culture of human vascular endothelial cells on a positively charged polystyrene surface, primaria: Comparison with fibronectin-coated tissue culture grade polystyrene. *Biomaterials* 1989;10:85–90.

25. Grinnell F, Geiger B: Interaction of fibronectin-coated beads with attached and spread fibroblasts: Binding, phagocytosis, and cytoskeletal reorganization. *Exp Cell Res* 1986;162:449–461.
26. Gristina AG, Oga M, Webb LX, et al: Adherent bacterial colonization in the pathogenesis of osteomyelitis. *Science* 1985;228:990–993.
27. Gristina AG, Kolkin J: Current concepts review: Total joint replacement and sepsis. *J Bone Joint Surg* 1983;65A:128–134.
28. Slusher MM, Myrvik QN, Lewis JC, et al: Extended-wear lenses, biofilm, and bacterial adhesion. *Arch Ophthalmol* 1987;105:110–115.
29. Ludwicka A, Jansen B, Wadström T, et al: Attachment of staphylococci to various synthetic polymers. *Zentralbl Bakteriol Mikrobiol Hyg [A]* 1984;256:479–489.
30. Hogt AH, Dankert J, Feijen J: Encapsulation, slime production and surface hydrophobicity of coagulase-negative *staphylococci. FEMS Microbiol Lett* 1983;18:211–215.
31. Knox KW, Hardy LN, Markevics LJ, et al: Comparative studies on the effect of growth conditions on adhesion, hydrophobicity, and extrracellular protein profile of *Streptococcus sanguis* G9B. *Infect Immun* 1985;50:545–554.
32. Simpson WA, Courtney HS, Ofek I: Interactions of fibronectin with streptococci: The role of fibronectin as a receptor for *Streptococcus pyogenes. Rev Infect Dis* 1987;9(suppl 4):S351–S359.
33. Vaudaux P, Suzuki R, Waldvogel FA, et al: Foreign body infection: Role of fibronectin as a ligand for the adherence of *Staphylococcus aureus. J Infect Dis* 1984;150:546–553.
34. Fröman G, Switalski LM, Faris A, et al: Binding of Escherichia coli to fibronectin: A mechanism of tissue adherence. *J Biol Chem* 1984;259:14899–14905.
35. Espersen F, Clemmensen I: Isolation of a fibronectin-binding protein from Staphylococcus aureus. *Infect Immun* 1982;37:526–531.
36. Proctor RA: Fibronectin: A brief overview of its structure, function, and physiology. *Rev Infect Dis* 1987;9(suppl 4):S317–S321.
37. Kuusela P: Fibronectin binds to *Staphylococcus aureus. Nature* 1978;276:718–720.
38. Speziale P, Höök M, Wadström T, et al: Binding of the basement membrane protein laminin to Escherichia coli. *FEBS Lett* 1982;146:55–58.
39. Gibbons RJ, van Houte J: Bacterial adherence and the formation of dental plaques, in Beachey EH (ed): *Bacterial Adherence. (Receptors and Recognition.* series B, vol 6.) London, Chapman & Hall, 1980, pp 63–104.
40. Rydén C, Maxe I, Franzén A, et al: Selective binding of bone matrix sialoprotein to Staphylococcus aureus in osteomyelitis, letter. *Lancet* 1987;2:515.
41. Gibbons RJ, Hay DI: Adsorbed salivary proline-rich proteins as bacterial receptors on apatitic surfaces, in Switalski L, Hook M, Beachey E (eds): *Molecular Mechanisms of Microbial Adhesion.* New York, Springer-Verlag, 1989, pp 143–163.
42. Voytek A, Gristina AG, Barth E, et al: Staphylococcal adhesion to collagen in intra-articular sepsis. *Biomaterials* 1988;9:107–110.
43. Speziale P, Raucci G , Visai L, et al: Binding of collagen to Staphylococcus aureus Cowan 1. *J Bacteriol* 1986;167:77–81.
44. Gristina AG, Costerton JW: Bacterial adherence and the glycocalyx and their role in musculoskeletal infection. *Orthop Clin North Am* 1984;15:517–535.
45. Gristina AG, Costerton JW: Bacterial adherence to biomaterials and tissue: The significance of its role in clinical sepsis. *J Bone Joint Surg* 1985;67A:264–273.

46. Schwarzmann S, Boring JR III: Antiphagocytic effect of slime from a mucoid strain of *Pseudomonas aeruginosa. Infect Immun* 1971;3:762–767.

47. Nichols WW, Dorrington SM, Slack MP, et al: Inhibition of tobramycin diffusion by binding to alginate. *Antimicrob Agents Chemother* 1988;32:518–523.

48. Nichols WW, Evans MJ, Slack MP, et al: The penetration of antibiotics into aggregates of mucoid and non-mucoid *Pseudomonas aeruginosa. J Gen Microbiol* 1989;135:1291–1303.

49. Costerton JW, Hoyle BD: The role of the glycocalyx in biofilm development. Presented at the International Conference on Multicellular Behavior of Bacteria in Nature, Industry, and the Laboratory, Marine Biological Laboratory, Woods Hole, Massachusetts, Oct 21–25, 1990.

50. Oga M, Arizono T, Sugioka Y, et al: In vivo colonization of surgical biomaterials by *Staphylococcus epidermidis. J Long-term Effects of Medical Implants*, in press.

Chapter 3

Microorganisms in Nature and Disease: The Surgeon's Perspective

Michael J. Patzakis, MD

Surgical Perspective

The two cardinal objectives in orthopaedic surgical procedures are to restore function and to prevent infection. Infection not only interferes with the restoration of function but often leads to increased morbidity, multiple surgical procedures, and increased socioeconomic costs. In addition, in the case of fracture healing, infection has a deleterious effect on osteogenesis by activating harmful enzymes, interfering with the differentiation of osteogenic cells, and retarding tissue maturation.

Through the use of preventive antibiotics and "clean" operating rooms, the infection rate for most surgery on noncontaminated wounds is generally accepted as being 1% or less. The infection rate in open fractures can vary from 1% to 50% depending on the type of fracture.[1-9]

Open Fractures

The management of open fractures includes taking of cultures, immediate antibiotic therapy, surgical debridement and irrigation, wound management and coverage, fracture stabilization, and, in specific cases, early bone grafting. Although surgical debridement is a well-recognized principle in the treatment of open fracture wounds, some surgeons question whether a type I open fracture requires formal surgical irrigation and debridement.

Classification of Wounds

Gustilo and associates[2-4] classified open fracture wounds into three major types, one of which has three subtypes. The rate of infection correlates directly with the type of fracture, which is based on the extent of soft-tissue damage.

A type I open fracture wound is less than 1 cm long, does not involve a crushing injury, and includes little soft-tissue damage and no significant contamination.

A type II wound is more than 1 cm long, involves little or moderate crushing, and is without extensive soft-tissue damage or loss.

A type III wound has extensive soft-tissue damage that includes muscle, skin, and neurovascular structures; often there is extensive contamination. Type IIIA open fracture wounds have extensive soft-tissue damage but the fractured bone is covered. This subtype includes a segmental or severely comminuted fracture regardless of wound size. Type IIIB open fracture wounds are associated with extensive soft-tissue loss or injury and with periosteal stripping and bone exposure. A type IIIC open fracture is one with an arterial injury that must be repaired regardless of the extent of soft-tissue damage.

It is important to point out that although gross contamination from dirt and other foreign material is apparent, extensive bacterial contamination can occur that is not apparent.

Cultures

As many as 70% of open fractures are contaminated when the initial culture is done.[9] Although both gram-positive and gram-negative organisms have been found, most of the organisms initially isolated from wounds are aerobic gram-positive cocci and aerobic gram-positive rods. Environmental contaminants such as clostridial species are more likely to be found around farms, stables, and soil.

My colleagues and I reported that infection occurred in 77 of 1,104 open fracture wounds we treated and that the infecting organism was found in the initial cultures in 51 of the 77 (66%). Of the remaining 26 infections, 18 (69.2%) occurred in type III open fractures. We believe this reflects secondary infection resulting from prolonged exposure. These findings reflect the need for early wound closure over bone.

Antibiotic Administration

Because open fractures are contaminated wounds, wide-spectrum antimicrobial agents effective against both gram-positive and gram-negative organisms should be administered. I routinely use a first- or second-generation cephalosporin in combination with an aminoglycoside. Cefamandole provides antistaphylococcal coverage and activity against strains of Enterobacter and is effective in combination with tobramycin or gentamicin.

In open fracture wounds where anaerobic contamination or vascular injury has occurred, I add penicillin. Other effective combinations include vancomycin with an aminoglycoside or with ciprofloxacin. Any antibiotic regimen that is effective against both gram-positive and gram-negative organisms will significantly reduce the infection rate.

The length of antibiotic therapy is arbitrary. My colleagues and I have used antimicrobial therapy for three days for type I and type II open fracture wounds and for five days for type III open fracture wounds. Although some wounds could be treated for shorter periods, our studies have shown that the majority of contaminated wounds require these periods of antibiotic therapy. In cases involving a secondary procedure, such as soft-tissue transfer, internal fixation, bone grafting, or any procedure involving the fracture site, an additional 72 hours of antimicrobial therapy is recommended.

Time of Soft-Tissue Transfer

Essentially all open fracture wounds are not closed primarily but are left open. For type I and type II open fracture wounds, I prescribe partial closure. This entails leaving the original wound open and closing only the portion that was extended to facilitate debridement. However, if the original wound overlies the fracture site, that portion of the original wound is closed over the fracture, and the remainder of the original wound and the wound lengthening for the purpose of debridement are left open.

Type III open fracture wounds are left open. Secondary wound closures are preferred within the first seven days. In type III open fracture wounds in which either a local muscle transfer or a free vascularized soft-tissue transfer is needed, the lowest incidence of infection and complications has been associated with wounds that were covered within the first seven days. Godina[10] reported an infection rate of 1.5% in type III open fracture wounds covered within the first 72 hours. Cierney and associates[11] reported a major complication rate of 4% in open fracture wounds covered within the first seven days and a 50% major complication rate when soft-tissue coverage was delayed until after seven days.

The most likely reason for the significant increase in the infection rate is that secondary contamination of these wounds occurs, as previously reported.[4] In addition, desiccation of the exposed bone occurs, which, together with the secondary contamination, leaves the wounds at higher risk for infection. Therefore, it is urgent to cover these wounds within the first three to seven days, provided the wound is free of infection and necrotic tissue. Otherwise, repeated debridements are advised.

Infected Wounds

Presence of Internal Fixation

Three problems that can cause infected fractures to continue to drain or to show signs of infection are nonunion of the fracture, the presence of sequestrum or dead bone, and the presence of a foreign body. The orthopaedic surgeon faced with the problem of internal fixation of an infected fracture must consider several factors, including the status of fracture healing, the location of the fracture, and the amount of time that has elapsed since fixation of the fracture. In the immediate postoperative period, if the internal fixation is needed, it should be left in place, provided that it is stable. If an intra-articular fracture has been internally fixed and the fracture is not united but the fixation is stable, then the fixation should be left in place. In cases in which fracture union has occurred, the internal fixation can be removed.

In an internally fixed infected fracture in which the internal fixation is not providing stability, it should be removed and the fracture stabilized. When plates are removed, an external fixation device should be used in its place for fracture stabilization. When an intramedullary rod is present in the face of an ununited infected fracture, it can be left in place, replaced with another rod, or replaced with an external fixation device. In certain instances, especially with femoral shaft fractures, it may be necessary to replace the intramedullary rod with another intramedullary rod following extensive surgical debridement.

Stability has a positive effect on infection in the presence of an ununited fracture. The improvement in the mechanical environment improves the biologic environment. Therefore, ununited infected fractures should be stabilized.

Gristina and Costerton[12] have reported that microorganisms grew in a biofilm or glycocalix that adhered to the surfaces of biomaterials. This exopolysaccharide glycocalix, by protecting the bacteria from host defense mechanisms and from antimicrobial therapy, can lead to resistance of treatment and persistence of infection.

Topical Antibiotic Delivery Systems

The three types of topical antibiotic systems commonly used are antibiotic-impregnated methylmethacrylate beads, antibiotic infusion pump, and high-volume, closed-suction antibiotic ingress and egress irrigation systems.

High volume closed suction antibiotic ingress and egress irrigation systems have been associated with a high incidence of secondary contamination.[13,14] My experience indicates that the longer this system is used, the more likely it is that secondary contamination with hydrophilic gram-negative organisms will occur. Because of this disadvantage, most orthopaedic surgeons have abandoned the use of this delivery system.

Perry and associates[15] advocated the use of an amikacin antibiotic infusion pump to treat chronic osteomyelitis. I have had no experience with this system. My colleagues and I have used methylmethacralate beads impregnated with gentamicin antibiotic in a multicenter study. This treatment was compared with a control group who received four to six weeks of intravenous antibiotic therapy followed by three months of oral antibiotic therapy. Gentamicin beads have been advocated by Klemm[16,17] for the treatment of chronic osteomyelitis.

Our results have been very encouraging. We have found this system to have great promise. The advantages are that it gives a high local concentration (five to 20 times that of conventional therapy), has minimal systemic effect because blood levels are low or negligible, and it has low toxicity. Also, it decreases the need for systemic antibiotic and oral therapy, decreases the length of hospitalization, and decreases the cost of treatment. When using the gentamicin beads in our prospective study, we either used no systemic antibiotics or limited their use to five days of therapy or less, and no oral antibiotics were given. The antibiotic beads do have some disadvantages. They have no effect on peripheral tissues, they are a foreign body, they require a closed wound, and their removal may require an additional surgical procedure. Also, they are not suitable for the treatment of all organisms and could cause development of resistant organisms, especially if the infection is not eradicated.

Until a more biologically degradable antibiotic system is available, we feel that gentamicin antibiotic-impregnated beads are a useful adjunct to good surgical debridement and surgical management of chronic osteomyelitis.

Dead Space Management

Bone defects are generally managed by use of muscle or soft-tissue transfers, cancellous bone grafting, or antibiotic-impregnated beads. After muscle transfers or antibiotic bead implantation for bone defects, I generally wait six weeks before performing cancellous bone grafting. Experience has shown that this time period allows infection control and decreases the risk that the bone graft will fail because of infection.

It would be advantageous to have a material with both antimicrobial and bone-stimulating properties that could be used to treat bone defects. Further research in this area may produce such a material.

Peripheral Teflon Catheters

Presently, plastic catheters are used routinely as peripheral vein conduits for the administration of fluids and medications. Contamination of these catheters has been found to increase in proportion to the length of time they are left in place. The predominant organisms isolated from the peripheral catheters are primarily those found on the skin and are considered normal flora.

Fitzgerald and associates[18] reported normal skin flora microorganisms in 21 of 49 (42.9%) infected isolates in their review of 41 infected total hips in 3,210 total hip arthroplasties. Salvati and associates[19] reported on 12 years of experience with joint reimplantation in infected hips. They reported that the normal skin flora organisms were the most common organisms causing infection.

Because it is possible that the presence of bacterial cells on a peripherally placed catheter could serve as a source for hematogenous seeding to a distant implant, Wilkins and Patzakis[20] recommended changing peripheral catheters within 24 hours to reduce the constant risk of occult bacteremia. Further attention and study is needed in this area.

References

1. Gustilo RB, Anderson JT: Prevention of infection in the treatment of one thousand and twenty-five open fractures of long bones: Retrospective and prospective analyses. *J Bone Joint Surg* 1976;58A:453–458.
2. Gustilo RB, Gruninger RP, Davis T: Classification of type III (severe) open fractures relative to treatment and results. *Orthopedics* 1987;10:1781–1788.

3. Gustilo RB; Mendoza RM, William DN: Problems in the management of type III severe open fractures: A new classification of type III open fractures. *J Trauma* 1984;24:742–746.

4. Gustilo RB, Merkow RL, Templeman D: Current concepts review: The management of open fractures. *J Bone Joint Surg* 1990;72A:299–304.

5. Patzakis MJ: The use of antibiotics in open fractures. *Surg Clin North Am* 1975;55:1439–1444.

6. Patzakis MJ, Harvey JP, Ivler D: The role of antibiotics in the management of open fractures. *J Bone Joint Surg* 1974;56A:532–541.

7. Patzakis MJ, Wilkins J, Moore TM: Use of antibiotics in open tibial fractures. *Clin Orthop* 1983;178:31–35.

8. Patzakis MJ, Wilkins J, Moore TM: Considerations in reducing the infection rate in open tibial fractures. *Clin Orthop* 1983;178:36–41.

9. Patzakis MJ, Wilkins J: Factors influencing infection rate in open fracture wounds. *Clin Orthop* 1988;243:36–40.

10. Godina M: Early microsurgical reconstruction of complex trauma of the extremities. *Plast Reconstr Surg* 1986;78:285–292.

11. Cierney G III, Byrd HS, Jones RE: Primary versus delayed soft tissue coverage for severe open tibial fractures: A comparison of results. *Clin Orthop* 1983;178:54–63.

12. Gristina AG, Costerton JW: Biomaterial-centered infections and bacterial adherence. *Infect Med* 1985;15:94.

13. Kelly PJ, Wilkowske CJ, Washington JA II: Musculoskeletal infections due to *Serratia marcescens*. *Clin Orthop* 1973;96:76–83.

14. Patzakis MJ, Dorr LD, Ivler D, et al: Early management of penetrating joint injuries. *J Bone Joint Surg* 1974;56A:1310–1311.

15. Perry CR, Davenport K, Vossen MK: Local delivery of antibiotics *via* an implantable pump in the treatment of osteomyelitis. *Clin Orthop* 1988;226:222–230.

16. Klemm K: Die Behandlung chronischer Knocheninfektionen mit Gentamycin-PMMA-Kugeln. *Unfallchirurgie* 1977;1:20.

17. Klemm K: Indikation und Technik zur Einlage von Gentamycin-PMMA-Kurgeln bei Knochen und Wechteilinfekten, in Burri C, Rutter A (eds): *Lokalbehandlung Chirurgischer Infektionen. Aktuelle Probleme in Chirurgie und Orthopedic.* Bern, Huber, 1979, vol 120.

18. Fitzgerald RH Jr, Nolan DR, Ilstrup DM, et al: Deep wound sepsis following total hip arthroplasty. *J Bone Joint Surg* 1977;59A:847–855.

19. Salvati EA, Chekofsky KM, Brause BD, et al: Reimplantation in infection: A 12–year experience. *Clin Orthop* 1982;170:62–75.

20. Wilkins J, Patzakis MJ: Peripheral Teflon catheters: A potential for bacterial contamination of orthopaedic implants? *Clin Orthop* 1990;254:251–254.

Chapter 4

Infectious Disease Perspectives on Musculoskeletal Sepsis

Barry D. Brause, MD

Introduction

Advances in medical science during the last two generations have often been marked by novel biotechnology, such as cardiac pacemaker implants and valvuloplasty, angioplasty, renal dialysis, and organ transplantation. These advances, in turn, require innovative solutions to clinical problems that would otherwise prevent the new techniques from being useful. Infection is one such problem, particularly in regard to the many treatment advances in musculoskeletal disorders.

Collaboration between clinicians and researchers from the different disciplines of orthopaedics, rheumatology, bioengineering, and infectious disease has led to the resolution of many clinical problems related to musculoskeletal sepsis. Although some principles of orthopaedics and infectious disease have been compromised in the course of clinical problem-solving, remarkably successful outcomes, such as in the treatment of prosthetic joint infections and infected fractures, as well as the development of antibiotic-impregnated acrylic cement, have resulted. Such coordination of activities among specialists should lead to further achievements. This chapter provides an overview from the perspective of the infectious disease specialist of the diagnosis, treatment, and prevention of musculoskeletal sepsis. In addition, arguments for and against prophylactic bacteremic procedures in patients with joint prostheses are presented.

Choice of Antibiotics

Antibiotic selection in the treatment of musculoskeletal infections can be separated into three stages: an initial, empiric stage followed by a definitive treatment stage and, finally, a phase of effectiveness confirmation. The type of initial therapy depends on pathogen predictability and the result of rapid diagnostic tests. A detailed patient history can identify likely pathogens in a particular setting. The patient's age and sexual activity are prime determinants in the bacteriology of septic native arthritis.[1,2] For example, staphylococci, streptococci, and *Haemophilus influenzae* account for 95% of pyarthroses in children less than 2 years of age, staphylococci cause 85% of such infections in older children and in adults more than 50 years old, and gonococci are responsible for 75% of septic joints in sexually active patients. Any history of contamination caused by trauma, penetrating wounds, recent surgery, overlying dermatitis or furunculosis is suggestive of infection by skin flora. In recent, potentially bacteremic procedures, or remote infections involving the skin, gingiva, or genitourinary or gastrointestinal tract, the microflora colonizing these reservoirs are probably involved in the patient's present illness. When bone infection develops in a patient with sickle cell hemoglobinopathy, *Salmonella* is the likely cause.

Physical examination supplements the data used to make a presumptive bacteriologic diagnosis. Sepsis limited to soft tissues, such as cellulitis, is generally caused by streptococci or staphylococci, and septic bursitis is usually staphylococcal in origin. The examination may reveal evidence of trauma or penetrating wounds, suggesting that skin flora may be causative factors. Identifying skin lesions typical of disseminated gonococcemia can be diagnostic in cases of septic arthritis. The association between any of these observations and the nature of the infection is always obvious in retrospect, but the determination of their presence and importance is critical in making an appropriate diagnosis and selecting the initial antibiotic therapy.

Further assistance in defining the pathogen involved is achieved by Gram staining available fluids or purulent material. Additional rapid diagnostic tests, including counterimmunoelectrophoresis and polymerase chain reaction techniques, identify antigens in blood, urine, and infected fluids. Counterimmunoelectrophoresis has been effective in diagnosing pneumococcal, meningococcal, and *Haemophilus* meningitis. Polymerase chain reaction methods appear to be more broadly applicable, but sensitivity and specificity both need to be refined.

The initial empiric antibiotic regimen is administered until additional clinical and laboratory data are available. Definitive antimicrobial therapy is designed on the basis of bacteriologic confirmation of the pathogen and the results of antibiotic susceptibility studies. The sensitivity of bacteria to antimicrobial agents is often determined by means of the Kirby-Bauer qualitative disk technique. Automated, microtiter, well-diluted methods have recently become popular because they provide quantitative data about the minimum inhibitory concentration. A tube-dilution technique to determine an organism's minimum bactericidal concentration is also available at many medical centers, but is labor intensive and costly. The minimum inhibitory concentration and minimum bactericidal concentration are useful in antibiotic selection because they allow quantitative comparisons of in vitro effectiveness between different antimicrobial agents and reveal how sensitive a pathogen is to a particular drug.

Converting this data to clinical use requires a knowledge of the anticipated antibiotic level in the infected tissue, which can vary markedly for different antibiotics. The minimum inhibitory concentration measures only the inhibitory (bacteriostatic) effect of the agent, whereas the minimum bactericidal concentration measures its bactericidal (killing) potency. Since the beginning of the antibiotic era, the usefulness of the bactericidal effect of antimicrobial therapy has been debated without resolution. For immunologically normal hosts with infections in tissues that allow plentiful diapedesis of phagocytic leukocytes (soft tissues and virgin joint spaces), a bacteriostatic agent may be sufficient, but, in most other circumstances, a bactericidal agent is preferred, if not mandatory. Therefore, bactericidal therapy is desirable for treating infections in osseous tissue (in which the number of phagocytes is limited), in tissue that has undergone surgery (the scar tissue interferes with diapedesis), and in infections associated with nonviable or foreign materials (such as grafts, prostheses, and acrylic cement).

Recent observations have revealed that infections associated with biofilms and biomaterials may require special studies to determine the efficacy of a particular antibiotic.[3-7] Testing for the minimum inhibitory and minimum bactericidal concentrations is performed routinely on suspensions of microorganisms in the logarithmic phase of growth. When the same bacteria are studied while they are adhering to biomaterials or during the stationary phase of growth, their resistance increases.[6] In a guinea pig model, drug potency on adherent and stationary-phase bacteria, but not the routine minimum inhibitory concentration, predicted the outcome of device-related infection.[7]

After a definitive antibiotic regimen has been designed on the basis of the previously mentioned in vitro tests, the effectiveness of the therapy should be confirmed. Serial clinical evaluations document the resolution of infections in superficial wounds and native articulations, but no physical or laboratory examination can confirm effectiveness during treatment for osteomyelitis and infected joint prostheses. However, gallium scanning techniques can determine the absence of bone infection. A gallium scan that is positive at the beginning of antibiotic therapy but negative at the conclusion of osteomyelitis treatment is reassuring, but this does not confirm the efficacy of a therapeutic regimen at the start of or during therapy. Because treatment regimens for osseous infections are protracted, costly, and potentially toxic, a test that predicts the potency of a chosen therapy is necessary. The serum bactericidal test, a labor-intensive and costly bioassay that is generally available only at medical centers, has been effective. A trough serum bactericidal test titer of 1:2 or more has been prognostically accurate in predicting eradication of infection in acute osteomyelitis and a titer of 1:4 or more predicts control of infection in chronic osteomyelitis.[8] A post-peak serum bactericidal test titer of 1:8 or more has been predictive of a successful outcome in prosthetic joint infections.[9-11] The methodology is not as yet standardized adequately, but the technique is potentially useful in prognosis and provides a means to compare the potency of two or more regimens as well as to confirm synergy or detect antagonism between antibiotics used in combination therapy.

Penetration of Antibiotics

Most intravenous antibiotics predictably penetrate soft tissue to eradicate the pathogens common in cellulitis, septic bursitis, and native joint septic arthritis.[12,13] Although synovial fluid aminoglycoside levels can vary, third-generation cephalosporins and other beta-lactam antibiotics attain very effective levels for treatment of gram-negative pyarthroses.[14]

Assessing the concentrations of antimicrobial agents in bone after systemic administration is problematic because antibiotic in the blood component of osseous tissue critically contaminates the sampling technique. If blood is cleansed from the bone too vigorously, some of the antibiotic may be siphoned from the tissue, lowering the antibiotic concentration, which in turn leads to inaccurate measurement of the antibiotic. Conversely, inadequate cleansing procedures result in falsely high levels of antibiotic in bone. Therefore, it is not surprising to find a great variability in different reports, and no standard for comparison exists. Hall and Fitzgerald[15] used isotopically labeled penicillin to measure the penetration of antibiotic into the interstitial fluid space of osteomyelitic canine bone. Their observations refuted the presence of a blood-bone barrier that controls the entrance of antibiotics into osseous tissue, and suggested that osseous levels of antimicrobial agents can be calculated from the total interstitial space concentration and from serum assays with correction for protein-binding of the specific drug.

Without a reliable technique to determine directly the amount of active antibiotic in osseous tissue, clinicians have used animal models of osteomyelitis and reports of the clinical successes and failures of various antimicrobial regimens. If important clinical decisions regarding antibiotic selection for osteomyelitis are to be made with confidence, pharmacokinetic data as well as data from animal models must be used to choose antibiotics for clinical trials in humans. Observations from these human studies would then provide the confidence needed to employ new antimicrobial agents.

Because of potential problems with bone penetration of systemically administered antimicrobial agents, various techniques have been developed to deliver antibiotics directly to the infected tissue. Antibiotics were initially used to irrigate septic joints, but this technique was associated with chemical synovitis; the potential for uncontrolled, occasionally toxic, serum levels; and superinfection.[16]

Depot administration of antimicrobials at the site of infection by means of antibiotic-impregnated polymethylmethacrylate cement or beads may be an ideal means of therapy. This technique offers protracted release of drugs, leading to high local concentrations of bioactive antibiotic, while serum levels are negligible, as seen in Table 1.[17-20] In this manner, antimicrobial potency is maximized and the risk of toxicity is minimized, producing an optimal delivery system. Antibiotic-impregnated polymethylmethacrylate has been used in exchange procedures to treat septic prosthetic joints successfully.[21,22] Similar mix-

Table 1 Pharmacokinetics of gentamicin release from polymethylmethacrylate

Site	Length of Time	Concentration (µg/ml)
Serum	0.5 hr.	1.5 to 2.0
	3 hrs.	1.0 to 1.6
	8 hrs.	0.5 to 0.9
	24 hrs.	0.1 to 0.2
Wound secretions (drainage fluid)	24 hrs.	41 to 118
Medullary bone	6 days	6 to 39
	12 days	3 to 12
	5.5 yrs.*	6.0
Cortical bone	6 days	0 to 34
	4.5 yrs.*	2.0

*Data based on a single patient.

tures of acrylic cement and antibiotic in bead form have been employed in large bone defects caused by osteomyelitis.

Implantable mechanical pumps also deliver antimicrobials directly to infected osseous tissue. These systems are designed to produce higher, more predictable, and more sustained local tissue concentrations of antibiotics than are obtained with antibiotic-loaded polymethylmethacrylate.[23] The potential for toxic serum levels is greater with this technique, but the infusion concentration can be altered easily to reduce this risk. Successful treatment of chronic osteomyelitis and septic nonunions has been reported.[24]

Duration of Antibiotic Therapy

In a soft-tissue infection, such as cellulitis, antibiotics are generally administered for ten to 14 days, a period that can be adjusted on the basis of the easily observable clinical improvement. Unfortunately, there is no opportunity to visualize or otherwise document the resolution of sepsis within joints and osseous tissue during or at the end of therapy. Although many reports have documented successful outcomes with a variety of treatment periods, there are no established minimum or maximum therapy durations for septic arthritis or osteomyelitis. Therefore, medical decisions are based on clinical judgment and a knowledge of usually successful regimens currently in use.

Native joint infections are generally treated for three to four weeks. Occasionally, longer courses of antibiotics are used in complicated cases. Gonococcal arthritis, an exception, is adequately treated in ten days. Uncomplicated acute osteomyelitis in adults usually receives four to six weeks of antimicrobial therapy, although childhood hematogenous osteomyelitis can be treated successfully in two to three weeks, depending on the pathogen. Because inadequately treated acute osteomyelitis can progress to chronic disease, it is difficult to perform the controlled studies needed to compare therapeutic courses of varying lengths. Chronic osteomyelitis can be controlled successfully with a four-week course of intravenous antibiotics (after any necessary sequestrectomy), often followed by protracted, suppressive oral therapy.

Table 2 Duration of intravenous antibiotic therapy for treatment of prosthetic joint infections

Method of Treatment	Length of Intravenous Therapy	Success Rate (%)
Exchange procedure	0	78
Re-implantation at 2 wks.	2	57
Re-implantation at 1 yr.	4	93
Re-implantation at 6 wks.	6	95

However, chronic bone infections have been treated with a variety of regimens without conclusive long-term results.

Infected prosthetic arthroplasties have been treated with several regimens with differing success rates, as seen in Table 2.[9–11,21,22,25,26] The best results are obtained with a six-week course of therapy followed immediately by reimplantation, or a four-week treatment period followed by reimplantation one year later. However, the data from these studies are not directly comparable because the patient populations were not the same and various elements in the regimens were not controlled. Therefore, treatment can be individualized by selecting the protocol that is most applicable to a particular clinical situation.

When circumstances prevent removal of an infected joint prosthesis, less successful suppressive regimens have been used. In selected patients with relatively avirulent pathogens in total hip replacements, protracted (for the life of the prosthesis) oral antibiotics preserve articular function in 63% of patients.[27] When similar suppressive oral therapy is employed in total knee replacements infected with a variety of microorganisms (both virulent and relatively avirulent), successful joint function is maintained in only 23%.[28]

The complexities of establishing adequate durations for antimicrobial therapy in bone infections are demonstrated in the many approaches used to manage infected nonunions in the presence of necessarily unremovable fixation devices. Fracture healing can be difficult when there is a coexisting infection, but infection cannot be eradicated in the presence of indwelling foreign materials. One method used to resolve this clinical dilemma is intravenous antibiotic therapy, initially given for one to two weeks to control systemic sepsis or local cellulitis, if present. Subsequently, oral therapy is used indefinitely to suppress the infection until osseous union occurs. Antibiotics are then discontinued. Approximately four weeks later, the fixation devices are removed and new cultures are obtained to reestablish the microbiologic diagnosis. At this point the fracture has healed and no foreign materials are present, allowing a routine course of antimicrobial therapy to eradicate any persistent osteomyelitis.

Prophylactic antibiotics are effective in reducing infection rates associated with orthopaedic surgery involving foreign materials.[29,30] The exact duration of prophylaxis is unknown. Antibiotic administration for a 24- to 48–hour period seems adequate, but it is possible that even shorter courses would be effective. Theoretically, a single preoperative antibiotic dose may be sufficient, but clinical studies are needed before this can be recommended.

Timing of Antibiotic Therapy

Premature institution of antimicrobial therapy can obscure the exact bacteriologic etiology of a septic process, and in some situations can make it difficult to determine if an infection is present. However, prompt administration of antibiotics can be lifesaving by reducing the spread of bacterial sepsis. Therefore, in treating acute, fulminant infections, antimicrobial therapy should be begun soon after cultures of blood and any other potentially involved fluids or tissues are obtained. Subacute and chronic infections should be fully defined, both anatomically and microbiologically, before treatment is begun. Knowledge of the tissue involved (synovium, bone) and the specific pathogen allows an appropriate therapeutic regimen to be selected. In addition, any necessary drainage or debridement procedures should be performed before antibiotics are started, in order to enhance the effectiveness of therapy and to reduce the risk of inducing resistant bacteria in sequestered and nonviable tissues.

Infections associated with open wounds represent a difficult clinical problem. Although antimicrobial therapy may stop the spread of sepsis in the exposed tissue, superinfection is more likely once antibiotics are started. Antiseptic dressings, applied locally, can prevent infection before pathogens invade wound tissue, but are ineffective in treating established infection. Wound closure should be done as soon as possible to reduce the risk of superinfection with sequentially more resistant microorganisms. Antibiotic therapy is necessary to treat most wound infections but drug therapy is not likely to be successful in a chronically open wound. In open wounds that are not definitely infected, the duration of antibiotic therapy should be limited to the period required to determine whether infection is truly present.

Delivery Systems for Antimicrobial Therapy

Intravenous Antibiotics

Bone and joint infections have been treated intravenously to provide the tissues with high levels of the antibiotic. As new oral antimicrobial agents with good enteric absorption and enhanced potency are developed, the need for parenteral treatment may decrease. Peripheral venous access is problematic with protracted intravenous therapy. As a result, central venous access devices (Broviac and Hickman-type catheters) have been designed to provide reliable long-term administration ports and reduce the risk of local cellulitis as well as chemical and septic phlebitis.[31]

Table 3 Aminoglycoside release from different polymethylmethacrylate cements

Site	No. of Hrs.	Gentamicin with Palacos	Tobramycin with Simplex
		(µg/ml)	
Hemovac	24	14.9	8.0 to 9.5
	48	10.0	5.0
Serum	24	0.06	1.1
Urine	24	0.8	4.2 to 5.0

Oral Antibiotics

Soft-tissue infections, septic bursitis, and gonococcal arthritis are easily treated with an oral antimicrobial agent.[32,33] Pediatric hematogenous osteomyelitis has recently been treated successfully with oral therapy.[34-36] Oral treatment of adult osteomyelitis has been limited; intravenous administration remains the mainstay of therapy.[37] With the advent of the quinolone group of antibiotics, potent, well-absorbed oral antimicrobial drugs are available. Early success in treating osteomyelitis with the oral fluoroquinolones, ciprofloxacin and ofloxacin, has been very encouraging.[38,39]

Suppressive antibiotic regimens for chronic osteomyelitis and certain prosthetic joint infections employ long-term oral antimicrobials. Oral therapy is also useful in special situations such as the treatment or suppression of infection in healing fractures that have undergone fixation.

Antibiotic-Impregnated Polymethylmethacrylate Cement

For antibiotic therapy to be effective, there should be high levels of antibiotic in the infected tissue and low, nontoxic levels systemically. Certain antibiotics diffuse from polymerized methylmethacrylate in vivo to produce such a situation. Pharmacokinetic studies of the release of gentamicin from bone cement show high levels of antibiotic in tissue and negligible levels in serum (Table 1).[17-20] The kinetics of the factory-homogenized cement-gentamicin mixture has been extensively evaluated, but because this product has not yet been approved by the Food and Drug Administration, a hand-mixed brand of cement impregnated with tobramycin is the most common combination in the United States. The release of different aminoglycosides from different brands of polymethylmethacrylate may vary. Table 3 illustrates the potentially significant higher and sustained serum levels observed with one brand of cement—tobramycin—compared with a different brand—gentamicin.[18,40,41] Additional studies are needed to determine which cement performs best with which antibiotic in vivo.

Antibiotic-impregnated polymethylmethacrylate has been used to treat joint replacement infections in a one-stage, prosthesis removal-reimplantation operation (exchange procedure). Although this approach is not as successful as two-stage procedures with an interval of intravenous antibiotic therapy, it requires minimum surgery and hospitalization.[21,22] The exchange procedure is successful in 78% of cases, whereas the two-stage technique is successful in 93% to 95% of patients (Table 2).[9–11,26] Additional studies are needed to determine the potential effectiveness of antibiotic-impregnated cement in the reimplantation stage of two-stage procedures.

Occasionally during therapy of infected total hip replacements, antibiotic-impregnated cement in the form of beads is placed in the femoral bone defect before reimplantation. During treatment of septic knee prostheses, joint spacers hand-molded with antibiotic-impregnated polymethylmethacrylate are occasionally inserted during prosthesis extraction to maintain the anatomic relationships in the surrounding tissues until reimplantation several weeks later. The effectiveness of these techniques has not been studied. Although these approaches provide potentially potent local antimicrobial therapy, the inserted cement (beads or spacer) acts as a foreign body adjacent to infected tissue, allowing the pathogen to remain. The usefulness of local therapy and the possible use of antibiotic-impregnated cement beads in large bone defects after sequestrectomies in osteomyelitis unassociated with prosthetic joints need to be evaluated. Problems in the clinical application of antibiotic-polymethylmethacrylate mixtures include (1) the loss of structural integrity of the cement; (2) the systemic toxicity of diffusing antibiotics; and (3) the potential for protracted hypersensitivity reactions to the sustained release of allergenic drugs.

Antibiotic Delivery by Pump Systems

Another means of achieving optimal antibiotic administration is a subcutaneous mechanical pump. An antimicrobial solution injected into the pump is transported to the distant infected tissue via tunnelled subcutaneous catheters. Specific aminoglycosides (amikacin and netilmicin) have been used in one such device for the successful treatment of osteomyelitis in a limited number of patients.[23,24] Tissue antibiotic levels are higher with this delivery system than with antibiotic-impregnated cement; however, serum levels are also higher. Potential toxic side effects from the systemic antibiotic levels can be avoided by decreasing the concentration of the infusion solution as necessary.

Provocative Issue

The Use of Prophylactic Antibiotics for Bacteremic Procedures in Patients With Joint Prostheses

Joint replacement surgery is common because of its magnificent success in restoring function to disabled arthritic individuals. Hundreds of thousands of prosthetic arthroplasties are performed annually worldwide, and millions of people have artificial joint implants.[42] Of indwelling prostheses, 1% to 5% become infected.[43] The cost of treating infected prostheses has been estimated conservatively at $40 million to $80 million per year in the United States alone.[44]

The patient faces protracted hospitalization, sizeable financial expense, and, most distressing, renewed disability.

Because of the catastrophic effects of prosthetic joint infection, prevention is important. It is wise to evaluate, before elective total joint replacement, for the presence of pyogenic dentogingival pathology, obstructive uropathy, and dermatologic conditions that might predispose the patient to infection and bacteremia. Perioperative antibiotic prophylaxis has been effective in reducing deep wound infections after total joint arthroplasty.[29,30] However, the use of prophylactic antibiotics in anticipated bacteremic events (eg, dental surgery, cystoscopy, colonoscopic biopsy, and surgical procedures on contaminated or infected tissues) remains controversial.

The rationale for recommending prophylactic antibiotics for procedures associated with substantial bacteremias is based on the accepted empiric use of preventative antimicrobials to reduce the risk of endocarditis in similar clinical settings, as outlined below:

(1) Prosthetic joint infection is associated with significant morbidity and, occasionally, death. Prosthesis removal, which is usually necessary to treat these infections, produces large skeletal defects, shortening of the extremity, and severe functional impairment.

(2) The patient population at risk is identifiable. Whereas approximately 50% of patients with underlying cardiac abnormalities at risk for endocarditis are identifiable, all patients with prosthetic articulations have a predisposition to infection.

(3) The pathogenic organisms are identifiable. Although the spectrum of microorganisms in prosthetic joint infection is far broader than that in endocarditis, the probable pathogens have been identified and are susceptible to many available antimicrobial agents.

(4) The procedures associated with bacteremia are identifiable. The procedures that place patients with joint prostheses and with intracardiac abnormalities at risk are identical.

(5) There is widespread belief that bacteremic procedures can cause prosthetic joint infection. A survey of 604 orthopaedic surgeons revealed that 67% believed a relationship exists between transient bacteremia of dental origin and prosthetic joint infection. Also, 93% recommended antibiotic prophylaxis before dental treatment for patients with prosthetic joints.[45] Animal models have proved that bacteremia can induce prosthetic joint infection.[46,47] Hematogenous infection of joint prostheses in humans has been reported.[11,48-53]

(6) It is not clear whether prophylactic antibiotics can reduce the risk of prosthetic joint infection or endocarditis. No controlled human trial has showed prophylaxis to be effective in treating endocarditis. Because of the large number of subjects required in such a study, there probably will never be an opportunity to validate effectiveness in patients with prosthetic joints. Animal models should be employed to study the relative potencies of various antibiotics in preventing hematogenous infection of joint prostheses.

As mentioned previously, the prophylactic use of antibiotics for bacteremia is not universal. The frequently stated arguments against recommending prophylaxis are outlined below:

(1) Whereas most cases of endocarditis are hematogenous in origin, a minority of prosthetic joint infections are blood-borne, and most of them are not associated with medical or dental procedures. Therefore, the risk of prosthetic joint infection represented by dental procedures, for example, is too low to justify the use of prophylactic antibiotics.

Comment: About 34% to 43% of prosthetic joints infections are hematogenous.[11,54,55] The risk of endocarditis from a tooth extraction has been estimated to be as high as 1 in 533 to as low as 1 in 115,500, or zero.[56] The risk of prosthetic joint infection from a dental procedure is also unknown, but has been estimated to be 1 in 3,333.[30] A national registry for prosthetic joint infections is warranted.

Whereas endocarditis is generally caused almost exclusively by aerobic, gram-positive cocci, joint prostheses are vulnerable to a much broader spectrum of microorganisms. Therefore, the risk of prosthetic joint infection may be substantially higher than that of endocarditis from similar bacteremic procedures. Also, the nature of dental bacteremia needs to be reexamined. Endocarditis prophylaxis is designed to reduce the risk of streptococcal bacteremia for abnormal, native cardiac valves, but *Staphylococcus epidermidis, Staphylococcus aureus,* and diphtheroids were the predominant organisms in many studies of dental bacteria.[57] It is possible that a substantial number of prosthetic joint infections caused by staphylococci and diphtheroids result from dental abnormalities and procedures. A national registry of total joint arthroplasty infections could quantitate the clinical significance of these events and provide convincing data that support the use of antibiotic prophylaxis for dental and other procedures.

(2) The potential toxicity of widespread antibiotic prophylaxis may outweigh the potential benefit.

Comment: The incidence of hypersensitivity reactions, a potential hazard, could be significantly reduced by selecting drugs other than the beta-lactam antibiotics (penicillins and cephalosporins).

(3) The financial cost of widespread antibiotic prophylaxis is not justifiable.

Comment: Cost-effectiveness and risk-benefit ratios cannot be calculated in the absence of data on the efficacy of prophylaxis. As stated previously, these data are not available and are not likely to be obtained for prosthetic joint infections or endocarditis because of the size of the study populations needed. The risk of endocarditis for any specific cardiac lesion or traumatic procedure is unknown. There have been no controlled trials showing efficacy of prophylaxis for endocarditis. The appropriateness of prophylaxis may need to be determined empirically, using the best clinical judgment.

(4) Recommendations for or against prophylaxis could create difficult medicolegal problems for the medical or dental practitioner.

Comment: This is an unfortunate issue. The American Dental Association and the American Academy of Oral Medicine have published noncommittal position papers suggesting that, in the absence of conclusive data, decisions regarding prophylaxis should be made by the individual dentists, physicians, and surgeons involved.[58,59] Separate groups of physicians (and dentists) have published their views and rationales in favor of prophylaxis with varied antibiotic regimens.[52,53,60] One solution to the present predicament would be for a multidisciplinary committee of orthopaedists, infectious disease specialists, and dentists to design prophylactic antibiotic schedules. Such recommendations could be used by those who favor preventative drugs in individual cases without supporting or rejecting prophylaxis in general. Such a committee could also meet at intervals to review current practices and modify guidelines.

It appears that the current controversy regarding the use of prophylactic antibiotics in patients with joint prostheses who are about to undergo procedures that may lead to infection will not be settled without further discussion. An animal model might help provide additional data for such discussions.

References

1. Fink CW, Nelson JD: Septic arthritis and osteomyelitis in children. *Clin Rheum Dis* 1986;12:423–435.
2. Cooper C, Cauley MID: Bacterial arthritis in an English health district: A 10–year review. *Ann Rheum Dis* 1986;45:458–463.
3. Farber BF, Kaplan MH, Clogston AG: *Staphylococcus epidermidis* extracted slime inhibits the antimicrobial action of glycopeptide antibiotics. *J Infect Dis* 1990;161:37–40.
4. Prosser BL, Taylor D, Dix BA, et al: Method of evaluating effects of antibiotics on bacterial biofilm. *Antimicrob Agents Chemother* 1987;31:1502–1506.
5. Dix BA, Cohen PS, Laux DC, et al: Radiochemical method for evaluating the effect of antibiotics on *Escherichia coli* biofilms. *Antimicrob Agents Chemother* 1988;32:770–772.
6. Gristina AG, Jennings RA, Naylor PT, et al: Comparative in vitro antibiotic resistance of surface-colonizing coagulase-negative staphylococci. *Antimicrob Agents Chemother* 1989;33:813–816.
7. Widmer AF, Frei R, Rajacic Z, et al: Correlation between in vivo and in vitro efficacy of antimicrobial agents against foreign body infections. *J Infect Dis* 1990;162:96–102.
8. Weinstein MP, Stratton CW, Hawley HB, et al: Multicenter collaborative evaluation of a standardized serum bactericidal test as a predictor of therapeutic efficacy in acute and chronic osteomyelitis. *Am J Med* 1987;83:218–222.
9. Windsor RE, Insall JN, Urs WK, et al: Two-stage reimplantation for the salvage of total knee arthroplasty complicated by infection. *J Bone Joint Surg* 1990;72A:272–278.
10. Salvati EA, Chekofsky KM, Brause BD, et al: Reimplantation in infection: A 12–year experience. *Clin Orthop* 1982;170:62–75.
11. Brause BD: Infected orthopaedic prostheses, in Bisno AL, Waldvogel FA (eds): *Infections Associated With Indwelling Medical Devices.* Washington, DC, American Society for Microbiology, 1989, pp 111–127.
12. Nelson JD: Antibiotic concentrations in septic joint effusions. *N Engl J Med* 1971;284:349–353.
13. Parker RH, Schmid FR: Antibacterial activity of synovial fluid during therapy of septic arthritis. *Arthritis Rheum* 1971;14:96–104.

14. Chow A, Hecht R, Winters R: Gentamicin and carbenicillin penetration into the septic joint. *N Engl J Med* 1971;285:178–179.

15. Hall BB, Fitzgerald RH Jr: The pharmacokinetics of penicillin in osteomyelitic canine bone. *J Bone Joint Surg* 1983;65A:526–532.

16. Argen RJ, Wilson CH Jr, Wood P: Suppurative arthritis. *Arch Intern Med* 1966;117:661–666.

17. Trippel SB: Antibiotic-impregnated cement in total joint arthroplasty. *J Bone Joint Surg* 1986;68A:1297–1302.

18. Salvati EA, Callaghan JJ, Brause BD, et al: Reimplantation in infection: Elution of gentamicin from cement and beads. *Clin Orthop* 1986;207:83–93.

19. Wahlig H, Dingeldein E: Antibiotics and bone cements: Experimental and clinical long-term observations. *Acta Orthop Scand* 1980;51:49–56.

20. Elson RA, Jephcott AE, McGechie DB, et al: Antibiotic-loaded acrylic cement. *J Bone Joint Surg* 1977;59B:200–205.

21. Buchholz HW, Elson RA, Engelbrecht E, et al: Management of deep infection of total hip replacement. *J Bone Joint Surg* 1981;63B:342–353.

22. Carlsson ÅS, Josefsson G, Lindberg L: Revision with gentamicin-impregnated cement for deep infections in total hip arthroplasties. *J Bone Joint Surg* 1978;60A:1059–1064.

23. Perry CR: Current status of local antibiotic delivery via an implantable pump. *Orthop Rev* 1989;18:626–645.

24. Perry CR, Davenport K, Vossen MK: Local delivery of antibiotics via an implantable pump in the treatment of osteomyelitis. *Clin Orthop* 1988;226:222–230.

25. Rand JA, Bryan RS: Reimplantation for the salvage of an infected total knee arthroplasty. *J Bone Joint Surg* 1983;65A:1081–1086.

26. McDonald DJ, Fitzgerald RH Jr, Ilstrup DM: Two-stage reconstruction of a total hip arthroplasty because of infection. *J Bone Joint Surg* 1989;71A:828–834.

27. Goulet JA, Pellicci PM, Brause BD, et al: Prolonged suppression of infection in total hip arthroplasty. *J Arthroplasty* 1988;3:109–116.

28. Schoifet SD, Morrey BF: Treatment of infection after total knee arthroplasty by debridement with retention of the components. *J Bone Joint Surg* 1990;72A:1383–1390.

29. Norden C: A critical review of antibiotic prophylaxis in orthopaedic surgery. *Rev Infect Dis* 1983;5:928–932.

30. Norden CW: Prevention of bone and joint infections. *Am J Med* 1985;78(suppl 6B):229–232.

31. Couch L, Cierny G, Mader JT: Inpatient and outpatient use of the Hickman catheter for adults with osteomyelitis. *Clin Orthop* 1987;219:226–235.

32. Ho G Jr, Tice AD, Kaplan SR: Septic bursitis in the prepatellar and olecranon bursae: An analysis of 25 cases. *Ann Intern Med* 1978;89:21–27.

33. Centers for Disease Control: Gonococcal infections, in *1989 Sexually Transmitted Diseases Treatment Guidelines*. Atlanta, U.S. Departmet of Health and Human Services, 1989, vol 38, pp 21–27.

34. Scoles PV, Aronoff SC: Antimicrobial therapy of childhood skeletal infections. *J Bone Joint Surg* 1984;66A:1487–1492.

35. Prober CG, Yeager AS: Use of the serum bactericidal titer to assess the adequacy of oral antibiotic therapy in the treatment of acute hematogenous osteomyelitis. *J Pediatr* 1979;95:131–135.

36. Kolyvas E, Ahronheim G, Marks MI, et al: Oral antibiotic therapy of skeletal infections in children. *Pediatrics* 1980;65:867–871.

37. Black J, Hunt TL, Godley PJ, et al: Oral antimicrobial therapy for adults with osteomyelitis or septic arthritis. *J Infect Dis* 1987;155:968–972.

38. Gentry LO, Rodriguez GG: Oral ciprofloxacin compared with parenteral antibiotics in the treatment of osteomyelitis. *Antimicrob Agents Chemother* 1990;34:40–43.

39. Gentry LO, Rodriguez-Gomez G: Ofloxacin versus parenteral therapy for chronic osteomyelitis. *Antimicrob Agents Chemother* 1991;35:538–541.

40. Turner RH, Miley GB, Fremont-Smith P: Septic total hip replacement and revision arthroplasty, in Turner RH, Scheller AD (eds): *Revision Total Hip Arthroplasty.* New York, Grune & Stratton, 1982, pp 291–314.

41. Soto-Hall R, Saenz L, Tavernetti R, et al: Tobramycin in bone cement: An in-depth analysis of wound, serum, and urine concentrations in patients undergoing total hip revision arthroplasty. *Clin Orthop* 1983;175:60–64.

42. Melton LJ III, Stauffer RN, Chao EYS, et al: Rates of total hip arthroplasty: A population-based study. *N Engl J Med* 1982;307:1242–1245.

43. Fitzgerald RH Jr: Problems associated with the infected total hip arthroplasty. *Clin Rheum Dis* 1986;12:537–554.

44. Salvati EA, Small RD, Brause BD, et al: Infections associated with orthopaedic devices, in Sugarman B, Young EJ (eds): *Infections Associated With Prosthetic Devices.* Boca Raton, CRC Press, 1984, pp 181–218.

45. Jaspers MT, Little JW: Prophylactic antibiotic coverage in patients with total arthroplasty: Current practice. *J Am Dent Assoc* 1985;111:943–948.

46. Blomgren G, Lindgren U: The susceptibility of total joint replacement to hematogenous infection in the early postoperative period: An experimental study in the rabbit. *Clin Orthop* 1980;151:308–312.

47. Blomgren G, Lindgren U: Late hematogenous infection in total joint replacement: Studies of gentamicin and bone cement in the rabbit. *Clin Orthop* 1981;155:244–248.

48. Rubin R, Salvati EA, Lewis R: Infected total hip replacement after dental procedures. *Oral Surg* 1976;41:18–23.

49. Stinchfield FE, Bigliani LU, Neu HC, et al: Late hematogenous infection of total joint replacement. *J Bone Joint Surg* 1980;62A:1345–1350.

50. Lindqvist C, Slatis P: Dental bacteremia: A neglected cause of arthroplasty infections? *Acta Orthop Scand* 1985;56:506–508.

51. Sullivan PM, Johnston RC, Kelley SS: Late infection after total hip replacement, caused by an organism after dental manipulation: A case report. *J Bone Joint Surg* 1990;72A:121–123.

52. Cioffi GA, Terezhalmy GT, Taybos GM: Total joint replacement: A consideration for antimicrobial prophylaxis. *Oral Surg Oral Med Oral Pathol* 1988;66:124–129.

53. Maderazo EG, Judson S, Pasternak H: Late infections of total joint prostheses: A review and recommendations for prevention. *Clin Orthop* 1988;229:131–142.

54. Inman RD, Gallegos KV, Brause BD, et al: Clinical and microbial features of prosthetic joint infection. *Am J Med* 1984;77:47–53.

55. Grogan TJ, Dorey F, Rollins J, et al: Deep sepsis following total knee arthroplasty: Ten-year experience at the University of Califrnia at Los Angeles Medical Center. *J Bone Joint Surg* 1986;68A:226–234.

56. Durack DT: Prophylaxis of infective endocarditis, in Mandell GL, Douglas RG Jr, Bennett JE (eds): *Principles and Practice of Infectious Diseases.* New York, John Wiley & Sons, 1985, pp 539–544.

57. Everett ED, Hirschmann JV: Transient bacteremia and endocarditis prophylaxis. *Medicine* 1977;56:61–77.

58. Eskinazi D, Rathbun W: Is systematic antimicrobial prophylaxis justified in dental patients with prosthetic joints? *Oral Surg Oral Med Oral Pathol* 1988;66:430–431.

59. Council on Dental Therapeutics: Management of dental patients with prosthetic joints. *J Am Dental Assoc* 1990;121:537–538.

60. Nelson JP, Fitzgerald RH Jr, Jaspers MT, et al: Prophylactic antimicrobial coverage in arthroplasty patients. *J Bone Joint Surg* 1990;72A:1.

Future Directions

The purpose of this section is to define the scope and impact of musculoskeletal infection from the standpoint of economics, including the epidemiology, direct and indirect costs, and quality of life issues; and from the perspective of the orthopaedic surgeon and infectious disease physician.

Classification Systems

At the present time there is no consensus on the terminology to be used in describing musculoskeletal sepsis. Several staging systems have been advocated over the years. None has been adopted by more than a few authors. Collaborative and epidemiologic studies hinge on the development of a system that would include: identification of the bone or tissue involved, location and extent of the infection within the bone or tissue, etiology, soft-tissue envelope quality, and general host status.

Epidemiology

How often does musculoskeletal sepsis occur in the United States in the absence of trauma or surgical intervention? What are the demographics of hematogenous osteomyelitis, postsurgical osteomyelitis, and septic arthritis in the 1990s? A National Registry for musculoskeletal sepsis and a uniform reporting scheme would be required to obtain the data. While many types of programs that monitor disability-causing injuries are in operation at local, state, and regional

levels, there is none for musculoskeletal infection.

Is there an increased risk to prosthetic joints from a second surgical procedure, distant infection, dental manipulation, or respiratory problem?

Economics

What does musculoskeletal infection prevention and care cost? What is the cost of orthopaedic care including hospitalization, rehabilitation, and indirect costs such as lost wages and lost earnings for personal family care givers? What is the cost/benefit ratio for adjunctive procedures such as hyperbaric oxygenation? Is the advantage of laminar air flow worth the expense in view of the other prophylactic measures taken during total joint arthroplasty?

Outcome Studies and Patient Satisfaction

Over the past decade, techniques for measuring health status, quality of life, and function have improved significantly. New functional assessments, many of which include self-administered questionnaires with excellent sensitivity and reproducibility, are able to determine the impact of musculoskeletal disorders. What are the patient's and the physician's expectations in terms of outcome in elective total joint arthroplasty? How would information concerning the risks of infection affect expectation and satisfaction? Can patient and family member quality of life be improved during the medical and surgical care of acute and chronic infection?

Orthopaedic Trauma Patient Decision Making

In the face of open fractures, under what circumstances is it safe to close the wound? How can we make it safer? Can wound debridement be performed with more precision? What is the optimal time for soft tissue transfers? Can the entity of chronic osteomyelitis be eradicated without excisional debridement? What is the role for aggressive debridement and subsequent bone replacement techniques such as allografting and distraction osteogenesis?

Infectious Disease Management of Established Infection

The optimal duration for antibiotic therapy of osteomyelitis has never been defined. If long-term suppressive therapy is the best that we have to offer, how should the dose and treatment interval be determined?

Section Two
Microorganisms and Microbial Adhesion

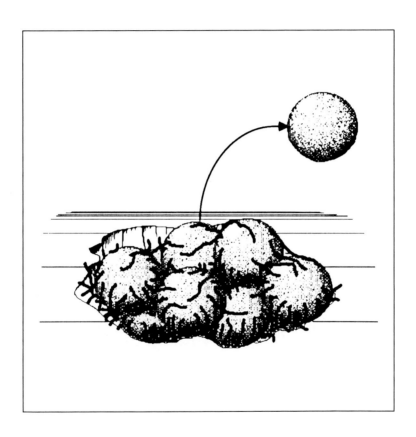

Introduction

John L. Esterhai Jr, MD
Jeffrey S. Gelb, BS

Orthopaedic infections are caused by microorganisms that include bacteria, fungi, viruses, and parasites. Much knowledge has been gained in recent years with regard to their cellular, molecular, and genetic structures and functions. It is clear that this knowledge, which continues to grow at a rapid pace, is essential for disease treatment and prevention. It is the aim of this section to present the current state of knowledge concerning some of the essential concepts in bacterial microbiology, especially those related to surgical infections. This section will make evident how much has been achieved in this area, and also what directions future research should pursue.

Bacteria are extremely complex organisms. They have traditionally been divided into gram-positive and gram-negative groups on the basis of differential staining. Gram-positive bacteria retain crystal violet dye after decolorization. Gram-negative bacteria do not. This phenomenon results from a difference in cell wall structure. Although gram-positive and gram-negative bacteria have many similarities, their differences determine some of their unique effects.

Gram-positive bacteria are protected by a cytoplasmic membrane surrounded by a cell wall composed of a peptidoglycan layer that provides rigidity and strength. The peptidoglycan structure is that of a polymer with repeating units of carbohydrates linked by peptide cross-bridges. Other cell wall components include teichoic acids, proteins, polysaccharides, and lipocarbohydrates. Many of these seem to serve simply as epidemiologic markers, at least to the best of our present understanding, whereas others, such as the M-protein in group A streptococci, provide virulence.

The cell walls of gram-negative bacteria consist of both outer and inner phospholipid bilayer membranes with an interposed peptidoglycan layer. The outer membrane, composed primarily of lipopolysaccharide, presumably serves as a protective barrier to toxins in the bacterial environment, preventing toxic compounds, such as intestinal bile salt, from entering the cell. Lipopolysaccharide, also known as endotoxin, provides virulence to gram-negative bacteria, leading to activation of the host immune system, causing fever, hypotension, and entities such as disseminated intravascular coagulopathy.

Gram-negative bacteria possess pili or fimbriae, hairlike protein structures that protrude outward from the cell surface. These pili make possible bacterial attachment to mucosal or epithelial cells on the host, thus permitting colonization and contributing to virulence.

Gram-positive and gram-negative bacteria share certain characteristics that contribute to their pathogenic potential. Capsular polysaccharide is an extremely common feature of invasive bacteria that allows them to evade nonspecific host immune responses, providing greater virulence. In fact, some bacteria that lose the ability to produce capsular polysaccharide become essentially incapable of causing disease. In the presence of encapsulated bacteria, the host must produce specific anticapsular antibodies that can be induced by natural infection or by specific vaccines such as those against pneumococci and meningococci.

The elaboration of exotoxins is another shared pathogenic characteristic. The toxin can act locally or can disseminate in the host, potentially causing systemic disease. Many of these toxins appear to stimulate or suppress host immune response, often to the benefit of the bacteria, furthering the disease process.

Antibiotic therapy revolutionized the practice of medicine during this century, allowing effective treatment of infectious diseases, especially those of bacterial origin. Antibiotics target important bacterial structural proteins or biochemical pathways that are not shared by the host cells. This difference between bacteria and host cells allows eradication of infection with little or no harm to the host. Antibiotic mechanisms of action typically focus on cell wall, protein, or DNA synthesis, altering the bacterial cell in such a way as to impair viability.

Unfortunately, with the widespread (and often injudicious) use of antibiotics, many bacteria have developed effective mechanisms of resistance.[1] This has necessitated development of new antibiotics, and in some cases has made certain infections, such as those caused by methicillin-resistant *Staphylococcus aureus*, difficult to treat. Antibiotic resistance can be either intrinsic or, more commonly, acquired. Intrinsic resistance essentially takes the form of mutations that alter antibiotic action, often by altering a binding protein critical to antibiotic effectiveness. Acquired resistance emerges in a population of bacteria previously sensitive to a given antibiotic, often by a mechanism that destroys the structural integrity of the antibiotic itself, as in the case of betalactamases and penicillin. This acquired resistance is obtained from other bacteria in the form of mobile genetic elements that include plasmids and transposons. Under selective pressure by antibiotic exposure, plasmids or transposons replicate and are transferred from resistant to sensitive bacteria, thus conveying antibiotic resistance. Of importance is that one plasmid often provides mechanisms of resistance for several antibiotics, which only serves to further complicate the problem. Essentially, bacterial resistance to

antibiotics represents a major challenge, both in clinical practice and in research.

Over the years, research has provided very detailed information about the behavior of bacteria in disease. The chapter on staphylococcal musculoskeletal infections by Christensen and Simpson defines the differences between *S aureus* and *Staphylococcus epidermidis* from both clinical and microbiologic viewpoints. Molecular characteristics of the extracellular matrix produced by *S aureus* appear critical for pathogenicity.

The next chapter, by Merritt, is devoted to gram-negative microorganisms. As a group, gram-negative bacteria are diverse, and their important, sometimes subtle, distinctions, are discussed. Special attention has been given to the interactions with both mammalian host cells and biomaterial implants. Finally, many of the specific infections seen in an orthopaedic setting are described, correlating basic science knowledge with the clinical features of gram-negative musculoskeletal infections.

Baseman and Tryon discuss mycoplasmal and spirochetal musculoskeletal infections. Special attention is given to animal models for disease, as well as laboratory analysis of these pathogens, including identification, antigen characteristics, and genetic information.

The fourth chapter recognizes the frequent presence of more than one organism in any given infection. Merritt discusses polymicrobial infections, that is, the various combinations of microorganisms, clinical situations, and mechanisms by which the organisms interact. Studies of the interrelationship of *S epidermidis*, biofilm production, and opportunistic infection with *Pseudomonas* and *Proteus* species have shown that biofilms formed by *S epidermidis* significantly increased adherence of *Pseudomonas*. Of note, the adherence of *Pseudomonas* was increased whether the biofilm was living or dead, with the greatest adherence being seen with autoclaved biofilm. Evaluation of gentamicin-impregnated polymethylmethacrylate samples showed that normal gentamicin-sensitive bacteria adhered to the specimens, and that this adherence was increased by the preincubation of the specimens with *S epidermidis* to allow formation of a biofilm.[2]

The chapter by Gibbons and Esterhai discusses adhesin-receptor interactions analogous to antibody-antigen or enzyme-substrate interactions. Adhesins, unlike most antibodies that can bind only to the terminal sequences of molecules, can also bind to internal sequences. There are three criteria for identifying an adhesin or receptor: the stereochemical-receptor interaction is saturable; adhesin receptor binding is reversible; and adhesins exhibit the same binding specificity as the bacteria. By recognizing only the novel segment of molecules, bacteria can avoid the cleansing activities of secretions and target the tissue surfaces.

The last chapter, by Schurman and Smith, defines the relationship between bacterial adherence to foreign bodies and the deposition of extracellular matrix by these bacteria.[3] In the past, investigators have found it difficult to quantify bacterial adherence and biofilm production. In this chapter, a new technique is described that quantifies extracellular matrix production by measuring the incorporation of glucose labeled with carbon 14. This information, correlated with the bacterial adherence data obtained by triated thymidine uptake microscopy, allows quantification of bacterial adherence, independent of the surfaces or materials being studied. This study concludes that the production and accumulation of biofilm is a specific characteristic of different strains of S epidermidis.[4]

References

1. Gentry LO: Bacterial resistance. *Orthop Clin North Am*, in press.
2. Chang CC, Merritt K: Effective of *Staphylococcus epidermidis* on adherence of *Pseudomonas aeruginosa* and *Proteus mirabilis* to polymethylmethacrylate (PMMA) and gentamicin-containing PMMA. *J Orthop Res* 1991;9:284–288.
3. VanPett K, Schurman DJ, Smith RL: Quantitation and relative distribution of extracellular matrix in *Staphylococcus epidermidis* biofilm. *J Orthop Res* 1990;8:321–327.
4. Barth E, Berg E, Gristina AG: Biomaterial specificity of *Staphylococcus aureus* and *Staphylococcus epidermidis* in orthopaedic infections. *Trans Orthop Res Soc* 1989;14:558.

Chapter 5

Gram-Positive Bacteria: Pathogenesis of Staphylococcal Musculoskeletal Infections

Gordon D. Christensen, MD
W. Andrew Simpson, PhD

The gram-positive bacteria have a unique predilection for infecting the musculoskeletal system. These infections include acute and chronic osteomyelitis, arthritis, myositis, and infections of implanted orthopaedic appliances. They may be spontaneous (hematogenous) in origin or secondary to contamination after accidental or surgical trauma. Common gram-positive pathogens include *Staphylococcus aureus*, the coagulase-negative staphylococci (predominantly *Staphylococcus epidermidis*), enterococci, and both aerobic and anaerobic streptococci; less common pathogens include *Clostridia, Bacillus*, diphtheroids, and *Listeria*.

Despite the variety of clinical syndromes and pathogenic etiologies, two organisms—*S aureus* and *S epidermidis*—are the preeminent pathogens of the musculoskeletal system. Although both these organisms are staphylococci, they produce entirely different clinical syndromes. Laboratory investigations during the last ten years have found major differences in the pathogenic mechanisms exhibited by the coagulase-positive and the coagulase-negative staphylococci. These different mechanisms provide a rationale for the different disease patterns exhibited by *S aureus* and *S epidermidis*. Further, these newly elucidated mechanisms also suggest new opportunities for the prevention, diagnosis, and treatment of staphylococcal musculoskeletal infections. This discussion focuses on staphylococcal virulence mechanisms and the pathogenic and clinical distinction between *S aureus* and *S epidermidis*.

Clinical Experience

S aureus is the leading individual cause of osteomyelitis[1] (Fig. 1, *left*) and nongonococcal bacterial arthritis[2] (Fig. 1, *right*). *S aureus* exhibits a remarkable tendency to infect traumatized tissue[3-5] such as wound and surgical incisions, to cause deep-tissue infections such as bacteremia, endocarditis, and abscess,[3,5] and to produce toxemia such as toxic shock syndrome, gastroenteritis, and scalded skin syndrome.[4]

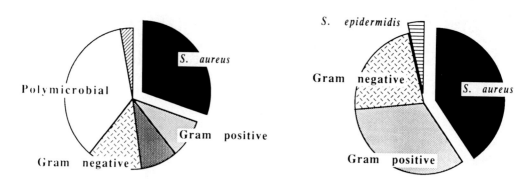

Fig. 1 *Left, Pie chart of microbial etiologies of osteomyelitis, demonstrating that S aureus is the primary cause (data from Gentry[1]). Right, A similar chart of microbial etiologies of infectious-nongonococcal arthritis, also demonstrating that S aureus is the primary pathogen (data from Goldenberg and Reed[2]).*

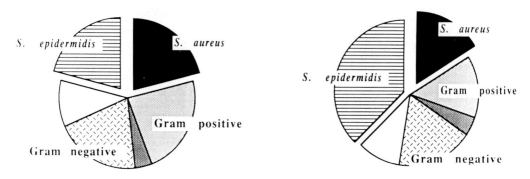

Fig. 2 *Left, Pie chart of microbial etiologies of prosthetic joint infection. Both S aureus and S epidermidis are prominent pathogens of orthopaedic devices. Right, S epidermidis is the primary etiology of prosthetic joint infections arising from contiguous foci (data from both charts is from Brause[6]).*

S aureus is also a prominent cause of prosthetic joint infection,[6] although *S epidermidis* apparently causes an equal number of such infections (Fig. 2, *left*).

When only infections arising from contiguous foci are considered,[6] *S epidermidis* causes more infections of orthopaedic devices than does *S aureus* (Fig. 2, *right*). Characteristically, *S epidermidis* virulence is essentially limited to infections of indwelling medical appliances (Table 1)[7,8] and causes more such infections than *S aureus* despite the greater tissue invasiveness of the latter. There is no immediate explanation for this distinction in virulence. It does not appear to be a function of the construction of the device, because all implanted med-

Table 1 Infections of indwelling medical devices*

Device	Most Common Pathogen	Next Most Common Pathogen
Intravascular catheters	S epidermidis	S aureus
Cerebrospinal fluid shunts	S epidermidis	S aureus
Peritoneal dialysis catheters	S epidermidis	S aureus
Aortofemoral grafts	S epidermidis	Gram-negative bacilli
Intraocular lenses	S epidermidis	S aureus
Prosthetic cardiac valves	S epidermidis	S aureus
Prosthetic joints	S epidermidis	S aureus

*Based on information in Christensen and associates.[7]

ical devices—regardless of material, design, or placement—exhibit a predisposition to infection with *S epidermidis*.[7]

Aside from the spectrum of staphylococcal infections, there is also a notable distinction in the clinical presentation of patients with *S aureus* foreign-body and deep-tissue infections and those with *S epidermidis* infections. *S aureus* characteristically causes an acute fulminant illness, with localized pain, erythema, swelling, and fever; frequently accompanied by bacteremia and systemic toxicity; and on occasion complicated by septic shock.[5] In contrast, *S epidermidis* typically causes an indolent—sometimes asymptomatic—infection. Although *S epidermidis* foreign-body infections may exhibit the signs and symptoms of an acute localized wound infection, the more common presentation is a subacute process. For orthopaedic prostheses the only initial complaint may be joint pain and the only initial finding may be loosening of the prosthesis.[8]

The indolent presentation could result from the capacity of the organisms to persist in a dormant state in wounds for a prolonged period. Dobbins and associates,[9] for example, intensively cultured 28 orthopaedic devices electively removed from 26 patients. The devices had been in place for an average of 15 months. Although none of the patients had any clinical evidence of infection, 77% of the cultures yielded bacteria, 75% of which were coagulase-negative staphylococci. Using plasmid pattern analysis, Archer and associates[10] investigated a cluster of *S epidermidis* prosthetic valve infections and determined that contamination of the valve with the infecting strain took place at the time of implantation. Clinical disease, however, was not manifested for as long as 13 months. It should be noted that on rare occasions *S aureus* may also persist in deep tissues in a dormant state. Musher and McKenzie,[5] for example, described a man who had had staphylococcal osteomyelitis for more than 15 years and whose illness was characterized by rare episodes of clinical disease interspersed with long periods (more than ten years) of quiescent disease.

Pathogenesis of Infections

Reservoir and Transmission

The primary reservoir for staphylococcal surgical infections is the patient's own skin. Both *S aureus* and *S epidermidis* are major elements

59

Table 2 Bacteria recovered from infected hip joints and from the air of a surgical suite*

Organism	Recovered From	
	Infections (% of Cases)	Air (% of Cases)
Anaerobic gram-positive cocci	40	34
Coagulase-negative staphylococci	40	97
Propionibacteria	10	26
Proteins	5	0
S aureus	24	23
Streptococci	14	0
Others	12	95

*Based on information from Lindberg.[14]

of the normal cutaneous microflora, although coagulase-negative staphylococci greatly predominate over *S aureus*.[11] Archer and Armstrong,[12] for example, cultured the skin of patients preparing for cardiac surgery; 92% of the cultures were positive and all of these yielded coagulase-negative staphylococci. Conversely, *S aureus* was recovered from the skin of only 34% of the patients.[12] Although contamination of the medical device or wound with the patient's cutaneous microflora undoubtedly takes place when the medical device is implanted, the surgical site can be contaminated with skin bacteria from other sources. It is well established that members of the surgical team can serve as sources of *S aureus* infection, and apparently they can also serve as sources of *S epidermidis* infection.[13] Cutaneous microflora from other patients and hospital staff may contaminate the surgical wound because of inadequate sterilization of the surgical instruments and equipment or by means of contaminated fluids and medications. The list of potential fomites includes air in the surgical suite, which can carry cutaneous microflora attached to floating desquamated skin particles. In one Swedish hospital, there was a remarkable concordance between bacteria recovered from infected prosthetic hip joints and bacteria recovered from the operating room air[14] (Table 2). Coagulase-negative staphylococci predominated in both sets of cultures.

Although exposure to cutaneous microflora explains part of the predilection of musculoskeletal surgical sites for staphylococcal infections, it is not the complete explanation. Other bacteria, specifically diphtheroids, micrococci, bacilli, and propionibacteria, are also prominent components of the skin microflora.[11] Nevertheless, as is evident from Figure 1, these organisms rarely cause musculoskeletal infections.

Musculoskeletal tissues are also susceptible to infection by the hematogenous route and once again the staphylococci—particularly *S aureus*—play a prominent pathogenic role (Fig. 3). We customarily distinguish between bacteremia that arises from an obvious peripheral focus, such as an abscess or contaminated intravascular catheter ("secondary bacteremia"), from bacteremia without an evident origin ("primary bacteremia"). Waldvogel and Papageorgiou[15] noted that *S aureus* caused between 60% and 90% of primary hematogenous osteomyelitis

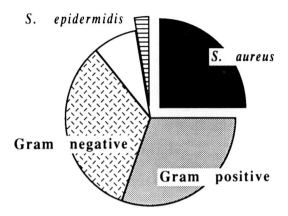

Fig. 3 S aureus *is the leading cause of prosthetic joint infections arising from a hematogenous source (data from Brause⁶).*

thought to arise from small, innocuous skin lesions.[3] These infections often occurred in previously traumatized bone.[5] Whether this represents the settling out of circulating organisms or the activation of resident but dormant deep-tissue bacteria is unclear. Coagulase-negative staphylococci also cause primary osteomyelitis,[16] but the incidence is extremely low.[14] Unlike *S aureus*, which rarely causes primary bacteremia,[3] the coagulase-negative staphylococci are frequently recovered from blood cultures of asymptomatic people. In a carefully controlled series of experiments, Zierdt[17] found *S epidermidis* in 6.8% of blood cultures, processed by the lysis-filtration technique, obtained from normal healthy blood donors; *S aureus* was not recovered from these cultures.[17] Secondary *S aureus* bacteremia leading to metastatic deep-tissue infection, including osteomyelitis and arthritis, is a relatively common complication of focal staphylococcal infections.[5] The precise frequency of this complication, however, is unknown. We now recognize that secondary bacteremia caused by coagulase-negative staphylococci can also lead to metastatic infection, including osteomyelitis and arthritis,[18,19] but these complications appear to be rare.

Musculoskeletal surgical sites are also susceptible to infection by the hematogenous route (Figs. 2 and 3). Brause,[6] reporting on prosthetic joint infections, found that the infections were contiguous in origin in 51% of cases and hematogenous in 34%; the source was unknown in 15%. *S aureus* was again the leading individual pathogen (25% of cases) with *S epidermidis* a minor etiologic agent (3% of cases). Nevertheless, the pathogenic role of the staphylococci in this situation was not as predominant as in the previously discussed clinical conditions. Gram-negative bacilli accounted for 30% of the infections and the grouping of enterococci with aerobic and anaerobic streptococci accounted for 43%. Many of these nonstaphylococcal infections were caused by secondary bacteremias from nosocomial infections or iatrogenic manipulations.[6]

Influence of the Foreign Body on the Effective Inoculum

The insertion of a foreign body into deep tissues has a profound effect on the immediate host defenses against infection. This effect is described elsewhere in this volume but can be briefly summarized as follows: Deep-tissue foreign bodies cause chronic inflammation; the chronic inflammation cripples the ability of the host to opsonize and phagocytose bacteria contaminating the surgical site. This impaired phagocytosis in turn potentiates the virulence of the contaminating bacteria, allowing small numbers of organisms to establish a foothold, resulting in infection. If the foreign body has an irregular surface or a surface that promotes bacterial attachment, the effective inoculum may be further increased by the trapping and sequestering of bacteria on the surface of the device. These individual factors dramatically reduce the minimal bacterial inoculum required to establish an infection.

This potentiating effect was demonstrated by Elek and Conen[20] in the late 1950s when they injected *S aureus* in the skin of human volunteers. They found that at least 10^6 bacteria were needed to establish an infection. When a silk suture was placed in the skin first, however, the number of organisms required to produce an infection was reduced to 100. More recently, Zimmerli and associates[21] used the relatively avirulent *S aureus* strain Wood 46, which is deficient in protein A, to challenge polymethylmethacrylate tissue cages implanted under the skin of guinea pigs. Only 10^3 organisms were required to produce an infection of the cage. When the cage was not present, however, even the injection of 10^8 bacteria failed to produce a subcutaneous infection. We reported similar results with coagulase-negative staphylococci.[22] We found that we could not produce a subcutaneous infection in mice with 10^6 organisms unless the animal had undergone subcutaneous implantation of a section of intravascular catheter. Ford and associates[23] recently reported similar results in mice with subcutaneous microcarriers.

Contrast in Virulence Factors Between *S aureus* and *S epidermidis*

Toxins and Extracellular Enzymes

Table 3 lists some of the toxins and extracellular enzymes produced by staphylococci and compares the production of these virulence factors by *S aureus* (defined as coagulase-positive staphylococci) and coagulase-negative staphylococci.[24-26] This list is incomplete and does not include many of the more recently described virulence factors, such as toxic shock toxin, for which the bacteriologic findings are poorly understood. Further, additional virulence factors that have yet to be identified almost certainly exist.

Table 3 Production of toxins and enzymes by *S aureus* and coagulase-negative staphylococci*

Substance	Produced by (% of Strains)	
	S aureus	Coagulase-Negative Staphylococci
DNAse	87	18
Fibrinolysin	90	11
Gelatinase	100	43
α-Hemolysin	43 to 95	2 to 21
β-Hemolysin	33 to 66	2 to 16
δ-Hemolysin	22 to 97	13 to 16
β-Lactamase	76	28
Leukocidin	99	1
Lipase	90 to 91	3 to 21
Phosphatase	98 to 100	20 to 52
Protease	89	13
Urease	90	13

*Based on information in Gemmell,[24] Marsik and Parisi,[25] and Selepak and Witebsky.[26]

Nevertheless, Table 3 illustrates three important points. (1) *S aureus* is a prototypic pathogen equipped with a diverse array of toxic factors for attacking the host. (2) In comparison with *S aureus*, the number of strains of coagulase-negative staphylococci that make these factors is small. (3) It is remarkable, however, that each of the virulence factors reported for *S aureus* can be made by individual strains of *S epidermidis*. Table 3 explains the fulminant toxic infections characteristic of *S aureus* and the indolent subacute infections characteristic of *S epidermidis* but does not explain the propensity for staphylococci in general to cause musculoskeletal infection or the tendency of the relatively avirulent coagulase-negative staphylococci—rather than the more virulent *S aureus*—to infect indwelling medical devices.

Antibiotic Resistance

Apparently there are few laboratory differences between *S aureus* and *S epidermidis* in regard to antimicrobial resistance. This has not always been true. Early in the antibiotic era the coagulase-negative staphylococci exhibited a greater range of antimicrobial resistance than *S aureus*; some strains had high-grade resistance.[8] By the 1980s, however, the distinction was less evident.[27] Hospital strains of both species are likely to exhibit high-grade resistance and to be multiply resistant.[27-29] The emergence of antimicrobial resistance in *S aureus* appears to have resulted in part from the acquisition of antimicrobial resistance genes from a reservoir of antimicrobial resistance in the coagulase-negative staphylococci. The transfer of genetic elements between *S aureus* and *S epidermidis* is evident from the discovery of identical gene sequences for macrolide resistance[30] and aminoglycoside resistance[27] in both organisms. The gentamicin-resistance gene is carried on a plasmid that promotes its conjugative transfer between *S epidermidis* and *S aureus*.[31]

Although *S aureus* and the coagulase-negative staphylococci exhibit similar antimicrobial resistance patterns, the organisms are quite different clinically. This clinical distinction reflects both the ubiquity of and the fundamental mechanisms peculiar to the coagulase-negative staphylococci. The clinical problem is that in patients given antimicrobial therapy—particularly antimicrobial prophylaxis—cutaneous microflora change from a generally susceptible form to multiply resistant coagulase-negative microflora.[21,32] The shift in microflora can include the supplantation of susceptible S aureus strains by resistant coagulase-negative strains.[12] The change in microflora appears to be the result of a selection for small resident populations of coagulase-negative staphylococci that happen to be resistant to the administered antibiotic, followed by overgrowth of the resistant organisms.[32] A similar process appears to apply to prosthetic joints using gentamicin-impregnated cement. Kristinsson and associates,[33] studying infected hip prostheses, reported that gentamicin-resistant coagulase-negative staphylococci were recovered from 88% of patients in whom gentamicin-impregnated cements was used but in only 15% of the patients in whom gentamicin-containing cement was not used (P<.001).

Capsules

The pathogenic role of staphylococcal capsules has been the subject of debate for many years. Highly encapsulated "mucoid" S aureus strains exhibit increased virulence in vivo and increased resistance to opsonization and phagocytosis in vitro.[34] Despite these apparent virulence attributes, mucoid strains are only rarely isolated from clinical sources, suggesting that the phenomenon is not pathologically relevant.[34] Karakawa and associates[35] reopened the issue of staphylococcal encapsulation with the publication of a scheme for serotyping S aureus.[35] Using polyclonal—and later monoclonal—antisera, they detected extracellular polysaccharide on nonmucoid strains, a phenomenon they called microencapsulation. More than 90% of S aureus strains were typeable by the Karakawa system, and 70% of the isolates were either type 5 or type 8.[36] Although the data are limited, there apparently is not an association between any particular clinical condition (including musculoskeletal infections) and any particular serotype.[36] The pathogenic role of the microcapsule is also subject to debate because microencapsulated strains appear to be no more pathogenic than unencapsulated strains.[34] Huycke and Proctor[37] reported a potential adherence function of staphylococcal microcapsules. Some strains of coagulase-negative staphylococci do produce capsules,[38] but their role in pathogenesis is undefined.

Protein Markers of Traumatized Tissue

On the molecular level, trauma causes dramatic changes in the topography of tissue surfaces. Trauma exposes normally buried inaccessible matrix proteins to the wound environment, and bleeding and serous drainage coat the wound with serum proteins. Implantation of medical devices into host tissues causes similar changes in the molecular topography of the device. Soluble host proteins are either pas-

Table 4 Human serum and extracellular matrix proteins important in the colonization of wounds and indwelling medical devices by staphylococci

Host Protein	S aureus		S epidermidis	
	Binds Soluble Protein	Binds Solid-Phase Protein	Binds Soluble Protein	Binds Solid-Phase Protein
Fibronectin	Yes[39–41]	Yes[42–45]	Yes[41–46]; no[47]	Yes[42]; low[48]; no[49]
Fibrinogen	Yes[50]	Yes[43]	No[51]	?
Collagen	Yes[52–54]	Yes[40,55]	Yes[41,54,56]	Yes[48]
Laminin	Yes[40,57]	Yes[42]	No[40,57]	No[42]
Vitronectin	Yes[58]; no[54]	Yes[42]	No[58]	No[42]
Sialoprotein II	Yes[41]	?	No[41]	?

sively adsorbed or actively deposited on the surface of the device. Although the degree to which host proteins coat the surface varies according to the physical and chemical conditions of the surface, all host proteins can become attached to all surfaces to some degree. Consequently, the surfaces of all wounds and medical devices are qualitatively similar.

From the viewpoint of the pathogen, host proteins are a convenient marker of a target tissue. Because proteins vary widely in form and function, the molecular configuration of each of the host proteins has topographic features, or "domains," that are unique to that protein. The pathogen recognizes these unique domains with a surface structure—the adhesin—that binds in a "lock-and-key" manner with the domain. This interaction between the bacterial adhesin and the host receptor anchors the free-floating microorganism to the targeted microenvironment. With this in mind, the tropism of staphylococci for wounds and indwelling medical devices could be explained by the selective ability of the staphylococci to recognize and become attached to wound proteins.

Table 4 lists the human serum and extracellular matrix proteins that are known to interact with staphylococci and are, therefore, the best candidates to serve as the receptors for the binding of staphylococci to wounds and indwelling medical devices. In constructing Table 4 we distinguished between the binding of soluble proteins to staphylococci and the binding of staphylococci to proteins in a solid phase because the transition from soluble phase to solid phase can result in a rearrangement of the three-dimensional structure of the molecule. This, in turn, can result in major functional distinctions between soluble- and solid-phase proteins.

Fibronectin

Fibronectin is a large glycoprotein found in soluble form in body fluids, particularly plasma, and in insoluble form in the extracellular matrix.[59] Soluble fibronectin exists in a dimeric folded globular form, and solid-phase fibronectin is a multimeric linear molecule.[59] The two chains of the soluble molecule are united at their carboxy terminus by a disulfide bond. Each chain contains three domains: a 120- to 140-

kd carboxy-terminal fragment that binds heparin and host cells, a 27-kd amino-terminal fragment that binds fibrin, and an intervening 40-kd fragment that binds collagen.[59]

A number of studies have been published on the interaction of staphylococci and other bacterial genera with fibronectin.[7] The principal finding that has emerged from these investigations applies to almost all other interactions attributed to fibronectin: fibronectin functions as a ligand, binding bacterial cells or host cells to other cell surfaces or extracellular matrices.[7]

The binding of heat-killed or living *S aureus* by fibronectin is saturable, specific, and essentially irreversible.[39,47,60] Fibronectin binding of staphylococci is strain-dependent, varying by as much as 30–fold or more in some studies.[39] Mosher and Proctor[61] reported that the primary domain on fibronectin for binding *S aureus* was contained within the 27-kd amino-terminal fragment. Kuusela and associates[62] later reported a second lower-affinity binding site in the 120- to 140-kd carboxy-terminal fragment.

The number of receptor sites for binding fibronectin has been estimated to range from fewer than 100 to more than 20,000 per staphylococcal organism.[39,60] The specific identity of these receptors is controversial. Huycke and Proctor[37] reported preliminary data indicating that serotype 8 exopolysaccharide binds fibronectin. Using transposon mutagenesis, Kuypers and Proctor[63] created mutants deficient in fibronectin binding and demonstrated a concordant decrease in virulence in an animal model of endocarditis. A number of investigators using an alternate approach—passing a variety of staphylococcal extracts over a fibronectin-Sepharose column—have reported the isolation of staphylococcal proteins that specifically bind fibronectin with a high affinity.[55,60] Whether these preparations represent variations of the same molecule and whether the fibronectin-binding protein functions as an adhesin have yet to be determined. Nevertheless, the production of a fibronectin-binding protein by *S aureus* can no longer be questioned. The staphylococcal fibronectin-binding protein has been cloned in *Escherichia coli* and purified.[64]

As already noted, blood and tissue fluids contain high concentrations of soluble fibronectin. These fluids bathe indwelling medical devices, resulting in the deposition of solid-phase fibronectin on the surface of the device.[45] Vaudaux and associates[45,65] convincingly demonstrated that fibronectin functions as an adherence receptor for the colonization of indwelling medical devices by staphylococci. Presumably, the adherence of staphylococci to surface-bound fibronectin promotes staphylococcal infection by increasing the number of bacterial cells attached to the device. Further, the fibronectin bond between the surface of the device and the staphylococci also renders the pathogens resistant to phagocytosis.[65] A problem arises, however, in considering this scenario. Because the staphylococci must pass through the fluid phase of the wound before encountering the medical device, one would expect the organism to become coated with soluble fibronectin before it has the opportunity to bind to solid-phase fibronectin. Nevertheless, Vaudaux and associates[45] demonstrated that staphylococci adhere to solid-phase fibronectin in the presence of soluble fibronectin.

One explanation for this apparent paradox is that staphylococci interact with fibronectin through two independent binding systems; one of which recognizes soluble fibronectin and the other solid-phase fibronectin. There is precedent for such a system. Soluble fibronectin binds to both *Streptococcus pyogenes* and *Streptococcus sanguis*.[66] *S sanguis*, however, adheres to solid-phase fibronectin in the presence of soluble fibronectin, whereas *S pyogenes* cannot.[66] The fibronectin-binding adhesin of *S sanguis* recognizes a binding site on solid-phase fibronectin that is hidden in soluble fibronectin.[66] In studies similar to those performed by Kuypers and Proctor,[63] transposon mutants of *S sanguis* deficient in binding to solid-phase fibronectin demonstrated a concordant decrease in virulence in an animal model of endocarditis.[67]

Extracellular Matrix and Serum Proteins and *S aureus*

S aureus   Because this is a new area of research, the other substances listed in Table 4 have not been as well studied as fibronectin. Nevertheless, it is both reasonable and consistent to presume that the specific adherence of staphylococci to these proteins is important to the pathogenesis of wound and foreign-body infections.

Soluble collagen binds to *S aureus*[52–54] and *S aureus* binds to solid-phase collagen.[40,55] This binding is strain-variable,[55] but when present it mediates the attachment of *S aureus* to plastic in vitro.[55] It also appears that for some strains collagen has an additional function as a co-factor for increasing the binding of *S aureus* to solid-phase fibronectin.[45] The staphylococcal agent responsible for collagen binding has recently been identified as a 15–kd protein.[68] The extracellular matrix proteins laminin,[40,57] vitronectin,[58] and sialoprotein II[41] bind to *S aureus* and *S aureus* binds to solid-phase laminin[42] and vitronectin.[42] Fibrinogen also binds to *S aureus*[50] and *S aureus* binds to fibrin[43]; further, *S aureus*-fibrin binding may function as a co-factor to increase the fibronectin-dependent adherence of staphylococci to plastic.[49] The earlier report that this binding was the result of a surface protein[69] has more recently been questioned.[70]

S epidermidis   Controversy exists regarding the association of *S epidermidis* with fibronectin. Some investigators[41,46] have reported the binding of fibronectin to *S epidermidis* but others have not.[47] Similarly, some investigators have observed the binding of *S epidermidis* to solid-phase fibronectin[42] whereas others have not.[48] Even at best, the association of fibronectin with *S epidermidis* is strain-variable[46,71] and of a lesser magnitude than that of *S aureus*.[46,48] The coagulase-negative staphylococci are also negative for clumping factor[51] and do not bind laminin,[40,42,57] vitronectin[42,58] or sialoprotein II.[41] *S epidermidis* does bind collagen[41,48,54,56] but to a lesser extent than does *S aureus*.[71] In summary, *S epidermidis* either lacks or expresses in low quantity all the factors that appear to promote *S aureus* wound and foreign-body infection.

The studies cited in Table 4 provide a rationale for the pathogenic tropism of *S aureus* for wound and foreign-body infections. They do not, however, explain the propensity of *S epidermidis* to infect indwelling foreign bodies.

Slime Production by *S epidermidis*

When grown in broth culture media, many strains of coagulase-negative staphylococci produce a thick viscid coat of bacteria on the culture-tube wall.[20] This "slime" production is currently the leading explanation for the association of coagulase-negative staphylococci with infections of indwelling medical devices.[7] When infected medical appliances, such as intravascular catheters,[73-75] cardiac pacemaker leads,[76,77] and peritoneal dialysis catheters,[78] are removed from patients and examined by a scanning electron microscope, thick sheets of bacteria are found cemented to each other and to the surface of the device by amorphous materials. The appearance of these naturally infected appliances is remarkably similar to the microscopic appearance of similar appliances incubated in vitro with slime-producing bacteria.[72,73,77,80,81] The association of slime production with pathogenicity has been reported in collections of strains from patients with intravascular catheters,[82,83] cerebrospinal fluid shunts,[84,85] and foreign-body infection.[86] Dobbins and associates[9] reported that all strains of coagulase-negative staphylococci recovered from asymptomatically infected orthopaedic appliances were slime producers.[9] When we examined a collection of strains from a hospital outbreak of sepsis associated with intravascular catheters,[28] strains associated with clinical disease demonstrated greater slime production (0.602) than blood culture contaminants (0.295; $P < .01$) and skin strains (0.371; $P < .05$).[82] Slime production has also been associated with increased resistance to antimicrobial agents in vitro[87,88] and in vivo[84,85] as well as with a greater frequency of clinical relapses.[84,85,89]

These studies have provided ample clinical and epidemiologic evidence for the association of slime production with pathogenicity. They have not, however, proven that slime itself is a virulence factor. Slime could just as easily serve as an incidental marker of pathogenic strains, that is, strains that were pathogenic for entirely different reasons, such as the production of a toxin or other adhesins. To resolve this issue we are currently pursuing a series of investigations to purify slime and to create mutants that do not produce slime. The first step in this investigation was to search for naturally occurring nonproducing variants of a slime-producing strain.

We found spontaneous nonproducing variants of a slime-producing strain of *S epidermidis* (RP62A).[90] Using these strains we were able to demonstrate a variation in slime production in vivo as well as the association of slime production with virulence in two animals with infected medical devices.[90] The association was, however, weak. There appeared to be only a threefold variation in virulence between the slime-producing and nonproducing strains.[90] This weak association may have reflected our crude methodology. Therefore, we refined our methods for discovering and maintaining strains with variable slime production. Although the issue of slime production as a virulence factor has yet to be resolved, our studies have shed light on a previously unsuspected system of phenotypic variation in the staphylococci.

Phenotypic Variation in Slime Production and Other Factors

The key to our observation of phenotypic variation was the development of a solid laboratory medium, Memphis agar,[91] that allowed us to recognize slime production in individual colonies or clones of *S epidermidis* (RP62A). With this medium we demonstrated that slime production was subject to reversible "phase variation" at a rate of 1.1 $\times$ 10^{-5} per bacterium per generation.[91] This rate is so rapid that, on the average, by the time a bacterial colony reaches 16,000 cells it includes at least two cells whose expression of slime production has changed. We also found that when a single slime-producing cell was mixed with 16,000 or fewer nonproducing cells, the resulting culture produced slime.[91] Finally, we found that the change in slime production represented a "pleiotropic" variation. In other words, extensive phenotypic characterization of slime-producing strains and nonproducing variants demonstrated that both strains were identical for all traits except one. The exception was methicillin resistance. The parent slime-producing strain was methicillin-resistant. After selecting first-generation nonproducing variants from the parent strain, we discovered that they were methicillin-sensitive. After selecting second-generation slime-producing strains from the nonproducing variants, we discovered that they had recovered resistance to methicillin.[91] Methicillin resistance is a well-known example of a heterotypic phenotype, that is, a methicillin-heteroresistant strain when cultured always includes a minor population of methicillin-resistant cells among a much larger population of methicillin-sensitive cells. For our strain, it appeared that methicillin resistance and slime production were genetically associated.

When we expanded our studies to include other staphylococci, we observed spontaneous phenotypic variation among all members of the genus *Staphylococcus*, but it was most pronounced for *S epidermidis*.[91] As in our slime-producing strain, the variation could be pleiotropic. For one strain studied in detail, the type strain for *Staphylococcus saprophyticus*, we found that methicillin resistance, β-glucosidase production, hemagglutination, and virulence were all subject to simultaneous variation.[91]

Previous investigators have reported the spontaneous pleiotropic variation of *S aureus*. Daughter strains can vary from the parent strain for a variety of factors, including production of protein A, hemolysins, and toxic shock toxin.[92,93] Recsei and associates[93] described and Peng and associates[94] cloned from *S aureus* a single gene, the accessory gene regulator gene (*agr*), responsible for the coordinate regulation of this panel of genes. The *agr* gene functions presumably by producing a

69

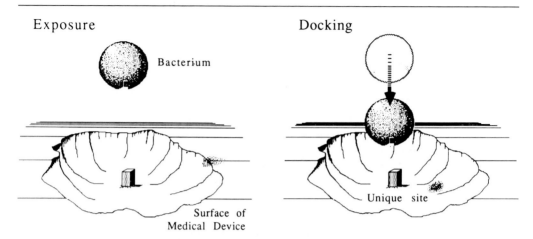

Exposure   Docking

Bacterium

Unique site

Surface of
Medical Device

Fig. 4 *Left, The setting for bacterial colonization of a foreign body (exposure). It includes exposure of a bacterium to the surface of the medical device. The bacterium may or may not exhibit specific binding structures (adhesins) on its surface, symbolized by the notch in the bacterial cell. The surface of the medical device will have unique sites in which chemical or topographic features promote bacterial attachment. These features are symbolized by the pit in the surface of the device. Implanted medical devices will also be coated by adsorbed host proteins, which may serve as receptors for adhesin specific attachment, symbolized here by the block in the pit. Right, The first stage of bacterial colonization of the medical device (docking). Bacteria are attracted to the surface by a variety of physical-chemical forces including Van der Waals forces, electrostatic charge, gravity, and hydrophobic interactions. These forces are universal and operate to a greater or lesser extent on all submerged particles in the immediate proximity of an immersed object. The sum of these interactions is to draw the organism into a close association with the surface of the device.*

factor that operates in trans to promote the expression of various products. Presumably this gene or a similar gene is responsible for the variation in slime production that we observed.

In addition to variation in slime production, we also observed a second system of variation that determined the size of the bacterial colony. Almost all strains from all species produced small numbers (1% or less) of small-colony variants.[91] Previous investigators have associated small-colony variants with low immunogenicity, slow growth, and persistence in deep tissues.[95] In foilow-up studies we found selection for the persistence of small-colony variant forms in cardiac vegetations recovered from experimentally infected rats.[96] The discovery of similar forms in the blood and vegetations from a patient with endocarditis[95] suggests that these forms may play an important role in the persistence of bacteria in deep tissues.

Colonization of Smooth Surfaces by Coagulase-Negative Staphylococci

Figure 4 shows our view of the four stages leading to colonization of indwelling medical devices by coagulase-negative staphylococci.

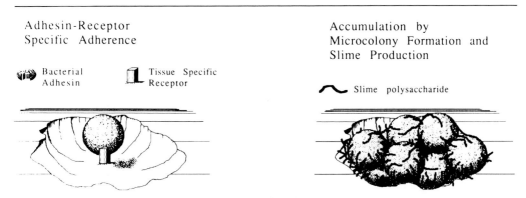

Adhesin-Receptor
Specific Adherence

Accumulation by
Microcolony Formation and
Slime Production

Bacterial
Adhesin

Tissue Specific
Receptor

Slime polysaccharide

Fig. 5 *Left, Adhesin-receptor specific adherence. If the bacterium exhibits a specific adhesin and the surface contains the corresponding tissue specific receptor, then the adhesin can bind the receptor when the bacterium docks on the surface. The result is a close permanent attachment to the surface.* **Right,** *The next stage of bacterial colonization. Following docking or adhesin-specific adherence, a slime-producing bacterium may multiply and accumulate on the surface of the medical device, producing a microcolony. Slime polysaccharides (indicated by the thick curvy lines) produced by the bacterial cells bind the cells to each other and to the surface, cementing the colony in situ.*

Colonization begins with the exposure of the device to bacteria (Fig. 4, *left*) and the inevitable nonspecific attachment of the bacteria to the surface of the device. This nonspecific attachment or "docking" (Fig. 4, *right*) occurs to some degree whenever free-floating microorganisms encounter a solid surface. The precise number of bacteria attaching to the surface varies depending on the concentration of bacteria in the bathing solution and the specific physicochemical properties of the bacteria and the surface. Hydrophobic bacterial surfaces in particular appear to promote the attachment of staphylococci to smooth surfaces.[97,98] Other mechanisms also play an important role in the immediate attachment of bacteria to smooth surfaces. Tojo and associates[99] described a capsular polysaccharide adhesin that mediates the immediate uptake of *S epidermidis* to medical devices by unknown mechanisms. Nevertheless, if the medical device is exposed to a reasonable number of microorganisms, a small proportion of those organisms inevitably becomes associated with the surface of the device.

The fraction of bacteria attached to the surface represents more than a simple mass effect. On the microscopic scale of the pathogen, local conditions can facilitate bacterial adherence to the device. All foreign bodies have microscopic surface irregularities.[73,74,80,100] Even if the surface of the device is designed to repel bacteria, these unavoidable surface variations create unique microscopic sites that allow or even promote bacterial attachment. These unique sites include local variations in the physicochemical characteristics of the surface, microscopic structural defects in the surface, and the deposition of host protein receptors on the surface.

71

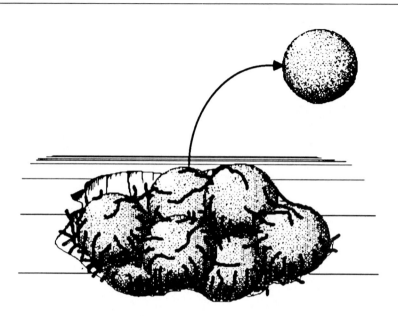

Fig. 6 *The final stage of bacterial colonization and the first stage of colonization of other sites. In order for the bacterial strain to maintain itself in the environment, individual bacterial cells must leave the colony and drift to new sites for bacterial colonization. This is accomplished by phenotypic variation, in which individual cells cease to produce adherence mechanisms. No longer adherent to the microcolony, these cells are released to spread to new sites.*

The deposition of host proteins onto medical devices appears to be essential to the colonization of the device with *S aureus*. As we have noted, *S aureus* is able to bind to a variety of host extracellular and serum proteins. The deposition of these proteins on the surface provides a large and varied number of specific receptors for the adherence of *S aureus* to the surface of the device (Fig. 5, *left*).

Many investigators[44,101,102] have demonstrated that adsorbed host proteins also promote the attachment of *S epidermidis* to implanted medical devices. Although this adherence must be important, the limited number and limited variety of protein adhesins on *S epidermidis* in comparison to *S aureus* make protein adherence an unlikely explanation for the foreign-body tropism demonstrated by *S epidermidis*. As demonstrated (Fig. 5, *right*) the capacity to produce slime probably explains this tropism. As slime-producing bacteria multiply at the original attachment site, they are bound to each other and to the surface by extracellular polysaccharides. We recently semipurified and characterized a polysaccharide antigen from *S epidermidis* that appears to be one of these slime polysaccharides.[103] Therefore, even if only a few organisms initially adhere to a surface, a slime-producing organism can successfully colonize the surface by virtue of cell-to-cell binding.

Figure 6 illustrates the final stage in the colonization process, which is the release of microorganisms from the colony. The existence of a rapid, reversible mechanism of spontaneous variation in slime production suggests that organisms can be released from a microcolony. The released bacterial cells can then drift to new sites to repeat the colonization and infection process.

In summary, the propensity of indwelling medical devices to become infected with coagulase-negative and coagulase-positive staphylococci, along with the propensity of wounds to become infected with *S aureus*, can be explained by the ability of *S aureus* to adhere to host proteins and the ability of *S epidermidis* to coat the surface of the device with a layer of slime.

Acknowledgment

These studies were supported by research funds from the US Veterans Administration.

References

1. Gentry LO: Osteomyelitis: Options for diagnosis and management. *J Antimicrob Chemother* 1988;21(suppl C):115–131.
2. Goldenberg DL, Reed JI: Bacterial arthritis. *N Engl J Med* 1985;312:764–771.
3. Sheagren JN: *Staphylococcus aureus*: Part 1. The persistent pathogen. *N Engl J Med* 1984;310:1368–1373.
4. Sheagren JN: *Staphylococcus aureus*: Part 2. The persistent pathogen. *N Engl J Med* 1984;310:1437–1442.
5. Musher DM, McKenzie SO: Infections due to *Staphylococcus aureus*. *Medicine* 1977;56:383–409.
6. Brause BD: Infected orthopedic prostheses, in Bisno AL, Waldvogel FA (eds): *Infections Associated with Indwelling Medical Devices*. Washington, DC, American Society for Microbiology, 1989, pp 111–127.
7. Christensen GD, Baddour LM, Hasty DL, et al: Microbial and foreign body factors in the pathogenesis of medical device infections, in Bisno AL, Waldvogel FA (eds): *Infections Associated with Indwelling Medical Devices*. Washington, DC, American Society for Microbiology, 1989, pp 27–59.
8. Lowy FD, Hammer SM: *Staphylococcus epidermidis* infections. *Ann Intern Med* 1983;99:834–839.
9. Dobbins JJ, Seligson D, Raff MJ: Bacterial colonization of orthopedic fixation devices in the absence of clinical infection. *J Infect Dis* 1988;158:203–205.
10. Archer GL, Vishniavsky N, Stiver HG: Plasmid pattern analysis of *Staphylococcus epidermidis* isolates from patients with prosthetic valve endocarditis. *Infect Immun* 1982;35:627–632.
11. Kloos WE, Musselwhite MS: Distribution and persistence of *Staphylococcus* and *Micrococcus* species and other aerobic bacteria on human skin. *Appl Microbiol* 1975;30:381–385.
12. Archer GL, Armstrong BC: Alteration of staphyococcal flora in cardiac surgery patients receiving antibiotic prophylaxis. *J Infect Dis* 1983;147:642–649.
13. Boyce JM, Potter-Bynoe G, Opal SM, et al: A common-source outbreak of *Staphylococcus epidermidis* infections among patients undergoing cardiac surgery. *J Infect Dis* 1990;161:493–499.

14. Lindberg, cited in Lidwell M: Airborne bacteria and surgical infection. *Am J Med* 1981;70:693–697.

15. Waldvogel FA, Papageorgiou PS: Osteomyelitis: The past decade. *N Engl J Med* 1980;303:360–370.

16. Paley D, Moseley CF, Armstrong P, et al: Primary osteomyelitis caused by coagulase-negative staphylococci. *J Pediatr Orthop* 1986;6:622–626.

17. Zierdt CH: Evidence for transient *Staphylococcus epidermidis* bacteremia in patients and in healthy humans. *J Clin Microbiol* 1983;17:628–630.

18. Hutton JP, Hamory BH, Parisi JT, et al: *Staphylococcus epidermidis* arthritis following catheter-induced bacteremia in a neutropenic patient. *Diagn Microbiol Infect Dis* 1985;3:119–124.

19. Bryan CS, Parisi JT, Strike DG: Vertebral osteomyelitis due to *Staphylococcus warneri* attributed to a Hickman catheter. *Diagn Microbiol Infect Dis* 1987;8:57–59.

20. Elek SD, Conen PE: The virulence of *Staphylococcus pyogenes* for man: A study of the problems of wound infection. *Br J Exp Pathol* 1957;38:573–586.

21. Zimmerli W, Waldvogel FA, Vaudaux P, et al: Pathogenesis of foreign body infection: Description and characteristics of an animal model. *J Infect Dis* 1982;146:487–497.

22. Christensen GD, Simpson WA, Bisno AL, et al: Experimental foreign body infections in mice challenged with slime-producing *Staphylococcus epidermidis*. *Infect Immun* 1983;49:407–410.

23. Ford CW, Hamel JC, Stapert D, et al: Antibiotic therapy of an experimental *Staphylococcus epidermidis* subcutaneous abscess in mice. *Zetralbl Bakteriol Mikrobiol Hyg* 1987ˡ6:247–255.

24. Gemmell CG: Extracellular toxins and enzymes of coagulase-negative staphylococci, in Easmon CSF, Adlam C (eds): *Staphylococci and Staphylococcal Infections*. London, Academic Press, 1983, vol 2, pp 809–827.

25. Marsik FJ, Parisi JT: Significance of *Staphylococcus epidermidis* in the clinical laboratory. *Appl Microbiol* 1973;25:11–14.

26. Selepak ST, Witebsky FG: Beta-lactamase detection in nine staphylococcal species. *J Clin Microbiol* 1984;20:1200–1201.

27. Schaberg DR, Zervos M: Plasmid analysis in the study of the epidemiology of nosocomial gram-positive cocci. *Rev Infect Dis* 1986;8:705–712.

28. Christensen GD, Bisno AL, Parisi JT, et al: Nosocomial septicemia due to multiply antibiotic-resistant *Staphylococcus epidermidis*. *Ann Intern Med* 1982;96:1–10.

29. Brumfitt W, Hamilton-Miller J: Methicillin-resistant *Staphylococcus aureus*. *N Engl J Med* 1989;320:1188–1196.

30. Lampson BC, Parisi JT: Naturally occurring *Staphylococcus epidermidis* plasmid expressing constitutive macrolide-lincosamide-streptogramin B resistance contains a deleted attenuator. *J Bacteriol* 1986;166:479–483.

31. Thomas WD Jr, Archer GL: Mobility of gentamicin resistance genes from staphylococci isolated in the United States: Identification of Tn4031, a gentamicin resistance transposon from *Staphylococcus epidermidis*. *Antimicrob Agents Chemother* 1989;33:1335–1341.

32. Kernodle DS, Barg NL, Kaiser AB: Low-level colonization of hospitalized patients with methicillin-resistant coagulase-negative staphylococci and emergence of the organisms during surgical antimicrobial prophylaxis. *Antimicrob Agents Chemother* 1988;32:202–208.

33. Kristinsson KG, Hope PG, Norman P, et al: Deep infections associated with total hip arthroplasties caused by coagulase-negative staphylococci: Pathogenesis and microbial diagnosis, in Wadström T, Eliasson I, Holder I, et al (eds): *Pathogenesis of Wound and Biomaterial-Associated Infections*. London, Springer-Verlag, 1990, pp 329–337.

34. Lee JC, Betley MJ, Hopkins CA, et al: Virulence studies, in mice, of transposon-induced mutants of *Staphylococcus aureus* differing in capsule size. *J Infect Dis* 1987;156:741–750.

35. Karakawa WW, Fournier JM, Vann WF, et al: Method for the serological typing of the capsular polysaccharides of *Staphylococcus aureus*. *J Clin Microbiol* 1985;22:445–447.

36. Arbeit RD, Karakawa WW, Vann WF, et al: Predominance of two newly described capsular polysaccharide types among clinical isolates of *Staphylococcus aureus*. *Diagn Microbiol Infect Dis* 1984;2:85–91.

37. Huycke M, Proctor R: New insights into encapsulation of *Staphylococcus aureus*: Implications for the development of vaccines. *Infect Dis Newslett* 1988;7:92–93.

38. Yamada T, Ichiman Y, Yoshida K: Possible common biological and immunological properties for detecting encapsulated strains of *Staphylococcus epidermidis*. *J Clin Microbiol* 1988;26:2167–2172.

39. Proctor RA, Mosher DF, Olbrantz PJ: Fibronectin binding to *Staphylococcus aureus*. *J Biol Chem* 1982;257:14788–14794.

40. Vercellotti GM, McCarthy JB, Lindholm P, et al: Extracellular matrix proteins (fibronectin, laminin, and type IV collagen) bind and aggregate bacteria. *Am J Pathol* 1985;120:13–21.

41. Rydén C, Maxe I, Franzén A, et al: Selective binding of bone matrix sialoprotein to *Staphylococcus aureus* in osteomyelitis. *Lancet* 1987;2:515.

42. Fuquay JI, Loo DT, Barnes DW: Binding of *Staphylococcus aureus* by human serum spreading factor in an in vitro assay. *Infect Immun* 1986;52:714–717.

43. Kuusela P, Vartio T, Vuento M, et al: Attachment of staphylococci and streptococci on fibronectin, fibronectin fragments, and fibrinogen bound to a solid phase. *Infect Immun* 1985;50:77–81.

44. Russell PB, Kline J, Yoder MC, et al: Staphylococcal adherence to polyvinyl chloride and heparin-bonded polyurethane catheters is species dependent and enhanced by fibronectin. *J Clin Microbiol* 1987;25:1083–1087.

45. Vaudaux PE, Waldvogel FA, Morgenthaler JJ, et al: Adsorption of fibronectin onto polymethylmethacrylate and promotion of *Staphylococcus aureus* adherence. *Infect Immun* 1984;45:768–774.

46. Switalski LM, Rydén C, Rubin K, et al: Binding of fibronectin to *Staphylococcus* strains. *Infect Immun* 1983;42:628–633.

47. Doran JE, Raynor RH: Fibronectin binding to protein A-containing staphylococci. *Infect Immun* 1981;33:683–689.

48. Miedzobrodzki J, Naidu AS, Watts JL, et al: Effect of milk on fibronectin and collagen type I binding to *Staphylococcus aureus* and coagulase-negative staphyloccci isolated from bovine mastitis. *J Clin Microbiol* 1989;27:540–544.

49. Toy PT, Lai LW, Drake TA, et al: Effect of fibronectin on adherence of *Staphylococcus aureus* to fibrin thrombi in vitro. *Infect Immun* 1985;48:83–86.

50. Kloczewiak M, Timmons S, Hawiger J: Reactivity of chemically cross-linked fibrinogen and its fragments D toward the staphylococcal clumping receptor. *Biochemistry* 1987;26:6152–6156.

51. Schumacher-Perdreau F, Ludwicka A, Pulverer G: Investigations on clumping factor, haemagglutinins and hydrophobicity of staphylococci. *Zentralbl Bakteriol Mikrobiol Hyg* 1982;253A:312–320.

52. Holderbaum D, Hall GS, Ehrhart LA: Collagen binding to *Staphylococcus aureus*. *Infect Immun* 1986;54:359–364.

53. Speziale P, Raucci G, Visai L, et al: Binding of collagen to *Staphylococcus aureus* Cowan 1. *J Bacteriol* 1986;167:77–81.

54. Wadström T, Erdei J, Paulsson M, et al: Fibronectin, collagen and vitronectin binding of coagulase-negative staphylococci, in Wadström T, Eliasson I, Holder I, et al (eds): *Pathogenesis of Wound and Biomaterial-Associated Infections.* London, Springer-Verlag, 1990, pp 339–347.

55. Maxe I, Rydén C, Wadström T, et al: Specific attachment of *Staphylococcus aureus* to immobilized fibronectin. *Infect Immun* 1986;54:695–704.

56. Watts JL, Naidu AS, Wadström T: Collagen binding, elastase production, and slime production associated with coagulase-negative staphylococci isolated from bovine intramammary infections. *J Clin Microbiol* 1990;28:580–583.

57. Lopes JD, dos Reis M, Brentani RR: Presence of laminin receptors in *Staphylococcus aureus*. *Science* 1985;229:275–277.

58. Chhatwal GS, Preissner KT, Muller-Berghaus G, et al: Specific binding of the human S protein (vitronectin) to streptococci, *Staphylococcus aureus*, and *Escherichia coli*. *Infect Immun* 1987;55:1878–1883.

59. Mosher DF, Furcht LT: Fibronectin: Review of its structure and possible functions. *J Invest Dermatol* 1981;77:175–180.

60. Rydén C, Rubin K, Speziale P, et al: Fibronectin receptors from *Staphylococcus aureus*. *J Biol Chem* 1983;258:3396–3401.

61. Mosher DF, Proctor RA: Binding and factor XIIIa-mediated cross-linking of a 27-kilodalton fragment of fibronectin to *Staphylococcus aureus*. *Science* 1980;209:927–929.

62. Kuusela P, Vartio T, Vuento M, et al: Binding sites for streptococci and staphylococci in fibronectin. *Infect Immun* 1984;45:433–436.

63. Kuypers JM, Proctor RA: Reduced adherence to traumatized rat heart valves by a low-fibronectin-binding mutant of *Staphylococcus aureus*. *Infect Immun* 1989;57:2306–2312.

64. Flock JI, Froman G, Jonsson K, et al: Cloning and expression of the gene for a fibronectin-binding protein from *Staphylococcus aureus*. *EMBO J* 1987;6:2351–2357.

65. Vaudaux PE, Zulian G, Huggler E, et al: Attachment of *Staphylococcus aureus* to polymethylmethacrylate increases its resistance to phagocytosis in foreign body infection. *Infect Immun* 1985;50:472–477.

66. Lowrance JH, Hasty DL, Simpson WA: Adherence of *Streptococcus sanguis* to conformationally specific determinants in fibronectin. *Infect Immun* 1988;56:2279–2285.

67. Lowrence JH, Baddour LM, Simpson WA: The role of fibronectin binding in the rat model of experimental endocarditis caused by *Streptococcus sanguis*. *J Clin Invest* 1990;86:7–13.

68. Switalski LM, Speziale P, Hook M: Isolation and characterization of a putative collagen receptor from *Staphylococcus aureus* strain Cowan 1. *J Biol Chem* 1989;264:21080–21086.

69. Espersen F, Clemmensen I, Barkholt V: Isolation of *Staphylococcus aureus* clumping factor. *Infect Immun* 1985;49:700–708.

70. Boden MK, Flock JI: Fibrinogen-binding protein/clumping factor from *Staphylococcus aureus*. *Infect Immun* 1989;57:2358–2363.

71. Wadström T, Speziale P, Rozgonyi F, et al: Interactions of coagulase-negative staphylococci with fibronectin and collagen as possible first step of tissue colonization in wounds and other tissue trauma. *Zentralbl Bakteriol Mikrobiol Hyg* 1987;16(suppl):83–91.

72. Christensen GD, Simpson WA, Bisno AL, et al: Adherence of slime-producing strains of *Staphylococcus epidermidis* to smooth surfaces. *Infect Immun* 1982;37:318–326.

73. Franson TR, Sheth NK, Rose HD, et al: Scanning electron microscopy of bacteria adherent to intravascular catheters. *J Clin Microbiol* 1984;20:500–505.

74. Marrie TJ, Costerton JW: Scanning and transmission electron microscopy of in situ bacterial colonization of intravenous and intraarterial catheters. *J Clin Microbiol* 1984;19:687–693.

75. Peters G, Locci R, Pulverer G: Microbial colonization of prosthetic devices: II. Scanning electron microscopy of naturally infected intravenous catheters. *Zentralbl Bakteriol Mikrobiol Hyg* 1981;173B:293–299.

76. Marrie TJ, Costerton JW: Morphology of bacterial attachment to cardiac pacemaker leads and power packs. *J Clin Microbiol* 1984;19:911–914.

77. Peters G, Saborowski F, Locci R, et al: Investigations on staphylococcal infection of transvenous endocardial pacemaker electrodes. *Am Heart J* 1984;108:359–365.

78. Marrie TJ, Noble MA, Costerton JW: Examination of the morphology of bacteria adhering to peritoneal dialysis catheters by scanning and transmission electron microscopy. *J Clin Microbiol* 1983;18:1388–1398.

79. Baddour LM, Smalley DL, Kraus AP Jr, et al: Comparison of microbiologic characteristics of pathogenic and saprophytic coagulase-negative staphylococci from patients on continuous ambulatory peritoneal dialysis. *Diagn Microbiol Infect Dis* 1986;5:197–205.

80. Locci R, Peters G, Pulverer G: Microbial colonization of prosthetic devices: III. Adhesion of staphylococci to lumina of intravenous catheters perfused with bacterial suspensions. *Zentralbl Bakteriol Mikrobiol Hyg* 1981;173B:300–307.

81. Peters G, Locci R, Pulverer G: Adherence and growth of coagulase-negative staphylococci on surfaces of intravenous catheters. *J Infect Dis* 1982;146:479–482.

82. Christensen GD, Simpson WA, Younger JJ, et al: Adherence of coagulase-negative staphylococci to plastic tissue culture plates: A quantitative model for the adherence of staphylococci to medical devices. *J Clin Microbiol* 1985;22:996–1006.

83. Ishak MA, Groschel DHM, Mandell GL, et al: Association of slime with pathogenicity of coagulase-negative staphylococci causing nosocomial septicemia. *J Clin Microbiol* 1985;22:1025–1029.

84. Diaz-Mitoma F, Harding GKM, Hoban DJ, et al: Clinical significance of a test for slime production in ventriculoperitoneal shunt infections caused by coagulase-negative staphylococci. *J Infect Dis* 1987;156:555–560.

85. Younger JJ, Christensen GD, Bartley DL, et al: Coagulase-negative staphylococci isolated from cerebrospinal fluid shunts: Importance of slime production, species identification, and shunt removal to clinical outcome. *J Infect Dis* 1987;156:548–554.

86. Davenport DS, Massanari RM, Pfaller MA, et al: Usefulness of a test for slime production as a marker for clinically significant infections with coagulase-negative staphylococci. *J Infect Dis* 1986;153:332–339.

87. Sheth NK, Franson TR, Sohnle PG: Influence of bacterial adherence to intravascular catheters on *in-vitro* antibiotic susceptibility. *Lancet* 1985;2:1266–1268.

88. Farber BF, Kaplan MH, Clogston AG: *Staphylococcus epidermidis* extracted slime inhibits the antimicrobial action of glycopeptide antibiotics. *J Infect Dis* 1990;161:37–40.

89. Deighton MA, Fleming VA, Wood CJ: Slime production by coagulase-negative staphylococci causing single and recurrent episodes of peritonitis, in Wadström T, Eliasson I, Holder I, et al (eds): *Pathogenesis of Wound and Biomaterial-Associated Infections*. London, Springer Verlag, 1990, pp 459–464.

90. Christensen GD, Baddour LM, Simpson WA: Phenotypic variation of *Staphylococcus epidermidis* slime production in vitro and in vivo. *Infect Immun* 1987;55:2870–2877.

91. Christensen GD, Baddour LM, Madison BM, et al: Colonial morphology of staphylococci on Memphis agar: Phase variation of slime production, resistance to β-lactam antibiotics, and virulence. *J Infect Dis* 1990;161:1153–1169.

92. Lee AC, Bergdoll MS: Spontaneous occurrence of *Staphylococcus aureus* mutants with different pigmentation and ability to produce toxic shock syndrome toxin 1. *J Clin Microbiol* 1985;22:308–309.

93. Recsei P, Kreiswirth B, O'Reilly M, et al: Regulation of exprotein gene expression in *Staphylococcus aureus* by *agr. Mol Gen Genet* 1986;202:58–61.

94. Peng HL, Novick RP, Kreiswirth B, et al: Cloning, characterization, and sequencing of an accessory gene regulator (*agr*) in *Staphylococcus aureus. J Bacteriol* 1988;170:4365–4372.

95. Baddour LM, Christensen GD: Prosthetic valve endocarditis due to small-colony staphylococcal variants. *Rev Infect Dis* 1987;9:1168–1174.

96. Baddour LM, Simpson WA, Weems JJ Jr, et al: Phenotypic selection of small-colony variant forms of *Staphylococcus epidermidis* in the rat model of endocarditis. *J Infect Dis* 1988;157:757–763.

97. Schadow KH, Simpson WA, Christensen GD: Characteristics of adherence to plastic tissue culture plates of coagulase negative staphylococci exposed to subinhibitory concentrations of antimicrobial agents. *J Infect Dis* 1988;157:71–77.

98. Hogt AH, Dankert J, de Vries JA, et al: Adhesion of coagulase-negative staphylococci to biomaterials. *J Gen Microbiol* 1983;129:2959–2968.

99. Tojo M, Yamashita N, Goldmann DA, et al: Isolation and characterization of a capsular polysaccharide adhesin from *Staphylococcus epidermidis. J Infect Dis* 1988;157:713–722.

100. Locci R, Peters G, Pulverer G: Microbial colonization of prosthetic devices: I. Microtopographical characteristics of intravenous catheters as detected by scanning electron microscopy. *Zentralbl Bakteriol Mikrobiol Hyg* 1981;173B:285–292.

101. Vaudaux P, Pittet D, Haeberli A, et al: Host factors selectively increase staphylococcal adherence on inserted catheters: A role for fibronectin and fibrinogen or fibrin. *J Infect Dis* 1989;160:865–875.

102. Chugh TD, Burns GJ, Shuhaiber HJ, et al: Adherence of *Staphylococcus epidermidis* to fibrin-platelet clots in vitro mediated by lipoteichoic acid. *Infect Immun* 1990;58:315–319.

103. Christensen GD, Barker LP, Mawhinney TP, et al: Identification of an antigenic marker of slime production for *Staphylococcus epidermidis. Infect Immun* 1990;58:2906–2911.

Chapter 6

Gram-Negative Microorganisms and Microbial Adhesion

Katharine Merritt, PhD

General Features

Structure of Gram-Negative Bacteria

The Gram stain is the first procedure used to identify organisms. Their size, shape, and other morphologic features and reaction to the Gram stain are often sufficient for a presumptive diagnosis. Gram-negative organisms, unlike gram-positive organisms, do not retain the crystal violet-iodine complex when rinsed with alcohol. After counter-staining with a contrasting dye, usually safranin O, the purple-staining gram-positive organisms can be distinguished from the gram-negative organisms that are counterstained pink.

In the attempt to understand the staining reaction, analyses have been done on the cell walls of these organisms and distinct differences have been noted.[1] The cell walls of gram-negative organisms do not have the teichoic acids associated with gram-positive organisms, but the organisms do have a lipoprotein core with an outer membrane similar to the cytoplasmic membrane but containing a lipopolysaccharide called endotoxin. This lipopolysaccharide is composed of a lipid called lipid A, and a polysaccharide structure containing unusual dideoxyhexoses. The molecular structure of the polysaccharide portion confers a unique antigenic structure that can be used in the identification of these organisms. This lipopolysaccharide is possessed by all gram-negative bacteria.

Mechanisms of Pathogenicity

Endotoxin has a set of unique biologic functions that can help or harm the host. The expression of endotoxin varies among the genera, but its presence is common to all. Many of the signs and symptoms of the diseases caused by gram-negative organisms can be attributed to the action of endotoxin.[2]

It can cause fever, cardiovascular shock, disseminated intravascular coagulation, tissue necrosis, increased susceptibility to stress, and death. Conversely, endotoxin is a potent stimulator of immune responses. It stimulates the production of cytokines by both monocytes and lymphocytes, stimulates the production of the various substances in the arachidonic acid pathways, increases nonspecific resistance in various ways, including the production of interferons, and is a potent stimulator of antibody production to other antigens.[3,4] It was clearly recognized in the 1930s that vaccines containing killed gram-negative organisms resulted in higher antibody titers to the protein components of the vaccine (such as diphtheria or tetanus toxoid). There have been decades of research on endotoxin as an immune adjuvant and a stimulator of nonspecific resistance and its use in humans is being explored. Nevertheless, it remains a potent toxin.

In addition, many of the gram-negative organisms secrete protein exotoxins that can act at some distance from the organism.[1,5] These include various enzymes and are often similar in action and structure to those associated with gram-positive organisms.

Finally, gram-negative organisms have also been the focus for much of the research on genetics and recombinant DNA activity since the observation of the transfer of resistance to antimicrobial agents. Some understanding of the mechanisms of transfer has now been attained. Much of the acquisition of resistance by previously sensitive bacteria is by way of transfer of plasmids or other cytoplasmic DNA. These are generally transferred by conjugative transfer of the genetic material from F+ piliated cells to F− cells. The F− cells then acquire resistance and become F+ and capable of further transfer. This transfer generally occurs between organisms of the same genus, but evidence of transfer between seemingly unrelated genera has been observed.[6]

Thus, gram-negative organisms often cause severe and debilitating disease that is difficult to treat. The mechanisms of pathogenicity are complex and multiple. Many of the signs and symptoms are related to endotoxin, some to the exotoxins, and some to other mechanisms peculiar to each species.

Classification Into Genus and Species

Classification is based on many components.[1,7] One is the shape of the organism shown by the Gram stain, that is, rod, coccus, or coccobacillary. There are no gram-negative spore-formers. A second is the organism's oxygen requirements, that is, whether it is an obligate aerobe, an obligate anaerobe, or facultative (can grow either aerobically or anaerobically), and special carbon dioxide or microaerophilic requirements. Some organisms have special growth medium requirements by which they can be classified, whereas others are inhibited by media supplements. Finally, the utilization of sugars, the fermentation of sugars to acid or acid and gas, and proteolytic activities are key issues in classification. Antigenic classification generally follows the initial classification by biochemical activities and growth requirements. This process is complex.[8] It is important for the clinician be aware of the subtle nature of some of these classifications and the errors that can be made. A difference in species reported on two separate days may reflect a small biochemical change rather than the acquisition of a new organism by the host. The results need careful interpretation and the laboratory should be consulted on the relationship of the two organisms isolated.

Although there are many genera of gram-negative organisms, this discussion is limited to those most important in orthopaedic infections. As a cause of infection, gram-negative organisms rank third after *Staphylococcus aureus* and *Staphylococcus epidermidis.*

The major group of organisms involved are those referred to as the enterics. This family, called Enterobacteriaceae, is composed of the gram-negative rods, which are facultative, normal flora in the gastrointestinal tract. The important genera are *Escherichia, Klebsiella, Proteus,* and *Enterobacter.* In addition, *Serratia, Citrobacter, Edwardsella, Erwinia,* and *Aeromonas* are found with less frequency.

Salmonella and *Shigella* are similar organisms but are not considered normal flora. Their presence is indicative of disease or potential disease. These organisms are generally identified, classified, and separated by biochemical tests; the fermentation of sugars is the most important of these. There are some 400 species of *Salmonella.*

The Pseudomonadaceae are gram-negative rods and obligate aerobes; they do not ferment sugars, but are often spoken of in the same breath as the enterics. The two genera of interest are *Alcaligenes* and *Pseudomonas.* The two species involved most are *Pseudomonas aeruginosa* and *Pseudomonas cepacia.* These organisms do not have complex growth requirements, and can survive in distilled water. They are very resistant to disinfectants. They are normal inhabitants of the gastrointestinal tract.

Other gram-negative rods with complex, demanding growth requirements (often including the addition of carbon dioxide or the diminution of oxygen levels) include the genera *Haemophilus, Brucella, Campylobacter, Bordetella, Yersinia, Pasteurella,* and *Francisella.*

The next group to be considered are the aerobic gram-negative cocci. These include the genera of *Neisseria, Branhamella, Moraxella,* and *Acinetobacter.* The *Branhamella* cause disease primarily in relationship to dental and oral manipulations. *Neisseria meningitidis* (meningococcus) and *Neisseria gonorrheae* (gonococcus) are important pathogens. The others are rare causes of disease.

The final group to be considered are the anaerobic gram-negative organisms. The most important of these are the gram-negative rods in the genera *Bacteroides* and *Fusobacterium.* The *Bacteroides* are a major, often unrecognized, cause of disease. The many species of *Bacteroides* vary in their ability to cause disease. *Bacteroides fragilis* and the black colony forms present the most problems.[9,10]

Bacteroides gracilis, Bacteroides urolyticus, and *Eikenella corrodens* are closely related organisms.[11,12] *Eikenella* organisms can grow aerobically, but the others cannot. All three types cause pitting of the agar surface on which they are grown. *E corrodens* does cause orthopaedic infections.[11,12]

Only a few of these organisms are major contributors to the disease process. Many are opportunists, causing hospital-acquired or nosocomial infections. Organisms that are part of the normal flora, such as *Escherichia coli* and *Proteus, Klebsiella,* and *Pseudomonas* organisms live in the gastrointestinal tract and on the skin or as part of the oral flora without causing harm. However, when medical manipulations force them out of their natural environment and they become residents of other sites, they cause disease. For example, the insertion of urinary catheters disturbs the perianal tissues, possibly causes trauma to the gastrointestinal tract, and alters urinary function, allowing these organisms to enter the blood stream. Fever, shock, and often death follow. In addition, these organisms are common contaminants of water and, therefore, can appear in any solution used for injection or irrigation unless strict aseptic precautions are taken. Contamination is often unavoidable.

Conversely, some organisms are not normal flora and are capable of establishing infection whenever they can gain access to the body. Such infections do occur more often in a compromised host such as a patient rendered immunodeficient by corticosteroid, antineoplastic, or antimicrobial therapy, or one compromised by extreme youth or old age.

Adhesion

Adhesion to Mammalian Cells

The adhesion of gram-negative bacteria to mammalian cells was recognized as an important pathogenicity mechanism long before the glycocalyx of the coagulase-negative staphyloccci was known. Most of these organisms adhere by means of the protein hairs or fimbriae or pili on the cells. Some types of pili (type 2, for example) seem to be more associated with adherence than others.[13-16] Prevention and therapy are being approached through the use of vaccines containing pili.[17] However, the efficacy of this technique remains to be evaluated. It is evident, however, that antibodies that interact with the pili, proteases that degrade the pili, and other alterations of the pili decrease adherence and thus decrease pathogenicity.

The production of a glycocalyx or slime by these organisms seems to be limited but is of extreme importance for at least one genus. *Pseudomonas* causes severe infection in patients who have cystic fibrosis. These organisms are found in a mass of bacteria, mammalian cells, mammalian secretions, and bacterial secretions. The glycocalyx formed by these organisms is apparently critical in the disease process.[18,19] The *Bacteroides* may also form a glycocalyx.[20,21]

The appearance of the colony growing on solid media in vitro gives some information as to whether or not these organisms are a cause of the disease. "Rough" colonies that are dry and irregular tend not to be formed by pathogenic organisms, whereas those that are "smooth and glistening" are formed by pathogenic organisms.[20-22] This results from the formation by the organism of a polysaccharide capsule. This capsule impairs host defense mechanisms, interferes with antimicrobial therapy, and increases virulence. The relationship between the capsule and the glycocalyx can be subtle. Rough organisms do not form the glycocalyx but smooth organisms can. Adhesion to mammalian cells, however, is achieved by means of protein structures, and the glycocalyx tends not to increase bacteria-cell interaction but may increase the tenacity of the mass.

Adhesion to Biomaterials

In general, the adhesion of bacteria to biomaterials is more pronounced with coagulase-negative staphylococci than with gram-negative organisms. However, many laboratory studies have indicated that these organisms can adhere to both polymeric and metallic materials.[23-25] The enterics adhere by means of the fimbriae. Scanning electron analysis of the material shows a uniform adherence in contrast with the clumpiness seen with *S epidermidis*. The adherence of *Pseudomonas* resembles that of *S epidermidis* more than it resembles that of other gram-negative organisms. *Pseudomonas* species, although adhering in fewer numbers, tend to form a glycocalyx-like structure and have a nonuniform adherence pattern.[26] However, it must be remembered that microscopic analyses for glycocalyx are difficult because the glycocalyx is often dissolved or disturbed by processing procedures. Thus, the contribution of the glycocalyx to adhesion and pathogenicity may be underestimated. The glycocalyx is apparently important in long-term adhesion to biomaterials, whereas the fimbriae are important in the initial adherence to biomaterials and in adherence to mammalian cells.

Orthopaedic Infections Caused by Gram-Negative Bacteria

Organisms of Special Concern

The organisms posing the greatest risk of infection in orthopaedic patients are the *Pseudomonas* species and the group classified as the enterics.[27] It is important to remember that *Pseudomonas*, *Proteus*, *Escherichia*, *Enterobacter*, and *Klebsiella* organisms are opportunistic, are frequently isolated from the skin, mouth, and feces of healthy individuals, and cause disease only when something has gone wrong— that is, they cause nosocomial infections. Most of the other organisms are of minor importance. However, each particular infection entity has a slightly different pattern.

Septic Arthritis

The opportunistic enterics and *Pseudomonas* organisms cause septic arthritis.[5,7,8] The disease generally results from surgical manipulations and penetrations of the joint with a break in aseptic technique. Thus, repeated joint taps to obtain fluid for cell counts or to isolate the organisms can result in the instillation of bacteria, producing an iatrogenic infection. These organisms can also spread to the joint from infections at other sites, especially when there is trauma. These organisms destroy the joint rapidly. Endotoxin is suspected of being one of the major causes of bone loss in this disease. Early aggressive therapy is mandatory. Animal models of *E coli* arthritis have been reported and allow excellent study of the problem.[28]

Haemophilus influenzae is a major cause of meningitis and pneumonia in infants and in the elderly. For unknown reasons, this organism often causes a concomitant arthritis. These organisms are fragile and difficult to grow, and thus their presence may be suspected rather than proven by culture. Rapid diagnostic techniques based on antigen-antibody reactions have proven helpful in early diagnosis.[29,30] Another organism causing septic arthritis is *N gonorrheae*. This organism too is difficult to isolate and grow in culture, and the diagnosis is often not proven by culture but rather suggested by the fact that the patient has had gonorrhea. *N meningitides* is also occasionally isolated from the joint fluid in arthritis. Whether this is a separate disease entity or merely a problem with the biochemical tests used to distinguish the two *Neisseria* species remains unknown. There are no animal models for these arthritides.

From time to time there are case reports of septic arthritis caused by other gram-negative bacteria. These are indicative of the low incidence of disease because a single case merits publication. Lyme disease, now a frequent diagnosis, is caused by a spirochete that is gram-negative (because it does not take up the crystal violet at all).

Septic arthritis is generally found in joints without implants and, thus, is not considered to be implant-related, but implants at other sites that can seed infection or the use of devices in the joint to explore, instill, or withdraw material are major factors influencing the disease. The bacteria may adhere to the collagen in the joint.[31] Infections associated with joint replacement are rarely caused by gram-negative bacteria. In almost all cases *Pseudomonas* species and the enterics are responsible.

Osteomyelitis

Gram-negative osteomyelitis is extremely rare in intact bone. This disease is almost always implant-related and follows the development of disease elsewhere such as contiguous wound infection, septicemia, or an extension of infection in an open fracture. The only exceptions to this are *Salmonella typhi* and *Salmonella typhimurium*, which can cause osteomyelitis without major recognized disease elsewhere.[32,33] This occurs more often, but not exclusively, in patients with sickle cell disease. Osteomyelitis has been produced in the rabbit with *Pseudomonas* species.[34] Animal models using the other gram-negative bacteria are not as reliable.

Wound Infections

The incidence of gram-negative wound infection is again not as large as that with *S aureus*, but remains a major cause of morbidity and prolonged hospital stays. The wound infections may follow surgery and are usually caused by the enterics or, especially, *Pseudomonas* species, which have a tendency to live in antiseptics such as the io-dofors. These infections are also apt to occur in patients with open fractures, with as many as 26% of the patients becoming infected. They tend to have a higher incidence than *S aureus* infections because the antimicrobial prophylaxis used in patients with open fractures sup-presses or kills gram-positive organisms but has little effect on the gram-negatives ones.[35-38] The animal models for this are limited.

Complications Altering Infection Risk

Sickle cell anemia seems to predispose to osteomyelitis by *Salmonella* organisms, presumably because of small infarcts and clots within the bone in these patients. The femur and tibia are the most common sites.

Open fractures have the highest risk of infection of any procedure in orthopaedic surgery. The patient is often compromised medically at other sites, many organisms of a variety of types have been intro-duced directly into the deep tissue and the bone as part of the injury, and the use of foreign bodies as internal fixation devices and/or sutures is frequent. There has been much discussion of the role of internal fixation devices in infection of open fractures. In the presence of good antimicrobial therapy and adequate operating facilities, the internal fixation device does not necessarily increase the risk of infection and may reduce the risk by preventing micromotion of the bone fragments that may lead to subsequent tissue damage. The use of sutures to close the wounds primarily is associated with a great increase in infection risk and is contraindicated,[39] but the role of gram-negative bacteria has not been separated from that of gram-positive bacteria. Animal models have been used extensively and successfully in this area. [40-43]

Almost all patients undergoing total joint replacement have an un-derlying bone disease of inflammatory or ischemic origin; the others have fractures. Both inflammation and ischemia can potentiate infec-tion, and a fracture also impairs blood supply and host defenses. Thus, these patients are at risk for infection. Infections caused by gram-negative bacteria at the site of total joint replacements are almost always delayed infections. That is, they are seeded from a gram-neg-ative infection elsewhere. The presence of the biomaterial, probably with adherent organisms with a biofilm including glycocalyx, increases the risk of infection. Animal models for the study of total joint infec-tion have been explored but tend to be expensive[44,45] and have not been entirely successful because hematogenous spread is difficult to achieve in a sufficient number of the animals.[46]

Thus, early infections in total joint replacements are generally caused by the gram-positive cocci. Delayed infections can be caused by these organisms or others, including gram-negative bacteria, and often come from exogenous sources such as pulmonary infections, gastrointestinal or genitourinary tract infections, wound infections near the implant, or dental manipulations.

References

1. Rice PA, Iglewski BH: The cell envelope of gram-negative bacteria: Structure and function. Summary of session. *Rev Infect Dis* 1988;10(suppl 2):S277–S278.
2. Morrison DC, Ryan JL: Endotoxins and disease mechanisms. *Annu Rev Med* 1987;38:417–432.
3. Morrison DC, Ryan JL: Bacterial endotoxins and host immune responses. *Adv Immunol* 1979;28:293–450.
4. Burrell R: Immunomodulation by bacterial endotoxin. *Crit Rev Microbiol* 1990;17:189–208.
5. Baron S (ed): *Medical Microbiology.* Menlo Park, Addison Wesley, 1982.
6. Stanier RY, Adelberg EA, Ingraham JL: *The Microbial World*, ed 4. Englewood Cliffs, Prentice-Hall, 1976.
7. Rose NR, Barron AL (eds): *Microbiology: Basic Principles and Clinical Applications.* New York, Macmillan, 1983.
8. Lennette EH, Balows A, Hausler WJ Jr, et al (eds): *Manual of Clinical Microbiology*, ed 3. Washington, DC, American Society for Microbiology, 1980.
9. Brook I: Encapsulated anaerobic bacteria in synergistic infections. *Microbiol Rev* 1986;50:452–457.
10. Brook I: Pathogenicity of the *Bacteroides fragilis* group. *Ann Clin Lab Sci* 1989;19:360–376.
11. Johnson CC, Reinhardt JF, Edelstein MAC, et al: *Bacteroides gracilis*, an important anaerobic bacterial pathogen. *J Clin Microbiol* 1985;22:799–802.
12. Flesher SA, Bottone EJ: *Eikenella corrodens* cellulitis and arthritis of the knee. *J Clin Microbiol* 1989;27:2606–2608.
13. Keith BR, Harris SL, Russell PW, et al: Effect of type 1 piliation on in vitro killing of *Escherichia coli* by mouse peritoneal macrophages. *Infect Immun* 1990;58:3448–3454.
14. Krogfelt KA, Bergmans H, Klemm P: Direct evidence that the FimH protein is the mannose-specific adhesin of *Escherichia coli* Type 1 fimbriae. *Infect Immun* 1990;58:1995–1998.
15. Kröncke KD, Orskov I, Orskov F, et al: Electron microscopic study of coexpression of adhesive protein capsules and polysaccharide capsules in *Escherichia coli. Infect Immun* 1990;58:2710–2714.
16. Sareneva T, Holthöfer H, Korhonen TK: Tissue binding affinity of *Proteus mirabilis* fimbriae in the human urinary tract. *Infect Immun* 1990;58:3330–3336.
17. Marx JL: Vaccinating with bacterial pili. *Science* 1980;209:1103–1106.
18. Inglis TJ, Millar MR, Jones JG, et al: Tracheal tube biofilm as a source of bacterial colonization of the lung. *J Clin Microbiol* 1989;27:2014–2018.
19. Saiman L, Cacalano G, Prince A: *Pseudomonas cepacia* adherence to respiratory epithelial cells is enhanced by *Pseudomonas aeruginosa. Infect Immun* 1990;58:2578–2584.
20. Lantz MS, Rowland RW, Switalski LM, et al: Interactions of *Bacteroides gingivalis* with fibrinogen. *Infect Immun* 1986;54:654–658.
21. Li J, Ellen RP: Relative adherence of *Bacteroides* species and strains to *Actinomyces viscosus* on saliva-coated hydroxyapatite. *J Dent Res* 1989;68:1308–1312.

22. Onderdonk AB, Cisneros RL, Finberg R, et al: Animal model system for studying virulence of and host response to *Bacteroides fragilis*. *Rev Infect Dis* 1990;12(suppl 2):S169–S177.

23. Jensen ET, Kharazmi A, Lam K, et al: Human polymorphonuclear leukocyte response to *Pseudomonas aeruginosa* grown in biofilms. *Infect Immun* 1990;58:2383–2385.

24. Kelly NM, Bell A, Hancock REW: Surface characteristics of *Pseudomonas aeruginosa* grown in a chamber implant model in mice and rats. *Infect Immun* 1989;57:344–350.

25. Slusher MM, Myrvik QN, Lewis JC, et al: Extended-wear lenses, biofilm, and bacterial adhesion. *Arch Ophthalmol* 1987;105:110–115.

26. Bisno AL, Waldvogel FA (eds): *Infections Associated With Indwelling Medical Devices*. Washington, DC, American Society for Microbiology, 1989.

27. Sherertz RJ, Sarubbi FA: A three-year study of nosocomial infections associated with *Pseudomonas aeruginosa*. *J Clin Microbiol* 1983;18:160–164.

28. Schurman DJ, Kajiyama G, Nagel DA: *Escherichia coli* infections in rabbit knee joints: The pharmacological and antibacterial effects of intramuscular antibiotics. *J Bone Joint Surg* 1980;62A:620–627.

29. Merritt K, Boyle WE Jr, Dye SK, et al: Counter immunoelectrophoresis in the diagnosis of septic arthritis caused by *Hemophilus influenzae*: Report of two cases. *J Bone Joint Surg* 1976;58A:414–415.

30. James K: Immunoserology of infectious diseases. *Clin Microbiol Rev* 1990;3:132–152.

31. Vercellotti GM, McCarthy JB, Lindholm P, et al: Extracellular matrix proteins (fibronectin, laminin, and type IV collagen) bind and aggregate bacteria. *Am J Pathol* 1985;120:13–21.

32. Govender S, Chotai PR: Salmonella osteitis and septic arthritis. *J Bone Joint Surg* 1990;72B:504–506.

33. *Salmonella* bone and joint infections, editorial. *J Infect* 1983;6:107–109.

34. Norden CW, Shinners E: Ciprofloxacin as therapy for experimental osteomyelitis caused by *Pseudomonas aeruginosa*. *J Infect Dis* 1985;151:291–294.

35. Marrie TJ, Costerton JW: Mode of growth of bacterial pathogens in chronic polymicrobial human osteomyelitis. *J Clin Microbiol* 1985;22:924–933.

36. Merritt K: Factors increasing the risk of infection in patients with open fractures. *J Trauma* 1988;28:823–827.

37. Clancey GJ, Hansen ST Jr: Open fractures of the tibia: A review of one hundred and two cases. *J Bone Joint Surg* 1978;60A:118–122.

38. Roth AI, Fry DE, Polk HC Jr: Infectious morbidity in extremity fractures. *J Trauma* 1986;26:757–761.

39. Hunt TK: Surgical wound infections: An overview. *Am J Med* 1981;70:712–718.

40. Merritt K, Dowd JD: Role of internal fixation in infection of open fractures: Studies with *Staphylococcus aureus* and *Proteus mirabilis*. *J Orthop Res* 1987;5:23–28.

41. Merritt K, Dowd JD: Fracture site motion and infection, in Perren SM, Schneider E (eds): *Biomechanics: Current Interdisciplinary Research*. Dordrecht, Martinus Nijhoff, 1985, pp 209–214.

42. Norden CW, Shaffer M: Treatment of experimental chronic osteomyelitis due to *Staphylococcus aureus* with vancomycin and rifampin. *J Infect Dis* 1983;147:352–357.

43. Dougherty SH: Pathobiology of infection in prosthetic devices. *Rev Infect Dis* 1988;10:1102–1117.

44. Petty W, Spanier S, Shuster JJ, et al: The influence of skeletal implants on incidence of infection: Experiments in a canine model. *J Bone Joint Surg* 1985;67A:1236–1244.

45. Fitzgerald RH Jr: Experimental osteomyelitis: Description of a canine model and the role of depot administration of antibiotics in the prevention and treatment of sepsis. *J Bone Joint Surg* 1983;65A:371–380.

46. Blomgren G, Lundquist H, Nord CE, et al: Late anaerobic haematogenous infection of experimental total joint replacement: A study in the rabbit using *Propionibacterium acnes*. *J Bone Joint Surg* 1981;63B:614–618.

Chapter 7

Microbial Adhesion and Arthritides: Other Pathogens

Joel B. Baseman, PhD
Victor V. Tryon, PhD

Bacterial pathogens have evolved multifaceted and sophisticated mechanisms by which they can interact with the host environment and cause disease. One of the most important is their ability to adhere to target cells and initiate the pathogenic process. Selective cytadherence permits individual microorganisms to colonize mucous membranes and other tissues, resist clearing mechanisms of the host, modify surface properties and other metabolic activities, and, occasionally, disseminate to other in vivo ecologic niches. Many of these host-pathogen interactions are mediated by microbial surface components, called adhesins, that seek out complementary stereospecific structures on the host, called receptors. In some instances, different classes of adhesins may be simultaneously or variably expressed by a single microorganism, thus providing biologic versatility and multiple host target sites. Further, adherence of microorganisms to surfaces can be influenced by electrostatic and hydrophobic forces, the physiochemical properties of the micro-environment, and the metabolic state of both host and pathogen.

The following discussion focuses on two important groups of pathogenic microorganisms and highlights aspects of their biology related to virulence and disease pathogenesis.

Mycoplasma

Natural infections with mycoplasmas in birds and nonhuman mammals can unquestionably result in acute and chronic arthritis. This observation, combined with occasional reports of the isolation of mycoplasmas from human joint tissues and fluid, the identification of mycoplasmal antigens in synovium from humans with acute polyarthritis, and the detection of anti-mycoplasmal antibodies in patients with rheumatoid arthritis, has driven the search for pathogenic mycoplasmas as the etiologic agents of acute and chronic rheumatoid arthritis in humans.

The mycoplasmas belong to an intriguing and heterogenous class of prokaryotes without cell walls, called Mollicutes ("soft skin") by taxonomists. The mycoplasmas properly represent only one of the families within this class of organisms, but most members of this class of bacteria continue to be referred to colloquially and collectively as the mycoplasmas. The Mollicutes are thought to be derived by chromosomal reductions from genomically more complex gram-positive ancestral bacteria.[1] The genus *Mycoplasma* contains many pathogenic species, including the human respiratory pathogen, *Mycoplasma pneumoniae*, and a recently described urogenital tract pathogen, *Mycoplasma genitalium*, which is believed to be the smallest free-living human pathogen. This organism was recently found to have only one eighth of the genetic coding capacity of *Escherichia coli*.[2]

The mycoplasmas have a number of special attributes that either obfuscate or reinforce their potential role in human disease. Swift and Brown[3] were the first to suggest that mycoplasmas were etiologic agents of rheumatoid arthritis. These organisms can be extremely difficult to cultivate outside the vertebrate host or away from eukaryotic cells in culture,[4,5] which makes diagnosis difficult. *M pneumoniae* and other *Mycoplasma* species can produce intense inflammatory reactions, perhaps through the activation of the alternate complement pathway[6] or the elaboration of potent T- and B-cell mitogens.[7,8] The mycoplasmas have a eukaryote-like, sterol-containing cell membrane without a cell wall. This may explain the propensity of these organisms to acquire host protein antigens.[9] This propensity to acquire antigens from the host or culture medium may in turn help explain the cross-reactions and autoimmune reactions that are part of the syndrome of mycoplasmal infections.[10–12]

Mycoplasma-Induced Arthritis in Animals

The mycoplasmas represent the most common etiologic agents of natural chronic joint inflammation and destruction in veterinary medicine. The arthritogenic activity of these agents in bovine, caprine, porcine, and avian infections was extensively reviewed by Cole and associates.[13] More than ten different *Mycoplasma* species are responsible for arthritis-like diseases in birds and mammals (Table 1). These organisms produce complex pathogenic and histopathologic features that mirror the manifestations of human rheumatoid arthritis.[8] These manifestations include immune complex deposition, altered lymphocyte reactivity (both increased and decreased), joint swelling, villous hypertrophy, formation of lymphoid nodules, and generalized, chronic inflammatory responses that are not limited to joints.

Spontaneous, natural arthritis in birds and mammals is a worldwide problem. One example is the avian arthritis caused by *Mycoplasma synoviae*. *M synoviae* is primarily a respiratory pathogen in chickens and turkeys, but outbreaks of infectious synovitis can result in high flock mortality. Similarly, *Mycoplasma bovis* (bovine) and *Mycoplasma hyorhinis* (swine) cause upper respiratory tract disease with arthritis as a common manifestation or occasional primary symptom.

Table 1 The arthritogenic mycoplasmas*

Organism	Usual Host	Natural Disease	Acute vs Chronic	Natural Disease Other Than Arthritis
M pneumoniae	Human	Yes	Acute†	Pneumonia
M genitalium	Human	Yes	Acute†	Genital tract, pneumonia
M arthritidis	Rat	Yes	Acute	Conjunctivitis, urethritis
	Mouse	No	Chronic	
	Rabbit	No	Chronic	
M pulmonis	Mouse	Yes	Chronic	Pneumonia, reproductive tract
	Rat	No	Acute	Pneumonia, reproductive tract
M hyorhinis	Swine	Yes	Chronic	Respiratory
M hyosynoviae	Swine	Yes	Chronic	Polyserositis
M synoviae	Fowl	Yes	Chronic	Sacculitis, hepatitis, endocarditis, anemia
M gallisepticum	Fowl	Yes	Chronic	Sacculitis, arteritis
M mycoides	Cattle	Yes	Chronic	Pleuropneumonia
M bovis	Cattle	Yes	Chronic	Mastitis, reproductive tract
M agalactiae	Sheep, goats	Yes	Chronic	Mastitis, conjunctivitis

*Adapted from Cole and Cassell.[8]
†See discussion in text and in Davis and associates.[45]

All of these *Mycoplasma*-induced diseases show greater morbidity and mortality in younger animals, are presumed to include hematogenous spread from the respiratory tract, incite high antibody levels in the synovial fluid of affected joints, show persistence of bacterial antigens in the joint tissues, and may result in erosive joint disease.

Much intensive experimental work has been done with *Mycoplasma arthritidis*, a causative agent of spontaneous polyarthritis in rats. *M arthritidis* is also used for the experimental induction of arthritis in rats, mice, and, after intra-articular injection, rabbits. The combined genetic studies done in rats by Cole and associates[14] and Kirchoff and associates[15] suggest a very complex interaction between pathogen and host with both susceptibility and sensitivity (that is, extent of disease) under polyallelic control. Binder and associates,[16] using inbred, congenic, and F1 hybrid rats, found similar results but also demonstrated a clear separation of the effects of heritable traits between acute and chronic arthritic disease states.

In behavioral studies on inbred rats, Gartner and associates[17] concluded that individuals of genetically mixed populations may be influenced in opposite directions with regard to their sensitivity to arthritic disease by their different inherited genotypes. These investigators concluded further that sensitivity to disease could be affected to some degree by "psychosomatic pathways" (that is, neuroendocrine events). These pathways may be influenced, for example, by stress.

Mycoplasmal Antigens in Joint Fluid and Tissue

Since the demonstration in 1967 by Schwab and associates[18] that streptococcal cell-wall components persisted in the joint spaces of rabbits, it has been suggested by many that *Mycoplasma*-induced rheumatoid arthritis may result from destructive host immune responses to persisting (and presumably nonviable) mycoplasmal antigens or *Mycoplasma*-altered self (host) antigens.

For example, Decker and Barden[19] found evidence for the production of IgG, IgM, and IgA in the synovia of Yorkshire swine for more than 12 months after a single intraperitoneal injection of *M hyorhinis*. One report suggested that the disease may have persisted because of a *M hyorhinis*-derived antigen in the synovia.[20] Interestingly, one other breed of pigs tested by Decker and Barden[19] was not susceptible to the *M hyorhinis*-induced arthritis. Washburn and associates[21,22] reported the induction of chronic arthritis and the local production of *Mycoplasma*-directed IgG, IgM, and IgA in rabbits after a single intra-articular injection of *M arthritidis*. Arthritis was reported to last for more than one year even though *Mycoplasma* organisms were detectable in joint tissue for only seven weeks.

Using the same experimental model, Cooke and Jasin[23] reported the persistence of mycoplasmal antigens in joint tissue. Cooke and associates[24] later detected immune complexes in the joint tissue of humans with rheumatoid arthritis. However, little correlation has been found between circulating or localized immune complexes and extent of disease in patients with rheumatoid arthritis.[25]

More recently, however, Clark and associates[26] reported the specific recognition of mycoplasmal antigens from *M pneumoniae*, *M arthritidis*, and *Mycoplasma hominis*, but not *Mycoplasma fermentans* or *Mycoplasma salivarium*, in immune complexes in synovial fluid obtained from three patients with rheumatoid arthritis. Immune complexes were isolated from the synovial fluid by affinity chromatography. Specific immunoglobulin was disaggregated and $F(ab')_2$ fragments were then immunoblotted to protein profiles of the reference mycoplasmas and a number of distinct bands were visualized from three of the five *Mycoplasma* species. The lack of mass standards in the published figures makes it difficult to determine if the peptides recognized in the immunoblot corresponded to identified and characterized *Mycoplasma* proteins, such as the immunodominant adhesin P1 of *M pneumoniae*.[27,28]

Clark and associates[26] concluded that their studies indicated the presence of mycoplasmal antigens or autosome-related (that is, cross-reactive) antigens within the joints of patients with rheumatoid arthritis. They further speculated that the mycoplasmal antigens found in the immune complexes are from mycoplasmas that originally colonized sites other than joints (for example, the respiratory tract or urogenital tract). In an immunologically competent host, these antigens are shed from the mycoplasmas to form an immune complex that is later sequestered in the joint space. Ultimately, the sequestered complex provokes a local inflammatory response in synovial tissues.[26]

Mycoplasmas Isolated From Human Joint Tissue and Fluid

The role of mycoplasmas in eliciting human joint disease is well documented with regard to hypogammaglobulinemia, a condition in which mycoplasmas have been isolated from acutely inflamed joints.[29] Also, *M hominis* has been isolated in septic arthritis in postpartum patients and in patients who underwent urogenital tract surgery.[30-32] A chronic, migrating polyarthritis has been reported after upper respiratory tract infection with *M pneumoniae*.[33-35]

Webster and associates[36] reported that an asymmetric, nonerosive polyarthritis develops in as many as 30% of patients with hypogammaglobulinemia. This resolves with long-term immunoglobulin therapy. Patients with hypogammaglobulinemia have also been reported to be at increased risk for pulmonary, urinary tract, and joint infections by mycoplasmas.[36] Both *M pneumoniae* and *Ureaplasma urealyticum* have been isolated from patients with hypogammaglobulinemia.[29,37-41] These results suggest that otherwise sterile joint effusions in patients with hypoglobulinemia should be cultured specifically for both *Ureaplasma* species and *Mycoplasma* species in laboratories with experience in isolating these fastidious pathogens. It is interesting to note that the arthritic disease associated with *M pneumoniae* was considered to be hyperplastic but nonerosive. This is in contrast to the report of Kraus and associates[39] concerning *U urealyticum*, in which they described a oligoarticular erosive arthritis in a single patient that involved both major and small joints and that evolved over a six-month period. Barile and associates[42] reported similar abnormalities in chimpanzees inoculated intra-articularly with large numbers of one strain of *M hominis* and *U urealyticum*, serovar II. No disease was elicited by intra-articular injection of the *M hominis* type strain PG21, or when the mycoplasmal and ureaplasmal strains were inoculated intravenously instead of intra-articularly. The mechanism of spread of these organisms from the respiratory tract or urogenital tract, the usual sites of colonization to the joints, is unknown but is presumably hematogenous.

Septic arthritis caused by *M hominis* has been associated with puerperal sepsis, abortion, trauma, and manipulation of the urogenital tract. There are at least two reports of the involvement of prostheses in *M hominis* septic arthritis.[43,44] Nylander and associates[44] reviewed the clinical findings associated with mycoplasmal septic arthritis (Outline 1).

Polyarthritis following upper respiratory infection with *M pneumoniae* occurred in approximately 1% of more than 1,200 patients with serologically proven infection.[33,34] Until recently, isolation of *M pneumoniae* from arthritic joint fluid was successful principally in patients with hypogammaglobulinemia.

The recent isolation of recognized human mycoplasmal pathogens from an apparently immunocompetent adult is an important development. Davis and associates[45] documented the isolation of *M pneumoniae* from synovial fluid from the wrist and knee of a single patient without hypogammaglobulinemia who had a history of degenerative joint disease. The acute polyarthritis followed an episode of atypical pneumonia. In addition, the synovial fluid from this patient contained both IgM and IgG antibody specific for *M pneumoniae*. The close

Outline 1 Risk factors for septic arthritis caused by mycoplasmas*

Hypogammaglobulinemia
Immunocompromise (organic or transient resulting from major trauma)
Atypical pneumonia
Genitourinary tract manipulation (surgery or even catheterization)
Postpartum or postabortal fever
Connective tissue disease
Synovial fluid
   White blood cell count > 80,000/mm^3
   Smear with more than 95% polymorphonuclear neutrophils
   Gram-negative stain but positive acridine-orange stain
Slow or absent growth in standard culture media

*Adapted from Nylander and associates.[44]

correlation of the acute upper respiratory tract disease and the isolation of *M pneumoniae* from the arthritic joints suggested a hematogenous dissemination of the pathogen. It was later discovered that both *M pneumoniae* and *M genitalium* existed in the original isolates from this patient (J.G. Tully, personal communication). *M genitalium*, which is serologically very closely related to *M pneumoniae*, was originally isolated from the male urogenital tract, but more recently has also been found in *M pneumoniae*-associated upper respiratory tract disease.[46]

Identification of *M pneumoniae* Proteinaceous Adhesins

The best studied of the mycoplasmas is *M pneumoniae*, the cause of a common, cold agglutinin-associated, usually self-limiting pneumonia in humans. Because the natural disease is rarely fatal, experimental models have been established that examine the dynamics of the host-parasite interaction. *M pneumoniae* has a unique flask shape and displays a distinct tip-like organelle (Fig. 1, *left*). This tip structure permits the highly oriented extracellular parasitism by mycoplasmas on respiratory epithelial cells,[47] followed by ciliostasis and progressive destruction of the epithelium.[48,49] Avirulent, noncytadhering mycoplasmas derived from the virulent parent strain do not cytadhere and are incapable of producing cytopathologic abnormalities.[50,51] It is clear that the ability of *M pneumoniae* to penetrate the network of host respiratory defenses, including ciliary motion and a mucous blanket, and to locate and adhere to appropriate receptors is necessary for the development of biochemical lesions and disease.

Brief protease pretreatment of *M pneumoniae* markedly reduces the adherence of mycoplasmas to respiratory cells and erythrocytes.[47,48,52] These observations suggest that specific mycoplasmal proteins may function as mediators of cytadherence. Gel electrophoretic analysis of trypsin-treated *M pneumoniae* revealed that the loss of a surface protein, designated P1, correlated directly with reduced surface parasitism and that resynthesis of this protein fully restored cytadherence capabilities.[47]

Other data further implicated P1 as a major adhesin. Antibodies

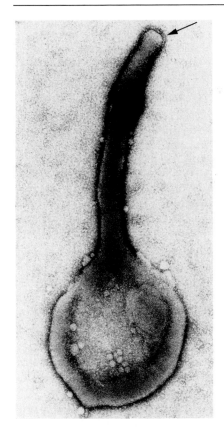 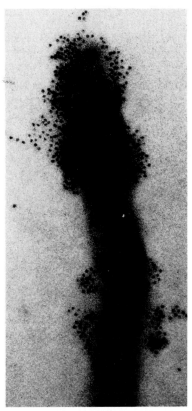

Fig. 1 *Left*, *Virulent* M pneumoniae *with its distinguishing nap and unique flask-like appearance.* ***Right***, *High-resolution electron microscopy of clusters of the* M pneumoniae *adhesin P1 at the tip region (× 150,000).*

generated against P1 inhibited mycoplasmal adherence to target cells without affecting the growth or metabolic state of *M pneumoniae*.[53-55] Even anti-P1 immunoglobulin Fab fragments and anti-P1 monoclonal antibodies blocked cytadherence.[56,57] Further, when immunoferritin labeling and electron microscopy were used to determine the membrane distribution of P1 on virulent *M pneumoniae*, P1 molecules were observed densely clustered at the tip organelle (Fig. 1, *right*), providing topographic evidence that P1 is structurally and functionally linked to cytadherence.[28] This was further substantiated by in vitro binding assays, using detergent-solubilized mycoplasmal preparations and chemically stabilized respiratory epithelium, that demonstrated the selective binding of P1 to host cell surfaces.[55]

Analysis of Cytadhering-Deficient Mutants of *M pneumoniae*

To further define the role of P1 and other mycoplasmal proteins in cytadherence, spontaneously arising noncytadhering *M pneumoniae*

Outline 2 Characterization of the P1 gene of *Mycoplasma pneumoniae*

Purification of the P1 adhesin by monoclonal antibody affinity chromatography and
   preparative gel electrophoresis
Determination of amino-terminal amino acid sequence by gas phase microsequencing
Generation of oligonucleotide probes (14-mer, corresponding to amino acids 1–5;
   18-mer, corresponding to amino acids 7–12) complementary to all possible mRNA
   combinations
Identification of a common DNA fragment by hybridization to both oligonucleotide
   probes
Cloning and sequencing of P1 gene with a 6-kb EcoRI genomic fragment

---

mutants were isolated.[51,56] Analysis of electrophoretic protein profiles
of these mutants revealed protein deficiencies not only in P1 but also
in other membrane proteins, permitting the categorization of mutants
into four classes. One class was deficient in the P1 protein whereas
another class synthesized the P1 protein but lacked a 30–kd surface
protein (P30) that was only moderately sensitive to protease.[57] This
second mutant class could not cluster P1 at the tip organelle, suggesting
that other membrane components, such as the 30–kd protein, are essential for P1 localization and function. Additional studies using anti-
30–kd antiserum and colloidal gold-labeling electron microscopic techniques revealed clustering of the 30–kd protein at the tip organelle of
M pneumoniae, apparently in juxtaposition with P1.[57] The remaining
mutant classes were deficient in other groups of proteins that appeared
to function as "accessory" proteins, mobilizing and clustering adhesins
P1 and P30 at the tip.

   After intranasal inoculation of hamsters, the noncytadhering mutants were cleared rapidly from the respiratory tract and other tissues
and were avirulent.[50,51,58] Spontaneous, cytadhering revertants were isolated from each mutant class and were shown to synthesize the full
complement of membrane proteins and to replicate and cause histopathologic changes in the hamster model of infection.[56] These data
indicated that *M pneumoniae* cytadherence is not mediated solely by
a single adhesin but requires a complex interaction of membrane proteins for successful surface parasitism and subsequent disease.

Cloning and Sequencing of the P1 and P30 Genes of *M pneumoniae*

   Initial attempts to introduce *M pneumoniae* DNA into *E coli* using
phage λ as the vector and to monitor expression of recombinant DNA
molecules were restricted by the unusual property of mycoplasmas to
use the universal stop codon UGA as a tryptophan codon.[59] Thus, *E
coli* prematurely terminated *M pneumoniae* proteins encoded by structural genes containing UGA codons. An alternate strategy was used
to characterize P1 that did not require expression of the P1 proteins
in *E coli* (Outline 2). Properties of the P1 adhesin gene and the deduced
amino acid sequence have been described.[28] One of the most interesting
aspects of the sequence is its homology to mammalian cytoskeletal
keratin and human fibrinogen, which may correlate with previous observations of autoimmune-like mechanisms in mycoplasmal disease.[11]

Whether this apparent antigenic mimicry plays a role in the inflammatory mechanisms and immunopathologic changes that might be associated with arthritides is undetermined.

Further analysis of the P1 structural gene revealed that it can be divided into several domains; some of these exist as single genomic copies and others exist as multiple copies, sharing homology with other *M pneumoniae* genes.[60] In other words, specific regions of the P1 gene hybridize to multiple bands of genomic DNA, indicating that extensive homologies occur among specific sequences of the P1 gene and other segments of the *M pneumoniae* genome.

Because repeated gene sequences of major surface antigens are associated with antigenic variation in pathogenic microorganisms,[61-64] the possibility existed that multiple P1–related gene copies could regulate the structural and functional properties of P1. If so, P1 could occur as a family of adhesin-related molecules with altered specificities and affinities for host target sites.[60] Consistent with this possibility was the existence of restriction fragment length polymorphisms (also called RFLPs or riflips) in the P1 structural gene of human clinical isolates of *M pneumoniae*,[65,66] reflected by sequence divergency in multiple-copy regions of the P1 gene.[67] These regions of sequence divergency in the P1 gene resulted in considerable amino acid changes in the P1 adhesin that could alter cytadherence and antigenic properties and influence the virulence potential of *M pneumoniae* strains.

Recently, the P30 adhesin-related gene of *M pneumoniae* was characterized,[68] and analysis of the sequence data revealed several interesting properties. For example, three types of repeat sequences were detected at the carboxy end, including an extensive proline-rich region. Unexpectedly, the P30 sequence data exhibited substantial homology with the proline-rich carboxy terminus of the P1 adhesin. In addition, homology was observed between the P30 protein and human vitronectin, myosin, and collagen, again implicating the role of antigenic mimicry in autoimmune abnormalities. The fact that P1 and P30 share structural and functional relationships may assist in defining the membrane polarity of these adhesin-related molecules at the differentiated tip organelle of virulent *M pneumoniae*. Whatever the case, the cytadherence of *M pneumoniae* is not a simple lock-and-key mechanism of recognition between a single mycoplasmal adhesin and host receptor but requires cooperation among several mycoplasmal membrane proteins, including P1 and P30.

Cytadherence Mechanisms Among Other Mycoplasmas

Adhesins of other human mycoplasmas are currently under investigation. Early observations revealed that *M genitalium*, like *M pneumoniae*, possesses a distinct tip organelle that mediates adherence to various eukaryotic cells.[69,70] In addition, several reports demonstrated antigenic cross-reactivity between the P1 adhesin of *M pneumoniae* and a 140–kd surface protein of *M genitalium*.[71,72] Therefore, the 140-kd protein may be functionally related to P1 and serve as the *M gen-*

italium adhesin. This possibility was confirmed by the observations that anti-140-kd antibodies are localized at the tip structure of *M genitalium*[73] and that specific anti-140–kd monoclonal antibodies blocked mycoplasmal adherence to target cells.[71] The recent discovery that *M genitalium*, which was originally isolated from the urethras of patients with nongonococcal urethritis in 1980, was detected in throat specimens from individuals with *Mycoplasma*-induced pneumonia[46] underscores the common cytadherence mechanisms and tissue tropisms associated with *M pneumoniae* and *M genitalium*.

The relationship between the adhesins of *M genitalium* and *M pneumoniae* was established definitively through the cloning and sequencing of the gene encoding the 140–kd protein[74] and through DNA-DNA hybridization data.[75] Specific parts of the P1 gene of *M pneumoniae* exhibited homology with the 140–kd gene, reinforcing their functional and immunologic similarities.[74,75] In addition, extensive homologies were observed between the DNA and protein sequences of these adhesins, which far exceeded the reported 6.5% to 8.0% total genomic DNA-DNA hybridization values shared by *M pneumoniae* and *M genitalium*.[76] Therefore, the two adhesin proteins of *M pneumoniae* and *M genitalium* are likely to exhibit similar conformational properties in the mycoplasmal membrane and to recognize identical or related host receptors.

Host Receptors Recognized by Mycoplasmal Adhesins

Much less information is available concerning the identification of corresponding receptor sites on host cells that bind mycoplasmal adhesins. *M pneumoniae* interactions with human erythrocytes are mediated by long-chain oligosaccharides of sialic acid linked $\alpha2$–3 to terminal galactose residues.[12] These studies were extended to show that similar long-chain sialo-oligosaccharides were concentrated at the human bronchial epithelium, establishing a biochemical basis for *M pneumoniae* adherence to respiratory sites.[77] Recent data further supported the role for $\alpha2$–3-linked sialic acid and implicated sulfatides and other sulfated glycolipids, which contain a terminal Gal ($3SO_4$) $\beta1$-residue, as receptors for *M pneumoniae* adherence.[78,79] Therefore, at least two distinct receptor-mediated specificities appear to be operative during *M pneumoniae* cytadherence. It is important to note that these receptors are not limited to the respiratory tract but occur on the surfaces of many eukaryotic cells and are associated with host macromolecules such as laminin and fetuin and various sulfated glycoconjugates. However, no evidence yet exists that these two categories of host receptors directly bind the *M pneumoniae* adhesins P1 and P30.

Lyme Disease and Arthritis

Lyme disease is a complex, zoonotic, infectious disease that Malawista and Steere[80] described as "infectious in origin and rheumatic in

Table 2 Manifestations of rheumatoid arthritis and Lyme arthritis*

Manifestation	Rheumatoid Arthritis	Lyme Arthritis†
Rheumatoid factor	Positive	Negative
Joint fluid		
Cryoglobulins	Elevated	Elevated
Total protein	Elevated	Elevated
Leukocytes (cell/mm)	5,000 to 50,000	500 to 100,000
Common HLA type	DR4	DR4‡
Symmetric involvement	Characteristic	Not common
Subcutaneous nodules	Characteristic	Do not occur
Morning stiffness	Common	Less common
Large joint involvement	Common	Common, more swelling than pain
Small joint involvement	Common	Not common
Erosive disease	Common	Occasionally reported

*Adapted from Tortorice and Heim-Duthoy.[124]
†There are no firm guidelines for the diagnosis of Lyme arthritis.
‡See text concerning the role of genetics in Lyme disease.

expression" (Table 2). Tick-mediated injection of the spirochete *Borrelia burgdorferi* in humans results in an immune-mediated multisystem disease that affects the skin, nervous system, heart (including conduction defects), and musculoskeletal system. The risk of spirochete transmission is thought to increase with the duration of tick attachment after the bite.[81] Lyme disease has been likened to syphilis in that it has been described as the latest great disease imitator or mimicker.[82,83]

Although the actual overall incidence in the United States is low, Lyme borreliosis has become the most frequently reported tick-borne infectious disease in the United States since it was first reported in 1977.[84,85] One recent epidemiologic study suggests that Lyme disease is still spreading geographically in Connecticut[86] where the disease was first identified by Steere and associates[85] after persistent urging by mothers alarmed by the increased frequency and clustering of juvenile arthropathies in local children. Laboratory data also suggest that the incidence of Lyme disease in this area is increasing.[86]

Although the course of Lyme disease varies greatly from patient to patient and in different geographic locations, the disease typically begins with a unique skin lesion, erythema chronicum migrans, at the bite site of the arthropod vector *Ixodes dammini* or other ticks.[87–89] The skin lesion may go unnoticed, especially in children, but is accompanied by headache, fever, myalgias, arthralgias, generalized lymphadenopathy, and vague symptoms such as malaise or fatigue. Localized, intermittent musculoskeletal pain or overt arthritis can begin early in the disease but is more generally seen at a later stage.[90]

Steere and associates[91] carefully documented the natural history of Lyme arthritis before the efficacy of antibiotic treatment was established. Fifty-five patients with erythema chronicum migrans were followed up for three to eight years before antibiotic therapy became standard. Twenty percent of the patients developed no further manifestations of the disease despite positive titers to *B burgdorferi*. The remaining 80% all had various symptoms of joint disease. Localized, intermittent musculoskeletal pain developed in approximately 50% and transient arthritis in more than 5%. The arthritis episodes were separated by months, and sometimes even years, of complete remission. Individual episodes of musculoskeletal pain lasted for hours to days.[90,91] Chronic arthritis lasting for a year or longer in one to three large joints (most commonly the knee) developed in 11% of the cohort. Transient arthritis generally preceded the development of chronic symptoms, which began as long as 48 months after the initial skin lesion. Erosive joint disease (cartilage and bone) was seen in less than 5% of patients.[90,91] Two studies suggested that children with Lyme disease were more likely to have arthritis as the initial symptom of the disease.[86,92]

B burgdorferi and Spirochetal Antigens in Joint Fluid and Tissue

When synovial lesions from patients with Lyme arthritis were first examined histologically, they were found to be very similar to those in other chronic inflammatory diseases such as rheumatoid arthritis. One difference was the visualization by silver stain of spirochetes in microangiopathic lesions in two of eight samples.[93]

When this question was examined later in a separate study, Steere and associates[94] also described the synovial lesions in Lyme disease as almost identical to synovium from patients with rheumatoid arthritis and typical of a chronic hypersensitivity immune response. The hypersensitivity reaction by the host was thought to be provoked by the localization of a small number of intact spirochetes and additional antigen deposits within the synovia. Synovia from six of the 12 patients in whom Lyme arthritis was diagnosed were reactive with immunoperoxidase-labeled monoclonal antibodies to flagellar and outer membrane *B burgdorferi* antigens.[94] The organisms were reported as scarce and described as difficult to find despite the examination of many sections. After a diligent search, Duray and Steere[95] found a few spirochetes in two of 17 samples examined by silver staining and light microscopy.

In two separate reports apparently concerning the same patient, Lastavica and associates[96] and Snydman and associates[97] reported the isolation of *B burgdorferi* from synovial fluid aspirated from one knee of a man with chronic Lyme arthritis. Synovial fluid was positive for anti-*B burgdorferi* IgG by immunofluorescence. Steere[98] reported negative results for cumulative attempts to culture the spirochete from synovial specimens from 18 patients with Lyme arthritis.

Supporting the impression of residual spirochetal antigens eliciting a destructive immune response is the proposal by McLaughlin and associates[99] to remove the provoking antigen physically by synovectomy. Surgical treatment of the knee was reportedly successful in two patients, although inflammatory symptoms continued in the untreated joints of one of the patients. At least one failure of a similar surgical strategy has been reported.[100]

Craft and associates[101] found serologic reactivity to at least 11 different *B burgdorferi* antigens in patients with Lyme disease. Mensi and associates[102] found that antibodies in synovial fluid from one patient recognized four different proteins from *B burgdorferi*. A comparison of amino terminal sequencing of the identified proteins demonstrated limited sequence homology to several proteins, including endoflagella from *Treponema pallidum*, mammalian myosin, and one GroEL-like protein common to bacteria, humans, and plants.[103] The authors suggested that antigenic mimicry and the subsequent immune response to cross-reactive antigens may therefore play a role in the pathogenesis of Lyme arthritis.

Host Genetic Factors and Lyme Arthritis

Steere and associates[104] reported an increased frequency of the B-cell alloantigen HLA-DR2 in patients with severe, chronic Lyme arthritis. Seven of ten patients with chronic arthritis had the alloantigen DR2 and four were positive for DR4. (Alloantigens are codominant in that each inherited allele may be expressed on the cell surface.) Bianchi and associates[105] reported inconclusive findings with regard to DR2 antigen expression in ten patients with Lyme arthritis.

In a follow-up study of 125 patients with a spectrum of Lyme disease manifestations that included arthritis in only 76 patients (61%), Steere[98] did not find an increased frequency of expression of a D locus antigen. When the 76 patients were segregated by severity of disease, however, a statistically significant increased number of patients (14 of 22 or 64%) with chronic Lyme arthritis showed expression of DR4 compared with 31% of a normal population. Because the frequency of DR4 expression is also increased in patients with rheumatoid arthritis, Steere speculated that similar mechanisms may predispose the host to chronic forms of both diseases.

What these "similar mechanisms" are has yet to be answered. Zabriskie and Gibofsky[106] suggested that cross-reactions between host tissues and microbial antigens may be involved because they detected heart-binding antibodies in the sera of patients with Lyme disease. Speculation on the mechanisms of disease involving cross-reactive antibodies is complicated by recent reports of late manifestations of Lyme disease found in seronegative patients.[107,108]

Malawista[109] has postulated that the host's individual immunogenetic "make-up" determines the type of immune response to infection with *B burgdorferi*, which in turn determines the clinical expression of the disease. In support of these observations, Schlesier and associates[110] suggested that chronic joint inflammation in both rheumatoid arthritis and Lyme arthritis may result from defective host suppression of autoreactive T cells in the inflamed joint.

Animal Models for Lyme Arthritis

As with other infectious diseases, progress in defining the fundamental mechanisms of Lyme borreliosis, and Lyme arthritis in particular, has been hampered by the lack of a suitable animal model. Vertebrate reservoirs for *B burgdorferi* include a variety of birds, rodents, carnivores, and ungulates. Clinical manifestations of Lyme disease, including rheumatoid arthritis subsequent to exposure to *B burgdorferi,* have been reported in dogs,[111] cattle,[112] and horses.[113]

Early in the study of Lyme borreliosis Krinsky and associates[114] used *I dammini* ticks to transfer *B burgdorferi* to rabbits and guinea pigs. The rodents developed characteristic erythema chronicum migrans, but no further clinical manifestations were observed. Similarly, Johnson and associates[115] showed that Syrian hamsters could be infected with the spirochetes but, despite prolonged persistence of the organism in different tissues, no clinical disease was observed.

Barthold and associates[116,117] reported that spirochetemia, multitissue infection, and a high prevalence of polyarticular arthritis developed in three different strains of rats that were inoculated intraperitoneally as neonates or weanlings with low-passage *B burgdorferi* isolates. These authors concluded that the development of Lyme-like arthritis in the young rats required inoculation of viable *B burgdorferi* (approximately 10^6 organisms injected intraperitoneally) and that polyarthritis was associated with the presence of spirochetes in joint tissues.

Heijka and associates[118] injected normal and gamma-irradiated (700 rads) inbred LSH/Ss Lak hamsters weighing 60 to 100 g with *B burgdorferi* in the hindpaw. A short-lived, acute inflammatory response developed in the tibiotarsal, intertarsal, and interphalangeal joints of the nonirradiated animals. As the inflammatory reaction resolved over a number of weeks, the number of visible spirochetes diminished. The joint disease was described as a chronic, mild synovitis.

In contrast, the sublethal gamma irradiation of hamsters prior to hindpaw inoculation resulted in a magnified and prolonged inflammatory response compared with the controls. An erosive and destructive arthritis of the knee joint consistently developed in the irradiated animals. The extent of disease appeared to be related to the presence of spirochetes (or more properly, inability to clear the spirochetes) and thus provided evidence that altered immune status plays a role in the development of disease.

Shortly thereafter, Schaible and associates[119] reported that a multisystem disease developed in mice with severe combined (impaired T- and B-cell functions) immunodeficiency disease (SCID) after inoculation with a low-passage tick isolate of *B burgdorferi.* Tissue involvement included brain, heart, lungs, kidneys, spleen, and, as in humans with Lyme disease, polyarthritis. The polyarthritis was progressive and characterized by synovial hyperplasia, cartilage destruction, and joint erosion. Development of disease depended on the inoculation of viable low-passage organisms. The high-passage strain B31 did not produce disease in the mice. Severe disease, then, was a product of both the virulence of the organism and the immunodeficiency of the mouse.

These reports were soon followed by continuing efforts to demonstrate successful protection by passive transfer of specific antibodies. Schmitz and associates[120] reported that immune sera obtained from hamsters inoculated three weeks previously with *B burgdorferi* strain 297 conferred complete protection on recipient irradiated LSH/Ss Lak hamsters that were subsequently challenged with 10^6 *B burgdorferi* organisms injected into the hindpaw. No histopathologic changes were observed in the hindpaw and knee joints, and no organisms were cultured from any tissue. In contrast, spirochetes were cultured from the urinary bladders, kidneys, and spleens of control, unprotected hamsters. Inflammatory responses were also observed in the joint tissues of unprotected controls and were associated with the presence of spirochetes.

An important observation made by these investigators was that immune antiserum, even in dilute form, was able to provide protection against arthritis and other manifestations of Lyme borreliosis in both naive, immunocompetent, and immunocompromised hosts even though the protective sera were obtained from donor animals with active disease. The observation that passive transfer of immune sera did not protect after the inception of disease had been made earlier by Johnson and associates.[121]

Schaible and associates[122] used the SCID mouse model to demonstrate that a monoclonal antibody (LA-2) to the *B burgdorferi* major outer surface antigen (OspA) or immune sera obtained from mice late in infection (68 days after inoculation with *B burgdorferi* ZS7), were able to prevent the development of overt signs of arthritis, carditis, and spirochetemia in SCID mice when passively transferred through intraperitoneal injection at the time of challenge and repeatedly at four-day intervals. However, monoclonal antibodies against endoflagella epitopes transferred similarly did not protect against the development of arthritis, and spirochetes were cultured from the blood of SCID mice receiving infusions of these nonprotective antibodies. The investigators also concluded that passive transfer of antibodies, even the monoclonal antibody previously shown to be protective, after the primary infection was not protective.

The encouraging recent data in animals models suggesting that Lyme arthritis in particular, and Lyme borreliosis more generally, can be prevented or ameliorated through the passive transfer of polyclonal and monoclonal antibodies must be tempered by at least two reports that the presence of antibodies in humans was not protective against naturally acquired disease.[101,123]

Schaible and associates[122] observed that in experimental infection of immunocompetent mice with *B burgdorferi*, antibodies to OspA (protective in SCID mice) were among the first detected.[123] In humans, however, antibodies to the 41–kd endoflagella antigen (not protective in SCID mice) were the dominant early response and antibodies to OspA did not develop until late in infection.[101]

These observations highlight the difficulties of extrapolating results from incompletely understood laboratory models to the pathogenesis of human disease. However, the development of animal models that reasonably mimic human disease such as Lyme arthritis is important

Table 3 Treatment of Lyme disease*

Treatment*	Stage 1	Stage 2	Stage 3
		Adults	
First-line	Tetracycline† (250 mg orally 4 times/day for 10 to 20 days)	Penicillin G (20 million units/day in 6 divided doses for 10 days) or ceftriaxone (1 g intramuscularly or intravenously every 12 hours for 14 days)	Ceftriaxone (1 to 2 g intramuscularly or intravenously every 24 hours for 14 days)
Alternative	Phenoxymethyl penicillin (200 to 500 mg orally 4 times/day)	Cefotaxime (2 g intravenously every 8 hours for 10 days)	Benzathine penicillin (2.4 million units intramuscularly every week for 3 weeks) or penicillin G (20 million units/day intravenously in 6 divided doses for 10 days)
		Children‡	
First-line	Phenoxymethyl penicillin (25 to 50 mg/kg/day orally in 4 divided doses for 10 days)	Penicillin G (250,000 units/kg/day intravenously in 6 divided doses for 10 days)	Penicillin G (250,000 units/kg/day intravenously in 6 divided doses for 10 days)
Alternative	Erythromycin (30 mg/kg/day orally in 4 divided doses for 15 to 20 days)	Benzathine penicillin (2.4 million units intramuscularly every week for 3 weeks) or ceftriaxone (50 mg/kg intravenously or intramuscularly every 12 to 24 hours for 14 days)	Benzathine penicillin (2.4 million units intramuscularly every week for 3 weeks) or ceftriaxone (50 mg/kg intravenously or intramuscularly every 12 to 24 hours for 14 days)

*Adapted from Tortorice and Heim-Duthay.[124]
See cautionary discussion in text
†This recommended treatment failed in five patients despite early administration.[130]
‡No randomized, controlled pediatric trials have been conducted.

so that questions such as the role of OspA in the pathogenesis of chronic arthritis can be answered.

Treatment Notes

The pharmacologic treatment of Lyme borreliosis has been extensively reviewed by Tortorice and Heim-Duthoy[124] (Table 3) and Luft and Dattwyler.[125] It is not the purpose of this discussion to recommend specific treatment strategies, but rather to identify some important conclusions drawn from the experimental literature.

First, it seems prudent to heed the cautionary note of Luft and Dattwyler.[125] That is, infection by *B burgdorferi* should be viewed as a chronic, potentially progressive infectious disease and treatment regimens should be designed to treat the systemic infection—and not just the symptomatic arthritis—adequately. The observations by Steere and associates[89,126] that early antimicrobial therapy may be associated with rapid resolution of the disease and lessening of other major complications should also be remembered. Early treatment with oral antibiotics was also associated with a positive response to later antibiotic treatment for arthritis symptoms.[127] These observations are consistent with the early treatment of erythema chronicum migrans with antibiotics since the 1950s by European physicians.[128]

Although Lyme borreliosis is the most commonly reported tick-borne illness in the United States, the overall incidence of the disease remains low.[84] Sigal[129] recently suggested that the improper overdiagnosis of Lyme disease appears to be common even in endemic areas because of the lack of strict diagnostic criteria and standardized laboratory tests. After reviewing the first 100 patients seen at a Lyme disease referral center in New Jersey, Sigal[129] concluded that about one half of the previously prescribed antibiotic therapies appeared to be unwarranted because of misdiagnosis or other factors.

In a double-blind, placebo-controlled antibiotic trial of a third-generation cephalosporin, ceftriaxone, in 60 adult patients with both inflammatory arthritis and increased antibody titers to *B burgdorferi*, Caperton and associates[127] concluded that the antibiotic promoted improvement in more than 50% of the treated patients. Extending their studies, these investigators further concluded that some patients with inflammatory arthritis may have undetected bacterial infections that respond to ceftriaxone and other antibiotics. Patients with low and high anti-*B burgdorferi* titers appeared to respond equally well to the antibiotic. However, the frequency of adverse side effects was severe in this study. Forty-seven of 60 patients reported a change in bowel habits and one-half had diarrhea. Four patients required treatment for diarrhea associated with *Clostridia difficile*.

Treatment failures with low-dose penicillin, tetracycline,[130] and erythromycin have been reported.[125] Besides the induction of multisystem symptoms, borreliosis may also share with syphilis the requirement for sustained and increased antibiotic levels for prolonged periods to eradicate the sequestered spirochetes successfully.

Treponema pallidum and Arthritis

The recent sharp increase in the incidence of syphilis among heterosexual adults and the predictable, devastating increase in congenital syphilis make it mandatory to consider syphilis in the differential diagnosis of arthralgias and arthritis. The worldwide epidemic of human immunodeficiency virus and attendant syndromes, including altered humoral immunity,[131] suggests that once again the physician will be faced with a diagnostic challenge when treating patients with rheumatic-like complaints.[132]

In 1926, Todd[133] published several clinical aphorisms; these included that rheumatism in any form should not be diagnosed until syphilis had been excluded as a possibility. A few years later Kling[134] summarized the whole literature on syphilis and arthritis from the time of the Middle Ages in one sentence: "Syphilitic arthritis can imitate every form of joint disease." That is, joint involvement can include large and small joints; be monoarticular, symmetric, or polyarticular;

and can vary from simple effusion to massive erosion of the synovial and articular surfaces.

Like the Lyme spirochete, the syphilis spirochete, *T pallidum*, appears to demonstrate a special tropism for joint fluid or tissue. Chesney and associates[135] were able to identify *T pallidum* from the joint fluid of three of ten patients examined over a five-year period who had serologic evidence of both syphilis and arthritis. Although the involvement of other sexually transmitted diseases such as gonorrhea was not ruled out, five of the ten patients showed immediate improvement (including the three positive for *T pallidum*) with antisyphilitic drug treatment. More recently, Reginato and associates[136] used light and electron microscopy to detect treponemes in the joint tissues of two of seven patients with secondary syphilis in whom polyarthritis developed over a 12–year period. The infectious basis of the polyarthritis was supported by the cultivation of treponemes after injection of affected joint fluid (1 to 2 ml) intratesticularly into rabbits and the rapid resolution of the arthritis after treatment with penicillin. The technique of rabbit passage of *T pallidum* remains the most satisfactory method of cultivation of this obligate parasitic bacterium. Our experience suggests that as many as three "blind" serial transfers in rabbits may be required to detect *T pallidum*.

Identification of *T pallidum* Proteinaceous Adhesins

The spirochetes in general, and *T pallidum* in particular, exhibit vigorous motility characterized by spinning, flexing, and translational and serpentine movements. However, during co-incubation with eukaryotic cells, treponemes adhere tip-first to host membranes and do not detach, yet remain actively motile (Fig. 2).[137] This obvious polarity of attachment was shown to be time- and temperature-dependent and regulated by properties of the host cell membrane.[137] In addition, avirulent treponemes were incapable of cytadherence. Taken together, these observations implicated adhesin-receptor mechanisms of recognition in treponemal surface parasitism on eukaryotic cells and in the virulence of *T pallidum*.

Because *T pallidum* cannot be satisfactorily grown in vitro and experimental approaches cannot be directly applied, alternate strategies were developed. Early studies showed that three major treponemal surface proteins (89.5, 37, and 32 kd) selectively bound to eukaryotic cell surfaces.[138] Competition assays using both radiolabeled and unlabeled *T pallidum* preparations indicated that these proteins bound to a finite number of protease-sensitive host membrane sites. In addition, the observation that antibodies generated against these treponemal proteins or against the eukaryotic cell surface blocked cytadherence reinforced the specificity of the host-*T pallidum* interaction.

Surface-Associated Host Proteins on *T pallidum*

Further characterization of the *T pallidum* surface demonstrated that various host macromolecules were either weakly or avidly associated

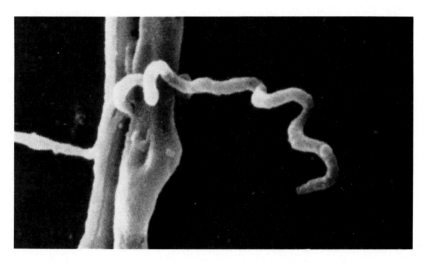

Fig. 2 *Scanning electron micrograph of* T pallidum *attaching to testicular cell. Note the orientation of the treponeme mediated by its tapered end (1 μ = 28 mm).*

with the treponemal outer membrane.[139] The avidly bound host proteins appeared to reside on noncompetitive sites, allowing the acquisition by *T pallidum* of host macromolecules in a nonrandom manner.

The role of specific and biologically important host proteins on the surface of *T pallidum* has been described.[139,140] For example, the binding of lactoferrin to virulent treponemes permits accumulation of iron by *T pallidum*, thus enhancing in vivo survival of the spirochete. The association of lipoproteins, sulfated proteoglycans, and ceruloplasmin with *T pallidum* may also serve as mechanisms by which treponemes acquire nutrients and cofactors, retain membrane integrity, mask themselves and major immunogens from host immune surveillance, and elicit autoimmune-like reactions.

Another of the biologically relevant host molecules that selectively and avidly adsorbed to the *T pallidum* surface was fibronectin. Fibronectin is a chemically well-defined dimeric glycoprotein with specific structural domains that function in eukaryotic cell adhesion and in the spatial organization of the extracellular matrix. Surprisingly, fibronectin-coated surfaces permit the tip-mediated adherence of *T pallidum*, similar to that previously observed in eukaryotic cells.[141] The relationship between treponemal adherence to fibronectin and adherence to eukaryotic cell surfaces was established when polyclonal and monoclonal antibodies reactive against fibronectin blocked treponemal adherence to both fibronectin and host cells.[141,142] Antibodies generated against laminin and collagen and other nonfibronectin proteins did not inhibit cytadherence.

Fibronectin Tetrapeptide

To define more precisely the mechanism by which fibronectin serves as an affinity matrix for tip-mediated treponemal adherence, fibronectin was fractionated into various domains to assess their adherence-promoting potential. Also, antibodies directed against these distinct domains were examined in the *T pallidum* adherence assay. The data clearly demonstrated that the cell-binding domain of fibronectin was the preferred site.[142] Fortunately, this domain, which mediates eukaryotic cell attachment and spreading, has been analyzed extensively. The cell-binding activity of the domain has been localized to the tetrapeptide, arginine-glycine-aspartate-serine; this tetrapeptide, and no other tetrapeptide, blocked treponemal cytadherence in competitive binding assays.[143] The specificity of the fibronectin-*T pallidum* interaction dramatically reinforces the fascinating relationships between the parasitic strategies of *T pallidum* and the physiologic environment of the host.

References

1. Woese CR, Maniloff J, Zablen LB: Phylogenetic analysis of the mycoplasmas. *Proc Natl Acad Sci USA* 1980;77:494–498.
2. Su CJ, Baseman JB: Genome size of *Mycoplasma genitalium. J Bacteriol* 1990;172:4705–4707.
3. Swift HF, Brown TM: Pathogenc pleuropneumonia-like microorganisms from acute rheumatic exudates and tissues. *Science* 1939;89:271–272.
4. Furness G, Whitescarver J: Adaptation of *Mycoplasma hominis* to an obligate parasitic existence in monkey kidney cell culture (BSC-1) (38821). *Proc Soc Exp Biol Med* 1975;149:427–432.
5. Hopps HE, Meyer BC, Barile MF: Problems concerning "noncultivable" mycoplasma contaminants in tissue cultures. *Ann NY Acad Sci* 1973;225:265–276.
6. Bredt W, Bitter-Suermann D: Interactions between *Mycoplasma pneumoniae* and guinea pig complement. *Infect Immun* 1975;11:497–504.
7. Cole BC, Taylor MB, Ward JR: Studies on the infectious etiology of human rheumatoid arthritis: II. Search for humoral and cell-bound antibodies against mycoplasmal antigens. *Arthritis Rheum* 1975;18:435–441.
8. Cole BC, Cassell GH: Mycoplasma infections as models of chronic joint inflammation. *Arthritis Rheum* 1979;22:1375–1381.
9. Wise KS, Cassell GH, Action RT: Selective association of murine T lymphoblastoid cell surface alloantigens with *Mycoplasma hyorhinis. Proc Natl Acad Sci USA* 1978;75:4479–4483.
10. Bayer AS, Galpin JE, Theofilopoulos AN, et al: Neurological disease associated with *Mycoplasma pneumoniae* pneumonitis: Demonstration of viable *Mycoplasma pneumoniae* in cerebrospinal fluid and blood by radioisotopic and immunofluorescent tissue culture techniques. *Ann Intern Med* 1981;94:15–20.
11. Biberfeld G: Antibodies to brain and other tissues in cases of *Mycoplasma pneumoniae* infection. *Clin Exp Immunol* 1971;8:319–333.
12. Loomes LM, Uemura K, Childs RA, et al: Erythrocyte receptors for *Mycoplasma pneumoniae* are sialylated oligosaccharides of Ii antigen type. *Nature* 1984;307:560–563.

13. Cole BC, Washburn LR, Taylor-Robinson D: Mycoplasma-induced arthritis, in Razin S, Barile MF, (eds): *The Mycoplasmas.* New York, Academic Press, 1985, pp 107–160.

14. Cole BC, Thorpe RN, Hassell LA, et al: Toxicity but not arthritogenicity of *Mycoplasma arthritidis* for mice associates with the haplotype expressed at the major histocompatibility complex. *Infect Immun* 1983;41:1010–1015.

15. Kirchhoff H, Binder A, Runge M, et al: Pathogenetic mechanisms in the *Mycoplasma arthritidis* polyarthritis of rats. *Rheumatol Int* 1989;9:193–196.

16. Binder A, Gärtner K, Hedrich HJ, et al: Strain differences in sensitivity of rats to *Mycoplasma arthritidis* ISR 1 infection are under multiple gene control. *Infect Immun* 1990;58:1584–1590.

17. Gärtner K, Kirchhoff H, Mensing K, et al: The influence of social rank on the susceptibility of rats to *Mycoplasma arthritidis*. *J Behav Med* 1989;12:487–502.

18. Schwab JH, Cromartie WJ, Ohanian SH, et al: Association of experimental chronic arthritis with the persistence of group A streptococcal cell walls in the articular tissue. *J Bacteriol* 1967;94:1728–1735.

19. Decker JL, Barden JA: *Mycoplasma hyorhinis* arthritis of swine: A model for rheumatoid arthritis? *Rheumatology* 1975;6:338–345.

20. Ennis RS, Johnson JS, Decker JL: Persistent *Mycoplasma hyorhinis* (MH) antigen in chronic mycoplasmal arthritis of swine, abstract. *Arthritis Rheum* 1972;15:108.

21. Washburn LR, Cole BC, Gelman MI, et al: Chronic arthritis of rabbits induced by myocoplasmas: I. Clinical, microbiologic, and histologic features. *Arthritis Rheum* 1980;23:825–836.

22. Washburn LR, Cole BC, Ward JR: Chronic arthritis of rabbits induced by mycoplasmas: II. Antibody response and the deposition of immune complexes. *Arthritis Rheum* 1980;23:837–845.

23. Cooke TD, Jasin HE: The pathogenesis of chronic inflammation in experimental antigen-induced arthritis: I. The role of antigen on the local immune response. *Arthritis Rheum* 1972;15:327–337.

24. Cooke TD, Hurd ER, Jasin HE, et al: Identification of immunoglobulins and complement in rheumatoid articular collagenous tissues. *Arthritis Rheum* 1975;18:541–551.

25. Theofilopoulos AN, Wilson CB, Dixon FJ: The Raji cell radioimmune assay for detecting immune complexes in human sera. *J Clin Invest* 1976;57:169–182.

26. Clark HW, Coker-Vann MR, Bailey JS, et al: Detection of mycoplasmal antigens in immune complexes from rheumatoid arthritis synovial fluids. *Ann Allergy* 1988;60:394–398.

27. Baseman JB, Cole RM, Krause DC, et al: Molecular basis for cytadsorption of *Mycoplasma pneumoniae*. *J Bacteriol* 1982;151:1514–1522.

28. Su CJ, Tryon VV, Baseman JB: Cloning and sequence analysis of cytadhesin gene (P1) from *Mycoplasma pneumoniae*. *Infect Immun* 1987;55:3023–3029.

29. Taylor-Robinson D, Gumpel JM, Hill A, et al: Isolation of *Mycoplasma pneumoniae* from the synovial fluid of a hypogammaglobulinaemic patient in a survey of patients with inflammatory polyarthritis. *Ann Rheum Dis* 1978;37:180–182.

30. Verinder DGR: Septic arthritis due to *Mycoplasma hominis*: A case report and review of the literature. *J Bone Joint Surg* 1978;60B:224.

31. Ti TY, Dan M, Stemke GW, et al: Isolation of *Mycoplasma hominis* from the blood of men with multiple trauma and fever. *JAMA* 1982;247:60–61.

32. McDonald MI, Moore JO, Harrelson JM, et al: Septic arthritis due to *Mycoplasma hominis*. *Arthritis Rheum* 1983;26:1044–1047.

33. Pönkä A: Arthritis associated with *Mycoplasma pneumoniae* infection. *Scand J Rheumatol* 1979;8:27–32.

34. Pönkä A: The occurrence and clinical picture of serologically verified *Mycoplasma pneumoniae* infections with emphasis on central nervous system, cardiac and joint manifestations. *Ann Clin Res* 1979;11(suppl 24):1–60.

35. Cimolai N, Malleson P, Thomas E, et al: *Mycoplasma pneumoniae* associated arthropathy: Confirmation of the association by determination of the antipolypeptide IgM response. *J Rheumatol* 1989;16:1150–1152.

36. Webster ADB, Loewi G, Dourmashkin RD, et al: Polyarthritis in adults with hypogammaglobulinaemia and its rapid response to immunoglobulin treatment. *Br Med J* 1976;1:1314–1316.

37. Stuckey M. Quinn PA, Gelfand EW: Identification of *Ureaplasma urealyticum* (T-strain Mycoplasma) in patient with polyarthritis. *Lancet* 1978;2:917–920.

38. Webster ADB, Taylor-Robinson D, Furr PM, et al: Mycoplasmal (ureaplasma) septic arthritis in hypogammaglobulinaemia. *Br Med J* 1978;1:478–479.

39. Kraus VB, Baraniuk JN, Hill GB, et al: *Ureaplasma urealyticum* septic arthritis in hypogammaglobulinemia. *J Rheumatol* 1988;15:369–371.

40. Johnson CLW, Webster ADB, Tayor-Robinson D, et al: Primary late-onset hypogammaglobulinaemia associated with inflammatory polyarthritis and septic arthritis due to *Mycoplasma pneumoniae*. *Ann Rheum Dis* 1983;42:108–110.

41. Burdge DR, Reid GD, Reeve CE, et al: Septic arthritis due to dual infection with *Mycoplasma hominis* and *Ureaplasma urealyticum*. *J Rheumatol* 1988;15:366–368.

42. Barile MF, Snoy PJ, Miller LM, et al: Mycoplasma-induced septic arthritis in chimpanzees. *Zentralbl Bakteriol Mikrobiol Hyg* 1990;20:299–393.

43. Sneller M, Wellborne F, Barile MF, et al: Prosthetic joint infection with *Mycoplasma hominis*, letter. *J Infect Dis* 1986;153:174–175.

44. Nylander N, Tan M, Newcombe DS: Successful management of *Mycoplasma hominis* septic arthritis involving a cementless prosthesis. *Am J Med* 1989;87:348–352.

45. Davis CP, Cochran S, Lisse J, et al: Isolation of *Mycoplasma pneumoniae* from synovial fluid samples in a patient with pneumonia and polyarthritis. *Arch Intern Med* 1988;148:969–970.

46. Baseman JB, Dallo SF, Tully JG, et al: Isolation and characterization of *Mycoplasma genitalium* strains from the human respiratory tract. *J Clin Microbiol* 1988;26:2266–2269.

47. Hu PC, Collier AM, Baseman JB: Surface parasitism by *Mycoplasma pneumoniae* of respiratory epithelium. *J Exp Med* 1977;145:1328–1343.

48. Powell DA, Hu PC, Wilson M, et al: Attachment of *Mycoplasma pneumoniae* to respiratory epithelium. *Infect Immun* 1976;13:959–966.

49. Hu PC, Collier AM, Baseman JB: Interaction of virulent *Mycoplasma pneumoniae* with hamster tracheal organ cultures. *Infect Immun* 1976;14:217–224.

50. Hansen EJ, Wilson RM, Clyde WA Jr, et al: Characterization of hemadsorption-negative mutants of *Mycoplasma pneumoniae*. *Infect Immun* 1981;32:127–136.

51. Krause DC, Leith DK, Wilson RM, et al: Identification of *Mycoplasma pneumoniae* proteins associated with hemadsorption and virulence. *Infect Immun* 1982;35:809–817.

52. Kahane I, Pnini S, Banai M, et al: Attachment of mycoplasmas to erythrocytes: A model to study mycoplasma attachment to the epithelium of the host respiratory tract. *Isr J Med Sci* 1981;17:589–592.

53. Krause DC, Baseman JB: Inhibition of *Mycoplasma pneumoniae* hemadsorption and adherence to respiratory epithelium by antibodies to a membrane protein. *Infect Immun* 1983;39:1180–1186.

54. Morrison-Plummer J, Leith DK, Baseman JB: Biological effects of anti-lipid and anti-protein monoclonal antibodies on *Mycoplasma pneumoniae*. *Infect Immun* 1986;53:398–403.

55. Krause DC, Baseman JB: *Mycoplasma pneumoniae* proteins that selectively bind to host cells. *Infect Immun* 1982;37:382–386.

56. Krause DC, Leith DK, Baseman JB: Reacquisition of specific proteins confers virulence in *Mycoplasma pneumoniae*. *Infect Immun* 1983;39:830–836.

57. Baseman JB, Morrison-Plummer J, Drouillard D, et al: Identification of a 32–kilodalton protein of *Mycoplasma pneumoniae* associated with hemadsorption. *Isr J Med Sci* 1987;23:474–479.

58. Leith DK, Hansen EJ, Wilson RM, et al: Hemadsorption and virulence are separable properties of *Mycoplasma pneumoniae*. *Infect Immun* 1983;39:844–850.

59. Yamao F, Muto A, Kawauchi Y, et al: UGA is read as tryptophan in *Mycoplasma capricolum*. *Proc Natl Acad Sci USA* 1985;82:2306–2309.

60. Su CJ, Chavoya A, Baseman JB: Regions of *Mycoplasma pneumoniae* cytadhesin P1 structural gene exist as multiple copies. *Infect Immun* 1988;56:3157–3161.

61. Bergström S, Robbins K, Koomey JM, et al: Piliation control mechanisms in *Neisseria gonorrhoeae*. *Proc Natl Acad Sci USA* 1986;83:3890–3894.

62. Blake MS, Gotschlich EC: Gonococcal membrane proteins: Speculation on their role in pathogenesis. *Prog Allergy* 1983;33:298–313.

63. Meier JT, Simon MI, Barbour AG: Antigenic variation is associated with DNA rearrangements in a relapsing fever Borrelia. *Cell* 1985;41:403–409.

64. Stern A, Brown M, Nickel P, et al: Opacity genes in *Neisseria gonorrhoeae*: Control of phase and antigenic variation. *Cell* 1986;47:61–71.

65. Su CJ, Dallo SF, Baseman JB: Molecular distinctions among clinical isolates of *Mycoplasma pneumoniae*. *J Clin Micobiol* 1990;28:1538–1540.

66. Dallo SF, Horton JR, Su CJ, et al: Restriction fragment length polymorphism in the cytadhesin P1 gene of human clinical isolates of *Mycoplasma pneumoniae*. *Infect Immun* 1990;58:2017–2020.

67. Su CJ, Chavoya A, Dallo SF, et al: Sequence divergency of the cytadhesin gene of *Mycoplasma pneumoniae*. *Infect Immun* 1990;58:2669–2674.

68. Dallo SF, Chavoya A, Baseman JB: Cloning and sequence determination of the 30 kDa adhesin-related gene from *Mycoplasma pneumoniae*. *Infect Immun* 1990;58:4163–4165.

69. Tully JG, Taylor-Robinson D, Cole RM, et al: A newly discovered mycoplasma in the human urogenital tract. *Lancet* 1981;1:1288–1291.

70. Tully JG, Taylor-Robinson D, Rose DL, et al: *Mycoplasma genitalium*, a new species from the human urogenital tract. *Int J Syst Bacteriol* 1983;33:387–396.

71. Morrison-Plummer J, Lazzell A, Baseman JB: Shared epitopes between *Mycoplasma pneumoniae* major adhesin protein P1 and a 140–kilodalton protein of *Mycoplasma genitalium*. *Infect Immun* 1987;55:49–56.

72. Clyde WA Jr, Hu PC: Antigenic determinants of the attachment protein of *Mycoplasma* shared by other pathogenic *Mycoplasma* species. *Infect Immun* 1986;51:690–692.

73. Hu PC, Schaper U, Collier AM, et al: A *Mycoplasma genitalium* protein resembling the *Mycoplasma pneumoniae* attachment protein. *Infect Immun* 1987;55:1126–1131.

111

74. Dallo SF, Chavoya A, Su CJ, et al: DNA and protein sequence homologies between the adhesins of *Mycoplasma genitalium* and *Mycoplasma pneumoniae*. *Infect Immun* 1989;57:1059–1065.

75. Dallo SF, Horton JR, Su CJ, et al: Homologous regions shared by adhesin genes of *Mycoplasma pneumoniae* and *Mycoplasma genitalium*. *Microb Pathog* 1989;6:69–73.

76. Yogev D, Razin S: Common deoxyribonucleic acid sequences in *Mycoplasma genitalium* and *Mycoplasma pneumoniae* genomes. *Int J Syst Bacteriol* 1986;36:426–430.

77. Loveless RW, Feizi T: Sialo-oligosaccharide receptors for *Mycoplasma pneumoniae* and related oligosaccharides of poly-N-acetyllactosamine series are polarized at the cilia and apical-microvillar domains of the ciliated cells in human bronchial epithelium. *Infect Immun* 1989;57:1285–1289.

78. Roberts DD, Olson LD, Barile MF, et al: Sialic acid-dependent adhesion of *Mycoplasma pneumoniae* to purified glycoproteins. *J Biol Chem* 1989;264:9289–9293.

79. Krivan HC, Olson LD, Barile MF, et al: Adhesion of *Mycoplasma pneumoniae* to sulfated glycolipids and inhibition by dextran sulfate. *J Biol Chem* 1989;264:9283–9288.

80. Malawista SE, Steere AC: Lyme disease: Infectious in origin, rheumatic in expression. *Adv Intern Med* 1986;31:147–166.

81. Piesman J, Mather TN, Sinsky RJ, et al: Duration of tick attachment and *Borrelia burgdorferi* transmission. *J Clin Microbiol* 1987;25:557–558.

82. Stechenberg BW: Lyme disease: The latest great imitator. *Pediatr Infect Dis J* 1988;7:402–409.

83. Duray PH: Clinical pathologic correlations of Lyme disease. *Rev Infect Dis* 1989;11(suppl 6):S1487–S1493.

84. Ciesielski CA, Markowitz LE, Horsley R, et al: Lyme disease surveillance in the United States, 1983–1986. *Rev Infect Dis* 1989;11(suppl 6):S1435–S1441.

85. Steere AC, Malawista SE, Snydman DR, et al: Lyme arthritis: An epidemic of oligoarticular arthritis in children and adults in three Connecticut communities. *Arthritis Rheum* 1977;20:7–17.

86. Petersen LR, Sweeney AH, Checko PJ, et al: Epidemiological and clinical features of 1,149 persons with Lyme disease identified by laboratory-based surveillance in Connecticut. *Yale J Biol Med* 1989;62:253–262.

87. Burgdorfer W, Barbour AG, Hayes SF, et al: Lyme disease—a tick-borne spirochetosis? *Science* 1982;216:1317–1319.

88. Schulze TL, Bowen GS, Bosler EM, et al: *Amblyomma americanum*: A potential vector of Lyme disease in New Jersey. *Science* 1984;224:601–603.

89. Steere AC, Grodzicki RL, Kornblatt AN, et al: The spirochetal etiology of Lyme disease. *N Engl J Med* 1983;309:733–740.

90. Kolstoe J, Messner RP: Lyme disease: Musculoskeletal manifestations. *Rheum Dis Clin North Am* 1989;15:649–656.

91. Steere AC, Schoen RT, Taylor E: The clinical evolution of Lyme arthritis. *Ann Intern Med* 1987;107:725–731.

92. Steere AC, Taylor E, Wilson ML, et al: Longitudinal assessment of the clinical and epidemiological features of Lyme disease in a defined population. *J Infect Dis* 1986;154:295–300.

93. Johnston YE, Duray PH, Steere AC, et al: Lyme arthritis: Spirochetes found in synovial microangiopathic lesions. *Am J Pathol* 1985;118:26–34.

94. Steere AC, Duray PH, Butcher EC: Spirochetal antigens and lymphoid cell surface markers in Lyme synovitis: Comparison with rheumatoid synovium and tonsillar lymphoid tissue. *Arthritis Rheum* 1988;31:487–495.

95. Duray PY, Steere AC: The spectrum of organ and systems pathology in human Lyme disease. *Zentralbl Bakteriol Mikrobiol [A]* 1986;263:169–178.

96. Lastavica CC, Snydman DR, Schenkein DP, et al: Demonstration of *Borrelia burgdorferi* in a patient with chronic Lyme arthritis. *Zentralbl Bakteriol Mikrobiol [A]* 1986;263:288.

97. Snydman Dr, Schenkein DP, Berardi VP, et al: *Borrelia burgdorferi* in joint fluid in chronic Lyme arthritis. *Ann Intern Med* 1986;104:798–800.

98. Steere AC: Pathogenesis of Lyme arthritis: Implications for rheumatic disease. *Ann NY Acad Sci* 1988;539:87–92.

99. McLaughlin TP, Zemel L, Fisher RL, et al: Chronic arthritis of the knee in Lyme disease: Review of the literature and report of two cases treated by synovectomy. *J Bone Joint Surg* 1986;68A:1057–1061.

100. Cimmino MA, Trevisan G: Lyme arthritis presenting as adult onset Still's disease. *Clin Exp Rheumatol* 1989;7:305–308.

101. Craft JE, Fischer DK, Shimamoto GT, et al: Antigens of *Borrelia burgdorferi* recognized during Lyme disease: Appearance of a new immunoglobulin M response and expansion of the immunoglobulin G response late in the illness. *J Clin Invest* 1986;78:934–939.

102. Mensi N, Webb DR, Turck CW, et al: Characterization of *Borrelia burgdorferi* proteins reactive with antibodies in synovial fluid of a patient with Lyme arthritis. *Infect Immun* 1990;58:2404–2497.

103. Lindquist S, Craig EA: The heat-shock proteins. *Annu Rev Genet* 1988;22:631–677.

104. Steere AC, Gibofsky A, Patarroyo ME, et al: Chronic Lyme arthritis: Clinical and immunogenetic differentiation from rheumatoid arthritis. *Ann Intern Med* 1979;90:896–901.

105. Bianchi G, Rovetta G, Monteforte P, et al: Articular involvement in European patients with Lyme disease: A report of 32 Italian patients. *Br J Rheumatol* 1990;29:178–180.

106. Zabriskie JB, Gibofsky A: Genetic control of the susceptibility to infection with pathogenic bacteria. *Curr Top Microbiol Immunol* 1986;124:1–20.

107. Lavoie PE, Lane RS, Murray RH: Seronegative Lyme borreliosis in three Californians with late manifestations, abstract. *Arthritis Rheum* 1987;30(suppl 4):S36.

108. Dattwyler RJ, Volkman DJ, Luft BJ, et al: Seronegative Lyme disease: Dissociation of specific T- and B-lymphocyte responses to *Borrelia borgdorferi*. *N Engl J Med* 1988;319:1441–1446.

109. Malawista SE: Pathogenesis of Lyme disease. *Rheumatol Int* 1989;9:233–235.

110. Schlesier M, Haas G, Wolff-Vorbeck G, et al: Autoreactive T cells in rheumatic disease: I. Analysis of growth frequencies and autoreactivity of T cells in patients with rheumatoid arthritis and Lyme disease. *J Autoimmun* 1989;2:31–49.

111. Roush JK, Manley PA, Dueland RT: Rheumatoid arthritis subsequent to *Borrelia burgdorferi* infection in two dogs. *J Am Vet Med Assoc* 1989;195:951–953.

112. Burgess EC, Gendron-Fitzpatrick A, Wright WO: Arthritis and systemic disease caused by *Borrelia burgdorferi* infection in a cow. *J Am Vet Med Assoc* 1987;191:1468–1470.

113. Burgess EC, Gillette D, Pickett JP: Arthritis and panuveitis as manifestations of *Borrelia burgdorferi* infection in a Wisconsin pony. *J Am Vet Med Assoc* 1986;189;1340–1342.

114. Krinsky WL, Brown SJ, Askenase PW: *Ixodes dammini*: Induced skin lesions in guinea pigs and rabbits compared to erythema chronicum migrans in patients with Lyme arthritis. *Exp Parasitol* 1982;53:381–395.

115. Johnson RC, Marek N, Kodner C: Infection of Syrian hamsters with Lyme disease spirochetes. *J Clin Microbiol* 1984;2:1099–1101.

116. Barthold SW, Moody KD, Terwilliger GA, et al: Experimental Lyme arthritis in rats infected with *Borrelia burgdorferi*. *J Infect Dis* 1988;157:842–846.

117. Barthold SW, Moody KD, Terwilliger GA, et al: An animal model for Lyme arthritis. *Ann NY Acad Sci* 1988;539:264–273.

118. Hejka A, Schmitz JL, England DM, et al: Histopathology of Lyme arthritis in LSH hamsters. *Am J Pathol* 1989;134:1113–1123.

119. Schaible UE, Kramer MD, Museteanu C, et al: The severe combined immunodeficiency (*scid*) mouse: A laboratory model for the analysis of Lyme arthritis and carditis. *J Exp Med* 1989;170:1427–1432.

120. Schmitz JL, Schell RF, Hejka AG, et al: Passive immunization prevents induction of Lyme arthritis in LSH hamsters. *Infect Immun* 1990;58:144–148.

121. Johnson RC, Kodner C, Russell M, et al: Experimental infection of the hamster with *Borrelia burgdorferi*. *Ann NY Acad Sci* 1988;539:258–263.

122. Schaible UE, Kramer MD, Eichmann K, et al: Monoclonal antibodies specific for the outer surface protein A (OspA) of *Borrelia burgdorferi* prevent Lyme borreliosis in severe combined immunodeficiency (*scid*) mice. *Proc Natl Acad Sci USA* 1990;87:3768–3772.

123. Barbour AG, Burgdorfer W, Grunwaldt E, et al: Antibodies of patients with Lyme disease to components of the *Ixodes dammini* spirochete. *J Clin Invest* 1983;72:504–515.

124. Tortorice KL, Heim-Duthoy KL: Clinical features and treatment of Lyme disease. *Pharmacotherapy* 1989;9:363–371.

125. Luft BJ, Dattwyler RJ: Treatment of Lyme borreliosis. *Rheum Dis Clin North Am* 1989;15:747–755.

126. Steere AC, Malawista SE, Newman JH, et al: Antibiotic therapy in Lyme disease. *Ann Intern Med* 1980;93:1–8.

127. Caperton EM, Heim-Duthoy KL, Matzke GR, et al: Ceftriaxone therapy of chronic inflammatory arthritis: A double-blind placebo controlled trial. *Arch Intern Med* 1990;150:1677–1682.

128. Hollström E: Successful treatment of erythema migrans Afzelius. *Acta Derm Venereol* 1951;31:235–243.

129. Sigal LH: Summary of the first 100 patients seen at a Lyme disease referral center. *Am J Med* 1990;88:577–581.

130. Dattwyler RJ, Halperin JJ: Failure of tetracycline therapy in early Lyme disease. *Arthritis Rheum* 1987;30:448–450.

131. Radolf JD, Kaplan RP: Unusual manifestations of secondary syphilis and abnormal humoral immune response to *Treponema pallidum* antigens in a homosexual man with asymptomatic human immunodeficiency virus infection. *J Am Acad Dermatol* 1988;18:423–428.

132. Gerster JC, Weintraub A, Vischer TL, et al: Secondary syphilis revealed by rheumatic complaints. *J Rheumatol* 1977;4:197–200.

133. Todd AH: Syphilitic arthritis. *Br J Surg* 1926;14:260–279.

134. Kling DH: Syphilitic arthritis with effusion. *Am J Med Sci* 1932;183:538–549.

135. Chesney AM, Kemp JE, Baetjer FH: An experimental study of the synovial fluid of patients with arthritis and syphilis. *J Clin Invest* 1926;3:131–148.

136. Reginato AJ, Schumacher HR, Jimenez S, et al: Synovitis in secondary syphilis: Clinical, light, and electron microscopic studies. *Arthritis Rheum* 1979;22:170–176.

137. Hayes NS, Muse KE, Collier AM, et al: Parasitism by virulent *Treponema pallidum* of host cell surfaces. *Infect Immun* 1977;17:174–186.

138. Baseman JB, Hayes EC: Molecular characterization of receptor binding proteins and immunogens of virulent *Treponema pallidum*. *J Exp Med* 1980;151:573–586.

139. Alderete JF, Peterson KM, Baseman JB: Affinities of *Treponema pallidum* for human lactoferrin and transferrin. *Genitourin Med* 1988;64:359–363.

140. Alderete JF, Baseman JB: Serum lipoprotein binding by *Treponema pallidum*: Possible role for proteoglycans. *Genitourin Med* 1989;65:177–182.

141. Peterson KM, Baseman JB, Alderete JF: *Treponema pallidum* receptor binding proteins interact with fibronectin. *J Exp Med* 1983;157:1958–1970.

142. Thomas DD, Baseman JB, Alderete JF: Fibronectin mediates *Treponema pallidum* cytadherence through recognition of fibronectin cell-binding domain. *J Exp Med* 1985;161:514–525.

143. Thomas DD, Baseman JB, Alderete JF: Fibronectin tetrapeptide is target for syphilis spirochete cytadherence. *J Exp Med* 1985;162:1715–1719.

Chapter 8

Polymicrobial Infections

Katharine Merritt, PhD

Microorganisms live in a complex world and in general share territory. Very different organisms that seemingly should not survive in the same environment do well together. Each ecologic niche is filled with many types of organisms. The human body can be considered as an ecologic niche and any attempt to understand infection in humans must also consider normal flora. These organisms vary widely from site to site,[1,2] and to disturb them is to invite problems. Altering the ecologic niche may allow one organism to thrive at the expense of others and perhaps at the expense of the host. We must begin with the premise that the human body is polymicrobial.

Definitions

The interactions of organisms living in the same environment are complex and must be carefully defined. Parasitism means that one organism lives at the expense of the other. Mutualism means that two organisms survive well together as commensals, merely existing in the same site without affecting each other or the host environment. Synergism means that the two together do something that neither organism could do alone. Antagonism means that the organisms cannot exist together and one or both are inhibited. Antagonism was used to advantage in the early 20th century when it was easy to cure malaria but difficult to cure syphilis. Syphilitic patients were deliberately infected with malaria to create a fever of sufficient magnitude to kill the *Treponema* organisms causing syphilis; the malaria was then cured with quinine drugs. This treatment is no longer used because it is now somewhat easier to cure syphilis with drugs than it is to cure malaria.

The other entity that must be defined is a polymicrobial infection.[3,4] When two different organisms are isolated from the same blood sample, the infection is unquestionably polymicrobial. The problem arises when two different organisms are isolated from the same patient but at different blood drawings. Would the presence of *Staphylococcus aureus* on day 1 and *Escherichia coli* on day 2 indicate polymicrobial

117

bacteremia or two separate bacteremic incidents? What if the isolates are obtained two weeks apart? What if the *E coli* appeared after antimicrobial therapy for the *S aureus*? Would this be an iatrogenic infection and sequentially unimicrobial?

Polymicrobial Soft-Tissue Infections

Infections of the soft tissues and the cardiovascular system have been studied more extensively and in more controlled fashion than have those of hard tissues. Much has been learned but there are still tremendous gaps in our knowledge.

Infections Caused by Two Different Gram-Positive Organisms

There is good evidence that *S aureus* and group A β-hemolytic streptococci act synergistically, making an abscess or cellulitis more severe than would either acting independently.[5] Similarly, there is evidence that group B streptococci, which cause infections primarily in neonates, produce more severe disease when associated with *S aureus*.[6] The evidence for synergism among enterococci, group D streptococci, and *S aureus* is not as strong but this seems probable.[6]

The important issue considered here is the synergism between the two major groups of staphylococci. Whether there is synergism between coagulase-positive *S aureus* and coagulase-negative staphylococci may be difficult to answer. The colony morphology of the two organisms can be similar. If laboratory testing shows the organism to be coagulase-positive, it will be reported as *S aureus*. If it is coagulase-negative, a second and perhaps third colony will be tested before the organism is reported as coagulase-negative staphylococci. Thus, a culture containing a mix of coagulase-positive and coagulase-negative organisms will be reported as *S aureus* and a polymicrobial infection will be missed.

Infections Caused by Two Gram-Negative Bacteria

There is little evidence in the literature on the role of two gram-negative organisms in infection. Once again, laboratory testing is unlikely to identify a second colony on a culture plate containing an abundance of one type. This will happen only when the two colonies are distinctly different. Thus, a combination of a lactose fermenter such as *E coli* and a nonfermentative organism such as *Pseudomonas* will probably be reported. A combination of *E coli* and *Salmonella* organisms will probably be reported as a combination but the report will emphasize the presence of *Salmonella* organisms. Thus, some polymicrobial infections will be reported but many will be missed. Polymicrobial infections in this class are not known to be significantly worse than those caused by the more virulent organism alone except for the combination of *Pseudomonas aeruginosa* and *Pseudomonas cepacia*.[7]

Infections Caused by One Gram-Positive and One Gram-Negative Organism

This combination is likely to be detected. This combination usually consists of gram-positive *S aureus* and a gram-negative enteric or *Pseudomonas* organism. This occurs frequently in wound infections and is especially common in wounds associated with open fractures.[8,9] This combination is generally associated with a much more severe infection than would occur with either alone.

Infections Caused by an Aerobe and an Anaerobe

This combination seems unlikely. However, it is known that obligate aerobes and obligate anaerobes can be isolated from the same site. Clinicians are surprised by the abundance of anaerobes in the oral cavity and the isolation of obligate aerobes from the gastrointestinal tract. The oxidation-reduction potential is such that the environment is made amenable to both organisms and neither could live without the other. Indeed, a laboratory can take advantage of this and grow an aerobe as part of an anaerobic culture to hasten the formation of an anaerobic environment. However, this combination will never be noticed unless the request for culture includes the instruction, "culture for both aerobes and anaerobes." Anaerobic cultures are more difficult to do, and, therefore, are done only when requested. In addition, some anaerobes are aerotolerant and can survive in air for a few hours, but many do not tolerate air and die almost immediately. Cultures for isolation of anaerobic organisms must be collected very carefully.

There are reports of various infections involving aerobes and anaerobes; the best studied combination is *Bacteroides* organisms and *E coli*. Both these organisms are gram-negative and both reside in the gastrointestinal tract and in the oral cavity. *Bacteroides* organisms are obligate anaerobes but are somewhat areotolerant. *E coli* organisms are facultative and can grow under both conditions but favor the aerobic environment. *Bacteroides* organisms alone probably never cause an infection but in the presence of *E coli* can cause a severe abscess.[10,11] These infections have been reproduced in animal models.[12,13] These infections can sometimes can be treated by eradicating only one of the organisms,[14,15] but often the infection is not cured until both are eradicated.[16,17] The demonstration that *Bacteroides* organisms isolated in the presence of *E coli* are encapsulated whereas those isolated in the absence of *E coli* are rough is extremely important in understanding the pathogenicity.[18] The encapsulated organisms are much more capable of causing disease and much more resistant to antibiotics than are the nonencapsulated strains.

The question remains as to whether or not any anaerobe other than *Clostridia* is capable of causing an infection without being in a polymicrobial environment. It is possible that *Bacteroides* organisms are capable of causing infection alone, but this has not been proven, whereas the combination with *E coli* is known to be highly pathogenic.[12-19] It is also possible that *Eikenella* organisms alone can cause infection, but the infections are more likely to be polymicrobial.[20,21]

The best examples of polymicrobial infections are probably those associated with bites. Bites by humans and other animals are apt to cause severe polymicrobial infections. The other unfortunate aspect of animal bites is that they are most likely to occur on the hand or around the face. These locations are notoriously susceptible to infection, partly because of the ready availability of the vascular system. Because of the small amount of soft tissue, the chances of penetrating bone is also greater. Infections of the hand after bites are usually polymicrobial, and the organisms resemble the mouth flora of the biter. Thus, there may be a mixture of anaerobes and aerobes and a mixture of gram-positive and gram-negative organisms. Antimicrobial therapy is particularly difficult in this group of infections.

Polymicrobial Infections at the Site of Biomaterials

The isolation of more than one organism in the same sample is indicative of polymicrobial infection. Although one of the organisms may be considered to be nonpathogenic while the other is considered to be the real etiologic agent, the fact that more than one was isolated should not be ignored because the nonpathogen undoubtedly contributes to the pathogenicity of the other.

One mechanism by which pathogenicity is promoted is encapsulation. Another is by one especially adherent organism forming a biofilm that enhances the adherence of a less adherent organism. A third is coaggregation of two or more species. Thus, *Staphylococcus epidermidis* can promote the adherence of gram-negative organisms to biomaterials.[22-24] The coaggreagation of many different species has been observed in association with hydroxyapatite and the oral environment. These include such interactions as those between *Propionibacterium* and *Streptococcus* organisms,[25] *Streptococcus* and *Bacteroides* organisms,[26] *Bacteroides* and *Actinomyces* organisms,[27] *Streptococcus* and *Candida* organisms,[28] and placque-forming bacteria among themselves.[29] The combination of *Lactobacillus* and *E coli* organisms on urinary catheters may actually decrease rather than promote adherence.[30]

Polymicrobial Infections in Orthopaedic Surgery

Anaerobic infections are enhanced by the presence of an implant and by the presence of aerobic bacteria.[31,32] It is also evident from bacterial adherence and musculoskeletal sepsis that the biofilm on the implant or the adjacent tissues is composed of more than one type of bacterium.[33-35]

There are many reports on infection rates at the site of total joint replacements. The organisms isolated are usually predominantly the two staphylococci with the more numerous of the two varying from institution to institution. Gram-negative organisms, usually *Pseudo-*

monas, run a distant third, with polymicrobial infections listed fourth.[36-38]

At highest risk for polymicrobial infections are patients who have undergone trauma, particularly open fractures. Studies on colonization of wounds in these patients have clearly indicated the polymicrobial origins of the infections. Patients with mixed gram-positive and gram-negative flora have a poor outcome.[39-43]

It is important to remember that the bulk of the early literature on foreign bodies and infections described cases in which sutures were used. Much was gained from these studies, which defined the problem, the chemistry, and the configuration.[44-45] Today, most sutures used consist of single filaments and are synthetic. The suture remains a major site of initiation of infection. In an open fracture, primary closure of the wounds is clearly contraindicated.[46-48] Care should also be taken in the decision to close the wounds in revision arthroplasty in the presence of infection. The suture may form a nidus of colonization by one organism that may then enhance the growth of another.

The incidence of polymicrobial infections in orthopaedic surgery is probably underrecognized. It is clear from examining the biofilm on the implants,[33-35] and from other in vitro studies, that the film is firmly adherent. Thus, most organisms remain on the implant. The tissue may or may not reflect the composition of the biofilm on the implant. Culturing scrapings from the material or ultrasonic elution of the organisms followed by culturing may provide better information on the polymicrobial nature of the infection. Anaerobic as well as aerobic cultures should be done. The cost-effectiveness of this is also an issue to be considered. Should we enhance medical care by isolating and identifying each and every organism, or should we treat only the obvious cause?

Other issues include how we deal with an obviously infected patient for whom cultures are negative and how we deal with antimicrobial therapy. There is some evidence in the studies on open fractures that 48 hours of prophylactic antibiotic therapy is beneficial.[39-43] Extension beyond this time is associated with increased infection. Finally, changing the antibiotic each time a new organism is isolated may create a polymicrobial, antibiotic-resistant infection.

Polymicrobial Infections in Dental Surgery

There is, of course, a strong correlation between the problems in dental surgery and those in orthopaedic surgery because both deal with soft tissue and bone. The materials used are often similar. The dental surgeon is by definition operating in a polymicrobial environment. Although problems faced by the dental and the orthopaedic patient are different, much can be learned from reviewing the literature on dental infections and dental microbiology. Studies on microbial adherence[49] and the role of anaerobes in polymicrobial infections[50-53] are well documented in the dental literature.

121

Polymicrobial Infections in Other Specialties

The cardiovascular surgeon generally deals with a clean surgical area and infections tend to be caused by a single microbe, with *S aureus*, *S epidermidis*, and *Pseudomonas* species being the major etiologic agents. The adherence of *S epidermidis* to polymeric catheters or to the graft material is of extreme importance because this may increase the risk of an unrecognized polymicrobial infection. Contact lenses are made of polymeric materials to which bacteria can adhere. *Pseudomonas* is the prominent organism in such cases, partly because these organisms live in the saline and cleaning solutions. The biofilm formed by *Pseudomonas* on these lenses[54] could promote infection by other organisms.

Ear infections are often polymicrobial in origin because they result from an extension of the normal flora of the nasopharynx. In fact, cultures of the surrounding areas are rarely taken in middle ear infections because the culture will grow a mixture and may not be helpful. Fluid withdrawn from the middle ear may provide useful culture information in infections not responding to conventional broad-spectrum therapy. Ear implants will be subjected to a polymicrobial environment.

It is of interest that the use of urinary catheters is rarely associated with a polymicrobial infection. This may be because one predominant gram-negative organism colonizes the catheter, and does not form a glycocalyx to attract other organisms. This infection is probably caused by the first organism to come in contact with the catheter.

References

1. Rose NR, Barron AL (eds): *Microbiology: Basic Principles and Clinical Applications.* New York, Macmillan, 1983.
2. Rosebury T: *Life on Man.* New York, Viking Press, 1969.
3. Cooper GS, Havlir DS, Shlaes DM, et al: Polymicrobial bacteremia in the late 1980s: Predictors of outcome and review of the literature. *Medicine* 1990;69:114–123.
4. Roberts FJ: Definition of polymicrobial bacteremia, letter. *Rev Infect Dis* 1989;11:1029–1030.
5. White A, Brooks GF: Furunculosis, pyoderma, and impetigo, in Hoeprich PD (ed): *Infectious Diseases: A Modern Treatise of Infectious Processes*, ed 2. Hagerstown, Maryland, Harper & Row, 1977, pp 785–793.
6. Peter G, Smith AL: Group A streptococcal infections of the skin and pharynx. *N Engl J Med* 1977;297:311–317, 365–370.
7. Saiman L, Cacalano G, Prince A: *Pseudomonas cepacia* adherence to respiratory epithelial cells is enhanced by *Pseudomonas aeruginosa. Infect Immun* 1990;58:2578–2584.
8. Merritt K, Dowd JD: Role of internal fixation in infection of open fractures: Studies with *Staphylococcus aureus* and *Proteus mirabilis. J Orthop Res* 1987;5:23–28.
9. Waldvogel FA, Papageorgiou PS: Osteomyelitis: The past decade. *N Engl J Med* 1980;303:360–370.
10. Brook I: Enhancement of growth of aerobic, anaerobic, and facultative bacteria in mixed infections with anaerobic and facultative gram-positive cocci. *J Surg Res* 1988;45:222–227.

11. Brook I: Pathogenicity of the *Bacteroides fragilis* group. *Ann Clin Lab Sci* 1989;19:360–376.

12. Onderdonk AB, Cisneros RL, Finberg R, et al: Animal model system for studying virulence of and host response to *Bacteroides fragilis*. *Rev Infect Dis* 1990;12(suppl 2):S169–S177.

13. Bom-van Noorloos AA, van Steenbergen TJM, Burger EH: Direct and immune-cell-mediated effects of *Bacteroides gingivalis* on bone metabolism in vitro. *J Clin Periodont* 1989;16:412–418.

14. Bartlett JG, Gorbach SL, Tally FP, et al: Bacteriology and treatment of primary lung abscess. *Am Rev Respir Dis* 1974;109:510–518.

15. Finegold SM: *Anaerobic Bacteria in Human Disease*. New York, Academic Press, 1977.

16. Brook I: Management of infection following intra-abdominal trauma. *Ann Emerg Med* 1988;17:626–632.

17. Brook I: Encapsulated anaerobic bacteria in synergistic infections. *Microbiol Rev* 1986;50:452–457.

18. Onderdonk AB, Kasper DL, Cisneros RL, et al: The capsular polysaccharide of *Bacteroides fragilis* as a virulence factor: Comparison of the pathogenic potential of encapsulated and unencapsulated strains. *J Infect Dis* 1977;136:82–89.

19. Raahave D, Friis-Møller A, Bjerre-Jepsen K, et al: The infective dose of aerobic and anaerobic bacteria in postoperative wound sepsis. *Arch Surg* 1986;121:924–929.

20. Johnson CC, Reinhardt JF, Edelstein MAC, et al: *Bacteroides gracilis*, an important anaerobic bacterial pathogen. *J Clin Microbiol* 1985;22:799–802.

21. Flesher SA, Bottone EJ: *Eikenella corrodens* cellulitis and arthritis of the knee. *J Clin Microbiol* 1989;27:2606–2608.

22. Merritt K: Factors affecting bacterial adherence in biomaterials. Presented at the Annual Meeting of the American Society for Microbiology, Miami, Florida, May 1988.

23. Chang CC, Merritt K: Polymicrobial adherence on poly(methylmethacrylate) (PMMA) surface. *J Biomed Mater Res*, in press.

24. Chang CC, Merritt K: The effect of *Staphylococcus epidermidis* on the adherence of *Pseudomonas aeruginosa* and *Proteus mirabilis* to polymethylmethacrylate (PMMA) and PMMA containing gentamicin. *J Orthop Res*, 1991;9:284–285.

25. Ciardi JE, McCray GF, Kolenbrander PE, et al: Cell-to-cell interaction of *Streptococcus sanguis* and *Propionibacterium acnes* on saliva-coated hydroxyapatite. *Infect Immun* 1987;55:1441–1446.

26. Cimasoni G, Song M, McBride BC: Effect of crevicular fluid and lysosomal enzymes on the adherence of streptococci and *Bacteroides* to hydroxyapatite. *Infect Immun* 1987;55:1484–1489.

27. Li J, Ellen RP: Relative adherence of *Bacteroides* species and strains to *Actinomyces viscosus* on saliva-coated hydroxyapatite. *J Dent Res* 1989;68:1308–1312.

28. Branting C, Sund ML, Linder LE: The influence of *Streptococcus mutans* on adhesion of *Candida albicans* to acrylic surfaces in vitro. *Arch Oral Biol* 1989;34:347–353.

29. Gibbons RJ, Nygaard M: Interbacterial aggregation of plaque bacteria. *Arch Oral Biol* 1970;15:1397–1400.

30. Hawthorn LA, Reid G: Exclusion of uropathogen adhesion to polymer surfaces by *Lactobacillus acidophilus*. *J Biomed Mater Res* 1990;24:39–46.

31. Hall BB, Fitzgerald RH Jr, Rosenblatt JE: Anaerobic osteomyelitis. *J Bone Joint Surg* 1983;65A:30–35.

32. Lewis RP, Sutter VL, Finegold SM: Bone infections involving anaerobic bacteria. *Medicine* 1978;57:279–305.

33. Gristina AG, Costerton JW: Bacterial adherence and the glycocalyx and their role in musculoskeletal infection. *Orthop Clin North Am* 1984;15:517–535.

34. Gristina AG, Costerton JW: Bacterial adherence to biomaterials and tissues: The significance of its role in clinical sepsis. *J Bone Joint Surg* 1985;67A:264–273.

35. Gristina AG, Oga M, Webb LX, et al: Adherent bacterial colonization in the pathogenesis of osteomyelitis. *Science* 1985;228:990–993.

36. Dougherty SH: Pathobiology of infection in prosthetic devices. *Rev Infect Dis* 1988;10:1102–1117.

37. Wilde AH, Ruth JT: Two-stage reimplantation in infected total knee arthroplasty. *Clin Orthop* 1988;236:23–35.

38. Wilson MG, Kelley K, Thornhill TS: Infection as a complication of total knee-replacement arthroplasty: Risk factors and treatment in sixty-seven cases. *J Bone Joint Surg* 1990;72A:878–883.

39. Merritt K: Factors increasing the risk of infection in patients with open fractures. *J Trauma* 1988;28:823–827.

40. Roth AI, Fry DE, Polk HC Jr: Infectious morbidity in extremity fractures. *J Trauma* 1986;26:757–761.

41. Clough JFM, Meek RN, Crichton A: Infection following compound fractures: The significance of different risk factors, abstract. *J Bone Joint Surg* 1982;64B:260.

42. Lawrence RM, Hoeprich PD, Huston AC, et al: Quantitative microbiology of traumatic orthopedic wounds. *J Clin Microbiol* 1978;8:673–675.

43. Marrie TJ, Costerton JW: Mode of growth of bacterial pathogens in chronic polymicrobial human osteomyelitis. *J Clin Microbiol* 1985;22:924–933.

44. Alexander JW, Kaplan JZ, Altemeier WA: Role of suture materials in the development of wound infection. *Ann Surg* 1967;165:192–199.

45. Edlich RF, Panek PH, Rodeheaver GT, et al: Surgical sutures and infection: A biomaterial evaluation. *J Biomed Mater Res* 1974;8:115–126.

46. Clancey GJ, Hansen ST Jr: Open fractures of the tibia: A review of one hundred and two cases. *J Bone Joint Surg* 1978;60A:118–122.

47. Hunt TK: Surgical wound infections: An overview. *Am J Med* 1981;70:712–718.

48. Sugarman B: Infections and prosthetic devices. *Am J Med* 1986;81:78–84.

49. Mergenhagen SE, Rosan B (eds): *Molecular Basis of Oral Microbial Adhesion: Proceedings of a Workshop Held in Philadelphia, Pennsylvania, 5–8 June 1984.* Washington, DC, American Society for Microbiology, 1985.

50. Haapasalo M: *Bacteroides* buccae and related taxa in necrotic root canal infections. *J Clin Microbiol* 1986;24:940–944.

51. Moore WEC: Microbiology of periodontal disease. *J Periodont Res* 1987;22:335–341.

52. Nakou M, Mikx FHM, Oosterwaal PJM, et al: Early microbial colonization of permucosal implants in edentulous patients. *J Dent Res* 1987;66:1654–1657.

53. Williams RC: Periodontal disease. *N Engl J Med* 1990;322:373–382.

54. Slusher MM, Myrvik QN, Lewis JC, et al: Extended-wear lenses, biofilm, and bacterial adhesion. *Arch Ophthalmol* 1987;105:110–115.

Chapter 9

Bacterial Adhesion to Host Tissues

Ronald J. Gibbons, PhD
John L. Esterhai, Jr, MD

Introduction

Bacteria attach to tissues in a surprisingly specific way, and their attachment often correlates with colonization. Early studies led to the realization that in any environment subjected to a fluid flow, bacteria must attach to a surface if they are to persist and have an opportunity to grow. In the oral cavity, *Streptococcus sanguis*, which is dominant on the surface of teeth, attaches selectively to teeth. In contrast, *Streptococcus salivarius*, one of the species found on the dorsum of the tongue, attaches avidly to the tongue surface. Both organisms are indigenous to humans and they attach much better to human tissues than to tissues of laboratory animals. The bacterial cell surface must have a sophisticated recognition system to enable bacteria to differentiate teeth from tongue, and human from mouse. Because of the specificity of this process, the relative susceptibility or resistance of different tissues to infection is largely determined by whether or not the tissue is receptive to the attachment of a particular bacterium.

This selectivity of bacterial attachment has attracted considerable interest. Before 1970, about five to ten papers dealing with bacterial adhesion were published each year. Once it became known that attachment of bacteria was selective and that it was associated with colonization, activity continuously increased. In 1989, more than 500 papers were published on this topic.[1] The reason for this interest is that knowledge of the molecular mechanisms involved in the attachment of bacteria to tissue surfaces promises to provide molecular explanations for the tropisms of bacteria and for the innate resistance or susceptibility of different tissues to infection. Almost everyone studying bacterial adhesion believes that this information will lead to new and better ways of controlling infections in the future.

Freter[2] demonstrated that complex microbial communities can coexist for extended periods only if the organisms have specific adhesion sites. Stable populations of two or more bacterial strains that compete for the same limited nutrients can coexist if the metabolically less efficient strain has specific adhesion sites available for which it need not compete.

Adhesins

Bacterial cells possess a surface net negative charge and can become associated with surfaces by nonspecific electrostatic or hydrophobic forces. These may be of importance for the attachment of bacteria to biomaterials. However, many bacteria possess proteinaceous ligands, called adhesins, that bind stereochemically to complementary receptors on tissue surfaces.[3] Many adhesins are associated with fimbriae or pili. Until recently, it was thought that these surface appendages were simply aggregates of adhesin molecules. However, adhesins of some *Escherichia coli* strains are localized at the tip of a pilus. Many adhesins bind to saccharide receptors, and are thus considered lectins.

Adhesin-receptor interactions are analogous to antibody-antigen or enzyme-substrate interactions. Some adhesins may be derived from enzymes by proteolytic cleavage that removes the catalytic site while leaving the binding site intact. A single bacterial cell may possess several thousand adhesin molecules that can interact with several receptors to produce high-affinity bonding.

Although many adhesins are proteins, it has been suggested that polysaccharides and lipoteichoic acids function in the same manner. Lipoteichoic acid molecules are amphipathic. Lipoteichoic acid binds hydrophobically to a variety of cell surfaces, but the specificity of this binding differs from that of group A streptococci.[4] Thus, lipoteichoic acid does not appear to be the principal adhesin for these organisms. However, highly purified M-protein derived from these streptococci binds to human epithelial cells with a pattern of selectivity similar to that of intact bacteria. Also, streptococcal mutants lacking M-protein do not bind well. Such observations suggest a role for M-protein in the adhesion of group A streptococci, and interactions between lipoteichoic acid and M-protein may serve to hold the adhesin on the bacterial cell surface.

A single bacterial cell can contain more than one type of adhesin and fimbriae. Some fimbrial adhesins are encoded by plasmids. The nature of the plasmid and the adhesin that is expressed allow grouping of bacteria according to their patterns of adhesion and the types of clinical disease that they produce.[5]

Receptors

Investigations designed to identify and characterize the tissue receptors for bacterial adhesins are intensive. Most receptors are glycoproteins or glycolipids. The receptor region appears to reside in oligosaccharides and, thus, provides a basis for recognition specificity. The carbohydrate chains on mammalian cell surfaces contain an enormous amount of molecular information. A disaccharide can exist in more than 50 isomeric configurations. Glycoproteins, including fibronectin, have been identified as receptors for some bacteria. Also, bacteria may bind to basement membrane and connective tissue components such as collagen and laminin.

The receptors for bacterial adhesins are not restricted to tissue surfaces, but can also be present in components of body fluids and secretions.[6] The mucins of oral secretions are structurally related in their saccharides to components on tissue surfaces. Mucins may interact with bacterial adhesins and inhibit binding of these adhesins to the tissue surface. This is important. Secretions augment the mechanical cleansing action on tissues by binding to bacterial adhesins and inhibiting attachment to cells. The in situ attachment of a bacterium then becomes a function of the relative concentration of receptor molecules on the tissue surface and the number of competing molecules in the secretions or body fluids in which the bacteria are suspended. These adhesin-receptor interactions give the molecular biologist an opportunity to construct receptor analogues that may bind with higher affinity. Such potent inhibitors of attachment could be useful in controlling bacterial adhesion.

Most antibodies bind only to the terminal sequences of molecules. However, adhesins can also bind to internal sequences and, depending on the adjacent groupings of molecules, isoreceptors may exist. Therefore, adhesins have primary and secondary binding sites in molecules. Some of these adjacent groupings may enhance binding and increase affinity. Other adjacent groupings may decrease or even block binding. The ability of adhesins to bind to internal sequences may expand the range of possible hosts that a bacterium can colonize because the terminal saccharide residues account for the blood group antigens. If bacteria were limited to recognizing only terminal sequences, as antibodies are, they would be limited in their range of hosts.

Identifying Adhesins and Receptors

There are three useful criteria for identifying an adhesin or receptor[7]: (1) A stereochemical adhesin-receptor interaction is saturable. The number of receptors on a tissue surface is finite and, therefore, the tissue can be saturated. (2) Adhesin-receptor binding is reversible. The adhesin can be disassociated from the receptor. (3) The adhesin should exhibit the same binding specificity as the intact bacterial cell and antibodies to the adhesin should block adhesion of the bacterium to the tissue surface. The expression of an adhesin on the bacterial cell should correlate with its adhesive properties. Mutants defective in the synthesis of the adhesin should no longer attach.

For a component to be identified as a receptor, it should bind to the adhesin and its distribution on the tissue surface should correlate with the receptivity of that surface. Tissues with a high density of receptors should be more receptive than tissues with a low density. The isolated receptor should competitively inhibit adhesion of the bacterium to the tissue surface.

Many substrata have been used to study bacterial adhesion: natural tissue surfaces, epithelial cells scraped from these tissues, excised tissue segments, tissue-cultured cells, erythrocytes, other microbes, and substrata-treated solids such as hydroxyapatite disks exposed to body fluids or pure isolated proteins.

The behavior of a molecule on a surface may be quite different from its behavior when it is free in solution. Most biomaterials inserted into a systemic situation adsorb a film of macromolecules onto their surface from the fluids in the environment. For example, the enamel of teeth is primarily hydroxyapatite. The mineral adsorbs macromolecules from saliva and other oral fluids. The attachment of bacteria to such solid materials, therefore, involves interactions between the adhesins of the bacteria and immobilized molecules adsorbed onto the surface of the substratum.

Some of the salivary materials that adsorb onto hydroxyapatite and serve as receptors for prominent plaque bacteria have been studied. Gibbons and Hay[8] fractionated saliva chromatographically and exposed hydroxyapatite beads to the saliva fractions. Any uncoated areas of the mineral were blocked with albumin. The beads were then exposed to radioactively labeled bacteria. *Streptococcus mutans* bound to the high-molecular-weight mucinous material from saliva. In contrast, *Actinomyces viscosus* did not bind to the mucinous components, but it did bind to other eluting components. These studies illustrated the selectivity of bacterial interactions, and indicated that different salivary components promote the attachment of different bacteria.

Additional purification revealed that the adhesion-promoting material for *A viscosus* was associated with the family of salivary proline-rich proteins.[9] This family of closely related nonglycosylated phosphoproteins constitutes 20% to 40% of the protein in saliva. Their function is to stabilize the ionic environment of saliva. Saliva is supersaturated with respect to calcium and phosphate, and these proteins bind very avidly to calcium atoms and prevent crystal formation. Some proline-rich proteins have 150 amino acid residues and differ from each other only at residues 4 and 50. Other proline-rich proteins terminate at residue 106. These molecules are unusually asymmetric with respect to charged residues. All contain two phosphoserines (negatively charged residues) clustered at one end of the molecule. Several positively charged residues are distributed at the other end of the molecule. There is a tryptic cleavage point at residue 30, and residues 1 to 30 are primarily responsible for binding the protein to hydroxyapatite surfaces. Treating hydroxyapatite beads with 1 to 2 μg of one type of proline-rich protein (PRP-1), for example, promotes maximal binding of *A viscosus*.[8] This corresponds to 10,000 proline-rich protein molecules per square micron, and constitutes a binding site for a bacterial cell. This represents only about 10% coverage of the mineral surface. Evidently, a monolayer of material is not required for maximal binding because the bacteria attach by spatially separated fimbriae with the adhesins at the tip.[8] Studies with fimbriae-defective mutants have shown that the adhesin is associated with the type 1 fimbriae of *A viscosus*. The minimal receptor recognition site in the proline-rich proteins for the *A viscosus* adhesin is the Pro-Gln dipeptide.

Proline-rich Proteins

Salivary proline-rich proteins exhibit striking structural similarities to collagens. A computer search of a database containing 6,418 protein sequences revealed that the salivary proline-rich proteins were most closely related to collagen.[1] This seems important because a variety of oral bacteria, including strains of *A viscosus* and *Bacteroides gingivalis*, bind avidly to collagen. In the case of *A viscosus*, the same adhesin that mediates binding to proline-rich proteins mediates binding to collagen. The predilection of many indigenous bacteria for producing infections in surgical wounds in which collagen fibers are exposed may be mediated by adhesins that bind to structurally related sequences in collagen and perhaps to other molecules present in body fluids.

Although *A viscosus* and other bacteria bind well to adsorbed proline-rich proteins on hydroxyapatite, they do not seem to interact with these proteins in solution.[8] Concentrations of proline-rich proteins as high as 1,000 µg/ml do not inhibit binding of *A viscosus* cells to hydroxyapatite containing only 1 to 2 µg of adsorbed proline-rich protein. Also, radioactively labeled proline-rich protein in solution does not bind to *A viscosus* cells. The apparent explanation for this difference in behavior is that the proline-rich proteins undergo a major conformational change when they adsorb onto mineral surfaces. This was initially suggested by Bennick and associates,[10] who observed differences in the calcium-binding properties of adsorbed and soluble proline-rich proteins. Studies of the thermodynamics of the adsorption of the proline-rich proteins onto hydroxyapatite indicated that the polypeptide chain in solution is folded over on itself with the positively charged end interacting with the negatively charged end.[11] The adsorption of the protein to hydroxyapatite is an endothermic process driven by an increase in entropy. The high degree of asymmetry in charged residues in proline-rich protein molecules is thought to contribute to the folding of the polypeptide chain in solution. Evidently, when the negatively charged amino terminal segment of the molecule interacts with calcium atoms on hydroxyapatite surfaces, the polypeptide chain unfolds. Bacterial adhesins then bind to segments that are exposed only when the molecule is adsorbed onto a surface. Because the proline-rich proteins can constitute 40% of the protein in saliva, bacteria would have little chance to bind to adsorbed molecules on tissue surfaces if these molecules could interact with bacterial adhesins while in solution. By recognizing only the novel segments of surface-associated molecules, bacteria are able to avoid the cleansing activities of secretions. These observations provide a molecular explanation for that fact that the surface of human teeth is the primary habitat of *A viscosus*.

These hidden receptors have been named "cryptitopes" from the Greek *kryptos*, meaning hidden, and *topos*, meaning place. Shortly after the above studies were reported, Lowrance and associates[12] reported that *Streptococcus sanguis* would bind to fibronectin that was complexed with collagen but not with fibronectin in solution. They suggested that this could account for the ability of *S sanguis* cells to bind to damaged heart valves, which may have collagen-fibronectin complexes, and avoid interacting with the free fibronectin in serum. This suggests that cryptitopes become exposed on fibronectin after it interacts with collagen molecules.

Enzymes can also modify molecules and expose hidden segments. Trypsin cleaves peptide bonds and exposes arginine residues. Studies with *Pseudomonas* species indicate that this organism attaches poorly to untreated epithelial cells. However, mild treatment with trypsin results in greatly enhanced attachment, presumably through the generation of cryptitopes.[13] *Pseudomonas* organisms also attach in much higher numbers to buccal and pharyngeal epithelial cells from acutely ill patients or patients with cystic fibrosis. This attachment has been associated with increased levels of proteinases in the secretions from these patients. It has been suggested that the proteinases remove fibronectin from the epithelial cell surface and expose receptors for *Pseudomonas*.

Because many indigenous and pathogenic bacteria contain lectin-like adhesins on their surfaces, it is not surprising that bacterial cells of one species can bind to the surfaces of other organisms. Such interactions result in coaggregations that are highly specific and exhibit many of the features evident in host-bacteria tissue interactions.[14]

Inhibition of Adhesion

Inhibition of bacterial attachment may result from antibody molecules binding to bacterial adhesins, thus blocking their interaction with tissue receptors. For example, antibodies to the M-protein inhibit attachment of *Streptococcus pyogenes* cells to host tissues. Antibodies of the IgA isotype possess such adhesion-inhibiting activity, and this is one of the mechanisms by which they provide protective immunity without mediation of the complement or phagocytic systems in mucosal environments.

Antibodies agglutinate bacterial cells, and aggregated bacteria attach less effectively than well-dispersed bacteria. Thus, antibodies to surface components other than adhesins may be effective. These observations suggest a strategy for the possible development of vaccines.[15] Because adhesins are proteins that bind to host tissues, they usually elicit a strong antibody response. However, bacteria can produce many antigenic subtypes of adhesins that complicate vaccine development. Adhesin molecules contain a conserved region and a variable region. Antigenically distinct adhesin molecules may be functionally similar. Such antigenic variability seems to permit populations of indigenous bacteria to persist in a host for long periods. The adhesins undergo antigenic variation and evade the immune response of the host.

Because bacterial adhesins are proteins, even low concentrations of antimicrobial agents that interfere with protein synthesis can reduce the ability of bacterial cells to attach. Antibiotics at 25% to 50% of the minimal inhibitory concentration for growth can result in bacterial cells with impaired capacity to attach.[16] In some instances, antibiotic-grown bacteria have fewer fimbriae and exhibit reduced hydrophobicity. Antibiotic administration can eliminate bacteria by several mechanisms. Antibiotics may interfere with bacterial cell growth or cause cell lysis. These effects augment the host's immune defenses. The concentration of a systemically administered antibiotic is much lower in mucosal secretions than it is in serum. Yet, these concentrations often suppress bacterial colonization on the mucosal surfaces. It seems likely that such effects are the result of anti-adhesion activity. In the past, most antibiotics were evaluated with screening assays that monitored bacterial growth. Perhaps in the future new therapeutic compounds will also be evaluated for their effect on bacterial adhesion.

Bacterial infections often develop after viral infections. Some virus-infected host cells have different receptive properties for bacteria. One mechanism is seen in the hemagglutinin of influenza virus, which is a sialic acid-binding adhesin that becomes incorporated into the epithelial cell membrane of virus-infected cells. It can bind bacteria that possess capsules containing sialic acid on their surface. Also, tissue-cultured cells infected with influenza A virus contain the viral glycoprotein on their surface. Fibrinogen is able to bind to this glycoprotein and also to the adhesin on streptococcal surfaces, thereby serving as a bridge. *Streptococcus pneumoniae* organisms colonize tracheal cells infected with influenza A virus. Microscopic observations have shown that extensive desquamation of the epithelium, which exposes the basement membrane, occurs in virus-infected animals. Pneumococcal cells were observed on the exposed basement membranes of infected animals, but not on the tracheal cells of control animals.[17]

The role of adhesion in pathogenic bacterial colonization suggests new techniques for controlling infection. Vaccines consisting of immunogenic adhesins or the conserved regions of such molecules linked to a carrier, antibiotics and other chemotherapeutic agents that affect the synthesis of bacterial adhesins, and soluble receptor analogues aimed at preventing attachment should be investigated. As additional information is obtained about the molecular nature of adhesins and receptors, it may become possible to develop practical remedies to augment current treatment plans and assist in the eradication of infection.

References

1. Gibbons RJ: Bacterial adhesion to oral tissues: A model for infectious diseases. *J Dent Res* 1989;68:750–760.
2. Freter R: Mechanisms of bacterial colonization of the mucosal surfaces of the gut, in Roth JA (ed): *Virulence Mechanisms of Bacterial Pathogens.* Washington, DC, American Society for Microbiology, 1988, pp 45–60.
3. Jones GW, Isaacson RE: Proteinaceous bacterial adhesins and their receptors. *CRC Crit Rev Microbiol* 1983;10:229–260.
4. Tylewska SK, Fischetti VA, Gibbons RJ: Binding selectivity of *Streptococcus pyogenes* and M-protein to epithelial cells differs from that of lipoteichoic acid. *Curr Microbiol* 1988;16:209–216.

5. Levine MM: *Escherichia coli* that cause diarrhea: Enterotoxigenic, enteropathogenic, enteroinvasive, enterohemorrhagic, and enteroadherent. *J Infect Dis* 1987;155:377–389.

6. Dean EA, Whipp SC, Moon HW: Age-specific colonization of porcine intestinal epithelium by 987P-piliated enterotoxigenic *Escherichia coli*. *Infect Immun* 1989;57:82–87.

7. Schoolnik GKI, Lark DL, O'Hanley PD: Molecular approaches for the study of uropathogenesis, in Horwitz MA (ed): *Bacteria-Host Cell Interaction*. New York, Alan R Liss, 1988, pp 201–211.

8. Gibbons RJ, Hay DI: Human salivary acidic proline-rich proteins and statherin promote the attachment of *Actinomyces viscosus* LY7 to apatitic surfaces. *Infect Immun* 1988;56:439–445.

9. Gibbons RJ, Hay DI, Cisar JO, et al: Adsorbed salivary proline-rich protein 1 and statherin: Receptors for type 1 fimbriae of *Actinomyces viscosus* T14V-J1 on apatitic surfaces. *Infect Immun* 1988;56:2990–2993.

10. Bennick A, McLaughlin AC, Grey AA, et al: The location and nature of calcium-binding sites in salivary acidic proline-rich phosphoproteins. *J Biol Chem* 1981;256:4741–4746.

11. Moreno EC, Kresak M, Hay DI: Adsorption thermodynamics of acidic proline-rich human salivary proteins onto calcium apatites. *J Biol Chem* 1982;257:2981–2989.

12. Lowrance JH, Hasty DL, Simpson WA: Adherence of *Streptococcus sanguis* to conformationally specific determinants in fibronectin. *Infect Immun* 1988;56:2279–2285.

13. Woods DE, Straus DC, Johanson WG Jr, et al: Factors influencing the adherence of *Pseudomonas aeruginosa* to mammalian buccal epithelial cells. *Rev Infect Dis* 1983;5(suppl 5):S846–S851.

14. Kolenbrander PE: Intergeneric coaggregation among human oral bacteria and ecology of dental plaque. *Annu Rev Microbiol* 1988;42:627–656.

15. Isaacson RE: Molecular and genetic basis of adherence for enteric *Escherichia coli* in animals, in Roth JA (ed): *Virulence Mechanisms of Bacterial Pathogens*. Washington, DC, American Society for Microbiology, 1988, pp 28–44.

16. Reid G, Sobel JD: Bacterial adherence in the pathogenesis of urinary tract infection: A review. *Rev Infect Dis* 1987;9:470–487.

17. Plotkowski M-C, Puchelle E, Beck G, et al: Adherence of type I *Streptococcus pneumoniae* to tracheal epithelium of mice infected with influenza A/PR8 virus. *Am Rev Respir Dis* 1986;134:1040–1044.

Chapter 10

Bacterial Biofilm and Infected Biomaterials, Prostheses, and Artificial Organs

David J. Schurman, MD
R. Lane Smith, PhD

Introduction

Bacterial biofilm contributes to foreign-body infection and bacterial pathogenesis.[1,2] Localized infection leads to poor surgical outcome because of tissue destruction, impairment of device function, and systemic spread of pathogens. Approximately 59,000 individuals in the United States underwent unilateral or bilateral hip joint replacements in 1980.[3] More than 200,000 total hip and total knee replacements and several hundred thousand fracture fixations are performed in the United States each year. The current infection rate ranges from 0.1% to 3.5% for such procedures. The problem of foreign-body infection intensifies when all orthopaedic implants and surgical procedures, such as cardiovascular, genitourinary, and plastic surgery, are considered. Temporary invasive devices used during surgery and recovery, such as intravascular lines and urinary catheters, cause less frequent but similar problems with infection. The type of materials used in prosthetic devices are diverse and include such dissimilar materials as titanium alloy, cobalt-chromium-molybdenum alloy, and a series of complex polymers such as polyethylene and silastic. This chapter briefly reviews the concepts applicable to bacterial adherence to implants, discusses the quantitation of biofilm production, and outlines the clinical behavior of the bacteria in infection as sessile and planktonic organisms.

Bacterial Adherence

Bacterial adherence is categorized into four interactive phases: (1) transport of bacteria by diffusion or convective flow; (2) initial contact and binding, either reversible or irreversible; (3) attachment mediated by special anchoring structures such as fibrils or polymers; and (4) colonization characterized by newly formed cells remaining together and proliferating to form a biofilm.[4] The initial surface binding of bacteria may involve either electrostatic interactions or intramolecular

133

van der Waals forces. Colloid chemical theories describe the attractive forces for interactions across short distances ($<$ 1 nm) and longer distances (3 to 5 nm).[5] Consolidation of bacterial binding is facilitated by the presence of pili and the deposition of exopolysaccharides.[6] Elaboration of fibrous exopolysaccharides within thick biofilms containing the bacteria themselves has been termed formation of glycocalyx.[7] Glycocalyx deposition appears to form a selective barrier to biocides,[8] antiseptics,[9] and eukaryotic phagocytes.[10]

Orthopaedic Infections and Biofilm Production

Bacteria attach to bone, cartilage, skin, tendons, ligaments, and other tissues as well as to implant materials. Localization of adherent bacteria to bone contributes to development of osteomyelitis, and dead bone serves as an effective surface for bacterial colonization.[11] Direct scanning electron microscopy of material obtained during surgical debridement of osteomyelitic bone shows that infectious bacteria grow in coherent microcolonies in a biofilm that obscures the bone surface.[12] *Staphylococcus aureus* and *Staphylococcus epidermidis* are often found when metallic prostheses and polymeric materials are involved in bone, joint, and soft-tissue infections.[13] In polymicrobial infections, *S epidermidis* augments or is augmented by the other organisms.[14,15] Polymicrobial infections account for more than two thirds of adult osteomyelitis cases[16,17] and appear to be linked to substratum-induced infection.

Bacterial Biofilm and Glycocalyx

Electron microscopy demonstrates that surface bacteria are covered with a diffuse extracellular matrix.[18–20] Bacterial biofilms are also detected with carbohydrate-specific stains such as Alcian blue or toluidine blue, or nonspecific stains such as methylene blue and safranin that bind the deposited materials.[21–25] Many techniques for detecting biofilm are semiquantitative because of limitations for visualizing bound dye. Epifluorescence of bacteria present on a polypropylene reaction support stick showed a linear correlation with adherent organisms,[26] but the usefulness of the assay is limited by the presence of the support stick. Individual foreign materials also influence adherence and deposition of biofilm because of differential responsiveness of the bacteria. *S aureus* and *S epidermidis* are examples of organisms that adhere to both metallic and polymer-based implant devices.[27–29] Several studies suggest that differences in materials may contribute to bacterial infections.[11,13,14]

Because individual materials influence biofilm production, the first step in bacterial binding depends on molecular interactions, resulting from charge properties and van der Waals forces, between the bacteria and the tissue or implant surfaces. The free energy of bacterial cell surfaces is also postulated to influence initial binding, although the bacterial surfaces may not behave as a homogeneous hydrophobic or hydrophilic substance.[30] Once binding occurs, consolidation begins, depending on the genetics and metabolism of the bacteria. Dead bacteria do not form biofilm.

Interaction between different biomaterials and the bacteria probably results in specific gene expression analogous to changes observed with metabolites such as lactose and galactose. The consequence is that only those bacteria having a select genetic background proceed through the four stages of binding and consolidation, leading to successful colonization of a foreign body. During colonization, other attributes, such as antibiotic resistance, also become expressed.[31-33]

In infection, structured biofilms shed bacteria into the surrounding environment, which is composed of tissue fluids and the circulatory system.[34,35] Studies suggest that the pathogenic consequences of biofilm are caused by the isolation of the bacteria from host-defense mechanisms[36,37] and by altered immune cell activity.[38,39] Other factors, such as deposition of fibronectin, laminin, and other cellular adhesive materials such as cell-surface proteoglycans, are potential activators of bacterial colonization.[40-42]

In order to evaluate biofilm, specific antibodies are necessary, along with selective bacterial products that are involved in biofilm deposition.[43] Further, the specialized pili that permit bacterial attachment of gonococci and *Escherichia coli* verify the synthesis of specialized matrix proteins.[44,45] A capsular polysaccharide, adhesin, has been isolated from *S epidermidis*[46] and reflects elaboration of adhesion-related molecules. The specificity of bacterial attachment appears to be related to selective gene expression in the host tissue.[47,48] This is likely to have a bacterial counterpart, particularly between different strains of an organism such as *S epidermidis*, which undergoes changes that increase its pathogenicity when localized to surfaces. To date, little data exist regarding the genetics of biofilm production because specific markers are unavailable.

Further studies are needed to evaluate the sensitivity of individual strains of *S epidermidis* for biofilm production and antibiotic resistance in the presence of prosthetic materials. The kinetics of attachment (initial binding and proliferation) must be studied in vitro, which will eliminate host defense mechanisms, permit the use of a known inoculum size, and allow nutritional control of the environment. Our published experiments show that *S epidermidis* strains, which produce little or no biofilm, initially attach to surfaces as well as bacteria that produce biofilm. The bacteria producing biofilm, however, continue to adhere and colonize, and appear to lose their sensitivity to antibiotics.

Quantification of Bacterial Biofilm

Our studies of bacterial biofilm and attachment assessed the relative deposition of bacterial and extracellular matrix and provided sensitive

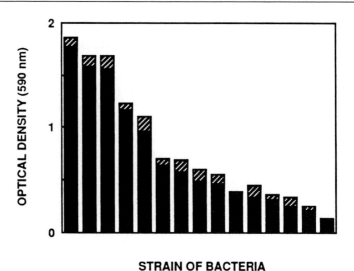

Fig. 1 *Optical density of biofilm produced wthin a 24-hour period on 15 glass culture tubes containing different strains of* S epidermidis. *Experiments were performed in quadruplicate. The data show the mean and the standard error of the mean. (Adapted with permission from Ching-Lin T, Schurman DJ, Smith RL: Quantitation of glycocalyx production in coagulase-negative* Staphylococcus. *J Orthop Res 1988;6:666–670.)*

and accurate methods of quantitating bacterial biofilm.[49] Initially, we developed a direct, accurate, and widely applicable procedure for quantifying biofilm by using toluidine blue binding and then solubilizing the dye-biofilm complex with sodium hydroxide before spectrophotometric analysis. In these studies, coagulase-negative staphylococci were cultured in trypticase soy broth, and slime production was evaluated by a variety of methods for fixation and staining.

Unlike previous techniques,[50] the amount of dye associated with the bacterial slime could be assessed spectrophotometrically after solubilization of the dye-biofilm complex with 0.2 M sodium hydroxide at 85 C for one hour. Carnoy's solution, an acidic alcohol-chloroform mixture, preserves the biofilm and, at the same time, leaves it reactive to toluidine blue for formation of a complex that could, in turn, be solubilized. A number of dyes and fixatives were screened and were less than optimal for solubilization of the matrix and quantitation of dye binding.

We analyzed 15 strains of *S epidermidis* and found a gradation in biofilm production ranging from high, to medium, to low levels. Biofilm production was strain-stable (Fig. 1). Regardless of the technique used, high, medium, and low producers of bacterial slime always remained in the same category and had optical density readings that were significantly different from each other. Thus, solubilization of the

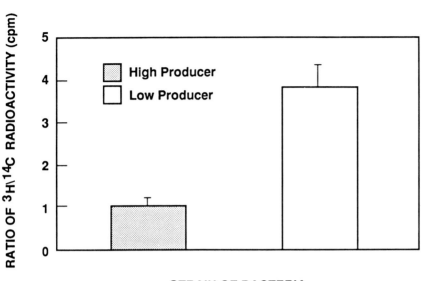

Fig. 2 *Relative incorporation ratios of tritiated thymidine and glucose labeled with radioactive carbon in two strains of* S epidermidis. *(Reproduced with permission from Van Pett K, Schurman DJ, Smith RL: Quantitation and relative distribution of extracellular matrix in* Staphylococcus epidermidis *biofilm.* J Orthop Res *1990;8:321–327.)*

toluidine blue bacterial biofilm complex provided a direct, simple, and efficient method for quantitating the glycocalyx. With this method, quantitation of biofilm production is rapid and can be done on any type of surface, and biofilm production in infection and in response to antibiotic therapy can be assessed.

In a second study, we sought to compare bacterial proliferation and extracellular matrix deposition. Attempts to label the extracellular matrix of coagulase-negative *Staphylococcus* radioactively by means of precursors specific for peptidoglycans such as alanine, acetate, and glucosamine were unsuccessful. To distinguish between bacteria and extracellular matrix in biofilms, we analyzed simultaneous uptake of glucose labeled with radioactive carbon and tritiated thymidine.[51] Strains of *S epidermidis* depositing biofilm exhibited a low ratio of tritiated thymidine to ^{14}C-glucose, and those strains showing no biofilm production had a high ratio of tritiated thymidine to ^{14}C-glucose. The tritiated thymidine was incorporated into the bacterial DNA and represented the actual number of bacteria present in the biofilm. The ^{14}C-glucose was more widely incorporated into bacterial products and accounted in part for extracellular matrix production.

Our results show that ^{14}C-glucose preferentially labeled bacteria strains in proportion to biofilm production. The ratio of tritium to

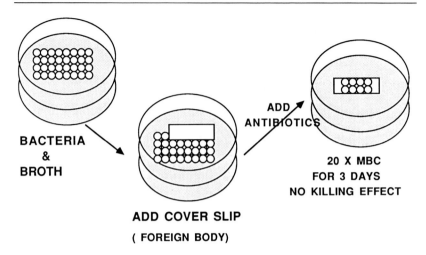

Fig. 3 *Effect of* S epidermidis *biofilm formation on antibiotic resistance.*

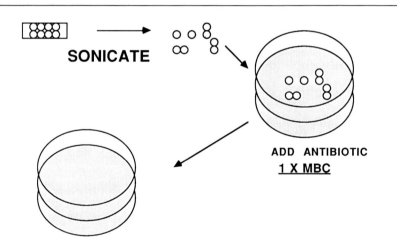

Fig. 4 *Effect of antibiotic on dissociated biofilm producing* S epidermidis. *Sonication and exposure to the minimum bactericidal concentration.*

[14]C-glucose in the high biofilm producers was 0.9; in the low producers, it was 3.7 (Fig. 2). Radioactive identification of organisms as high and low producers was confirmed by electron microscopy. Therefore, production and accumulation of biofilm over time is a stable characteristic of different strains of *S epidermidis.* The use of ratios reflecting radioactive labeling of bacteria and biofilm by tritiated thymidine and ^{14}C-glucose, respectively, provides a quantitative yet simple technique

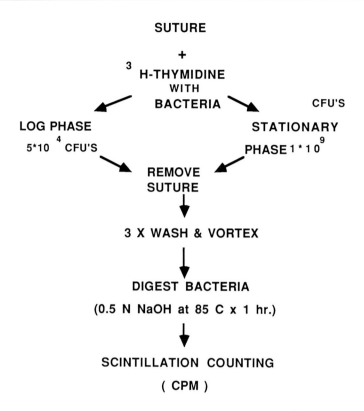

Fig. 5 *Quantitation of bacterial adherence and proliferation on prolene sutures.*

to assess extracellular matrix deposition in bacterial proliferations by different types of bacteria and to determine the relationship between adherence of the bacteria to foreign bodies and the deposition of extracellular matrix on different biomaterials.

Preliminary studies using this biofilm labeling technique have shown that bacteria rapidly adhere to suture material. These results are consistent with previous studies and show that the technology of double radioisotope labeling of biofilm-producing bacteria provides a direct quantitative assessment of both adherence and proliferation and an excellent base for study.

Biofilm, Bacterial Adherence, and Pathogenicity

The significance of a high slime producer can be demonstrated in a simple in vitro experiment (Figs. 3 and 4). We placed *S epidermidis* in standard growth medium and determined its minimal bactericidal concentration (Fig. 3). The experiment was repeated, only this time a glass coverslip was placed into the broth to represent a foreign body.

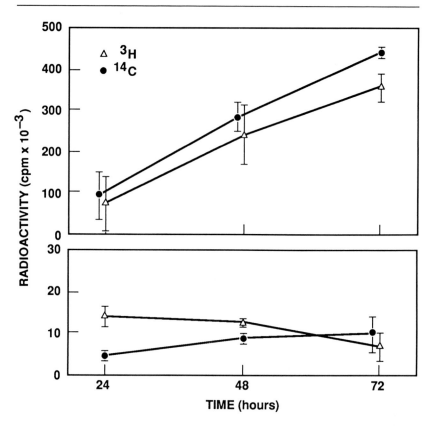

Fig. 6 *Relative incorporation over time of tritiated thymidine and glucose labeled with carbon 14 in two strains of* S *epidermidis, one, a high producer of biofilm,* **(top)** *and the other a low producer* **(bottom)**. *Radioactivity represents counts per minute per sample. (Reproduced with permission from Van Pett K, Schurman DJ, Smith RL: Quantitation and relative distribution of extracellular matrix in* Staphylococcus epidermidis *biofilm.* J Orthop Res *1990;8:321–327.)*

The broth was inoculated once again with 10^4 bacteria and incubated overnight with the glass coverslip. The next day, the coverslip was added to a new tube with broth containing 20 times the minimal bactericidal concentration of antibiotic. After 24 hours, approximately the same number of viable bacteria remained on the coverslip. We repeated this test, only this time we continued the antibiotics for three days, changing the broth and adding new antibiotic each day. There were no bactericidal effects. To prove that the bacteria on the coverslip were viable and had not changed their antibiotic resistance, we removed the bacteria from the coverslip by sonication. The minimal bactericidal concentration of the recovered bacteria had not changed (Fig. 4).

We also experimented with prolene sutures, 2.5 cm in length, exposing them to either log-phase or stationary-phase slime-producing

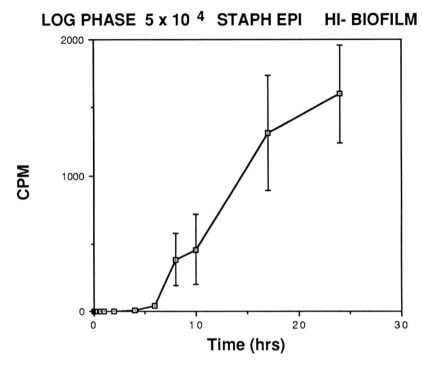

Fig. 7 *Rate of bacterial adherence of* S epidermidis *to prolene suture material. Bacterial attachment was quantified by analysis of organisms labeled with tritiated thymidine at designated time periods.*

S epidermidis (Fig. 5). Log-phase and stationary-phase organisms and their effect on attachment to the suture were studied. The sutures were exposed to different concentrations of bacteria for various times in the presence of tritiated thymidine and ^{14}C-glucose, removed from the solution, washed three times with broth, and vortexed. Next, bacteria were treated with 0.5 N sodium hydroxide at 85 C for one hour and the solution was placed in a scintillation counter.

The rate of bacterial growth on the sutures was measured at 24, 48, and 72 hours (Fig. 6). After 24 hours, with an initial inoculum of 10^4 bacteria, there were more adherent bacteria in the group producing high amounts of slime than in the group producing low amounts. After 48 hours, low-producing *S epidermidis* did not undergo a significant change in total numbers of bacteria or the quantity of slime produced. Conversely, the high-producing bacteria grew geometrically for the next 48 hours and maintained a steady ratio of slime per bacteria. We concluded from these experiments that the slime-producing organisms can grow on a suture and have a high affinity for it. The low-producing organisms appeared to have a rapidly reversible attachment with a low affinity to the suture.

141

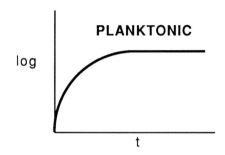

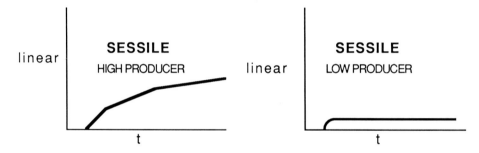

Fig. 8 *Kinetics of bacterial growth of planktonic or sessile organisms (t=time).*

The rate of bacterial adherence to the suture was measured for *S epidermidis* producing high amounts of slime starting with an inoculum of 5×10^4 bacteria. An excess of tritiated thymidine was maintained throughout the experiment. Sutures were then removed at intervals and counts per minutes measured. Under these circumstances, the bacteria did not show any definitive attachment to the suture until almost four hours later (Fig. 7). From that point on, geometric growth occurred until 20 hours, at which point the slope seemed to bend downward.

Similar experiments were carried out in which the sutures were exposed to overnight log-phase growth at a concentration of 10^9 bacteria. Under these circumstances, attachment took place within seconds. The results imply that high concentrations of seasoned, slime-rich bacteria are more likely to adhere to the suture, in much the same way paint clings to a brush that is dipped into a can of paint for a moment.

In contrast to bacterial growth in broth (so-called planktonic forms), which is exponential until it reaches log phase, bacteria that produce high amounts of slime and attach to foreign objects in vitro grow at a geometric rate (Fig. 8). Growth does slow with time. Sessile bacteria that produce low amounts of slime attach steadily after 24 hours, and their absolute numbers thereafter do not increase; different bacteria

HIGH PRODUCER   **LOW PRODUCER**

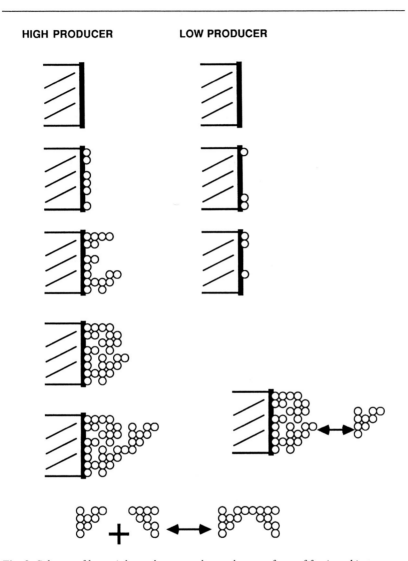

Fig. 9 *Schema of bacterial attachment and growth on surfaces of foreign objects or organisms producing high or low amounts of biofilm.*

may adhere as older bacteria detach. The hypothesis as to how bacterial growth takes place on the surfaces of foreign objects is depicted in Figure 9. Surface bacteria are more likely to grow at a two-dimensional rate, as opposed to bacteria growing in fluid, which grow in a space that is three-dimensional. Scanning electron micrograph pictures of high-producing bacteria show a progressive thickening of the surface layer. After the surface is saturated with bacteria, an outgrowth of bacteria occurs away from the surface. This biofilm space consists of bacteria within slime with interbacterial bonding. Complete saturation

143

and maximum bacterial density eventually occur. The bacteria that continue to grow thereafter are governed by the kinetics and biology of interbacterial attachment, which is somewhat different from the adhesion of bacteria to foreign objects.

Clinically, the more superficial bacteria (those farthest from the surface-bacteria interface) are more likely than the bacteria closer to the interface to continue multiplying. Moreover, the more superficial bacteria will break off at interbacterial connections and change from the sessile to the planktonic forms. Planktonic bacteria are sensitive to the effects of antibiotics, but bacteria in sessile form are seldom affected by antibiotics. One possible reason is that it is difficult for diffused antibiotics to permeate the inner layers of bacteria. A more likely explanation of antibiotic resistance is that the bacteria close to the interface no longer duplicate and metabolization is minimal. Recently, a gene has been found in *E coli* that is responsible for turning off bacterial multiplication. Bacterial interactions with nonbacterial objects are known to depend on bacterial genomic expressions, which in some instances are explicit and interactive.[52-58]

References

1. Blauth W, Hassenpflug J: Are unconstrained components essential in total knee arthroplasty?: Long-term results of the Blauth knee prosthesis. *Clin Orthop* 1990;258:86–94.
2. Wolfe SW, Figgie MP, Inglis AE, et al: Management of infection about total elbow prostheses. *J Bone Joint Surg* 1990;72A:198–212.
3. Melton LJ III, Stauffer RN, Chao EYS, et al: Rates of total hip arthroplasty: A population-based study. *N Engl J Med* 1982;307:1242–1245.
4. Marshall KC: Mechanisms of bacterial adhesion at solid water interfaces, in Savage DC, Fletcher M (eds): *Bacterial Adhesion: Mechanisms and Physiological Significance.* New York, Plenum Press, 1985, pp 133–161.
5. Gristina AG: Biomaterial-centered infection: Microbial adhesion versus tissue integration. *Science* 1987;237:1588–1595.
6. Costerton JC, Geesey GG, Cheng K-J: How bacteria stick. *Sci Am* 1978;238:86–95.
7. Costerton JW, Irvin RT, Cheng K-J: The bacterial glycocalyx in nature and disease. *Annu Rev Microbiol* 1981;35:299–324.
8. Costerton JW, Irvin RT, Cheng K-J: The role of bacterial surface structures in pathogenesis. *CRC Crit Rev Microbiol* 1981;8:303–338.
9. Marrie TJ, Costerton JW: Prolonged survival of *Serratia marcescens* in chlorhexidine. *Appl Environ Microbiol* 1981;42:1093–1102.
10. Dickinson GM, Bisno AL: Infections associated with indwelling devices: Concepts of pathogenesis. Infections associated with intravascular devices. *Antimicrob Agents Chemother* 1989;33:597–601.
11. Marrie TJ, Costerton JW: Mode of growth of bacterial pathogens in chronic polymicrobial human osteomyelitis. *J Clin Microbiol* 1985;22:924–933.
12. Pugsley MP, Sanders WE Jr: Infections of prosthetic joints, in Root RK, Trunkey DD, Sande MA (eds): *New Surgical and Medical Approaches in Infectious Diseases.* New York, Churchill Livingstone, 1987, pp 229–244.
13. Gristina AG, Hobgood C, Barth E: Biomaterial specificity, molecular mechanisms and clinical relevance of *S. epidermidis* and *S. aureus* in infections. *Surg Zentralbl Bakteriol* 1987;16:143–157.

14. Gristina AG, Costerton JW: Bacterial adherence to biomaterials and tissue: The significance of its role in clinical sepsis. *J Bone Joint Surg* 1985;67A:264–273.

15. Gristina AG, Price JL, Hobgood CD, et al: Bacterial colonization of percutaneous sutures. *Surgery* 1985;98:12–19.

16. Gristina AG, Oga M, Webb LX, et al: Adherent bacterial colonization in the pathogenesis of osteomyelitis. *Science* 1985;228:990–993.

17. Mayberry-Carson KJ, Tober-Meyer B, Smith JK, et al: Bacterial adherence and glycocalyx formation in osteomyelitis experimentally induced with *Staphylococcus aureus*. *Infect Immun* 1984;43:825–833.

18. Leake ES, Gristina AG, Wright MJ: Scanning and transmission electron microscopy as tools for the study of phagocytosis of bacteria adherent to hard surfaces. *J Leukocyte Biol* 1984;35:527–534.

19. Nickel JC, Gristina AG, Costerton JW: Electron microscopic study of an infected Foley catheter. *Can J Surg* 1985;28:50–51, 54.

20. Lambe DW Jr, Mayberry-Carson KJ, Ferguson KP: Morphological stabilization of the glycocalyces of 23 strains of five *Bacteroides* species using specific antisera. *Can J Microbiol* 1984;30:809–819.

21. Christensen GD, Simpson WA, Bisno AL, et al: Adherence of slime-producing strains of *Staphylococcus epidermidis* to smooth surfaces. *Infect Immun* 1982;37:318–326.

22. Christensen GD, Parisi JT, Bisno AL, et al: Characterization of clinically significant strains of coagulase-negative *Staphylococci*. *J Clin Microbiol* 1983;18:258–269.

23. Christensen GD, Simpson WA, Younger JJ, et al: Adherence of coagulase-negative *Staphylococci* to plastic tissue culture plates: A quantitative model for the adherence of staphylococci to medical devices. *J Clin Microbiol* 1985;22:996–1006.

24. Sheth NK, Rose HD, Franson TR, et al: In vitro quantitative adherence of bacteria to intravascular catheters. *J Surg Res* 1983;34:213–218.

25. Peters G, Pulverer G: Pathogenesis and management of *Staphylococcus epidermidis* "plastic" foreign body infections. *J Antimicrob Chemother* 1984;14(suppl D):67–71.

26. Dunne WM Jr, Sheth NK, Franson TR: Quantitative epifluorescence assay of adherence of coagulase-negative *Staphylococci*. *J Clin Microbiol* 1987;25:741–743.

27. Buxton TB, Horner J, Hinton A, et al: In vivo glycocalyx expression by *Staphylococcus aureus* phage type 52/52A/80 in *S. aureus* osteomyelitis. *J Infect Dis* 1987;156:942–946.

28. Caputy GG, Costerton JW: Morphological examination of the glycocalyces of *Staphylococcus aureus* strains Wiley and Smith. *Infect Immun* 1982;36:759–767.

29. Christensen GD, Simpson WA, Bisno AL, et al: Experimental foreign body infections in mice challenged with slime-producing *Staphylococcus epidermidis*. *Infect Immun* 1983;40:407–410.

30. van Loosdrecht MCM, Lyklema J, Norde W, et al: Influence of interfaces on microbial activity. *Microbiol Rev* 1990;54:75–87.

31. Anwar H, van Biesen T, Dasgupta M, et al: Interaction of biofilm bacteria with antibiotics in a novel in vitro chemostat system. *Antimicrob Agents Chemother* 1989;33:1824–1826.

32. Dix BA, Cohen PS, Laux DC, et al: Radiochemical method for evaluating the effect of antibiotics on *Escherichia coli* biofilms. *Antimicrob Agents Chemother* 1988;32:770–772.

33. Needham CA, Stempsey W: Incidence, adherence, and antibiotic resistance of coagulase-negative *Staphylococcus* species causing human disease. *Diagn Microbiol Infect Dis* 1984;2:293–299.

34. Franson TR, Sheth NK, Menon L, et al: Persistent in vitro survival of coagulase-negative *Staphylococci* adherent to intravascular catheters in the absence of conventional nutrients. *J Clin Microbiol* 1986;24:559–561.

35. Ishak MA, Gröschel DH, Mandell GL, et al: Association of slime with pathogenicity of coagulase-negative *Staphylococci* causing nosocomial septicemia. *J Clin Microbiol* 1985;22:1025–1029.

36. Costerton JW, Watkins L: Adherence of bacteria to foreign bodies: The role of the biofilm, in Root RK, Trunkey DD, Sande MA (eds): *New Surgical and Medical Approaches in Infectious Diseases.* New York, Churchill Livingstone, 1987, pp 17–30.

37. Vaudaux PE, Zulian G, Huggler E, et al: Attachment of *Staphylococcus aureus* to polymethylmethacrylate increases its resistance to phagocytosis in foreign body infection. *Infect Immun* 1985;50:472–477.

38. Gray ED, Regelmann WE, Peters G: Staphylococcal slime and host defenses: Effect on lymphocytes and immune function, in Pulverer G, Quie PG, Peters G (eds): *Pathogenicity and Clinical Significance of Coagulase-Negative Staphylococci.* Stuttgart, Gustav Fischer Verlag, 1987, pp 45–54.

39. Gray ED, Peters G, Verstegen M, et al: Effect of extracellular slime substance from *Staphylococcus epidermidis* on the human cellular immune response. *Lancet* 1984;1:365–367.

40. Kuusela P, Vartio T, Vuento M, et al: Attachment of *Staphylococci* and *Streptococci* on fibronectin, fibronectin fragments, and fibrinogen bound to a solid phase. *Infect Immun* 1985;50:77–81.

41. Akiyama SK, Yamada KM, Hayashi M: The structure of fibronectin and its role in cellular adhesion. *J Supramol Struct Cell Biochem* 1981;16:345–348.

42. Proctor RA: The staphylococcal fibronectin receptor: Evidence for its importance in invasive infections. *Rev Infect Dis* 1987;9(suppl 4):S335–S340.

43. Jacob E, Arendt DM, Brook I, et al: Enzyme-linked immunosorbent assay for detection of antibodies to *Staphylococcus aureus* cell walls in experimental osteomyelitis. *J Clin Microbiol* 1985;22:547–552.

44. Chan R, Acres SD, Costerton JW: Use of specific antibody to demonstrate glycocalyx, K99 pili, and the spatial relationships of K99+ enterotoxigenic *Escherichia coli* in the ileum of colostrum-fed calves. *Infect Immun* 1982;37:1170–1180.

45. Isaacson RE, Fusco PC, Brinton CC, et al: In vitro adhesion of *Escherichia coli* to porcine small intestinal epithelial cells: Pili as adhesive factors. *Infect Immun* 1978;21:392–397.

46. Tojo M, Yamashita N, Goldmann DA, et al: Isolation and characterization of a capsular polysaccharide adhesin from *Staphylococcus epidermidis*. *J Infect Dis* 1988;157:713–722.

47. Relman D, Tuomanen E, Falkow S, et al: Recognition of a bacterial adhesion by an integrin: Macrophage CR3 (alpha M beta 2, CD11b/CD18) binds filamentous hemagglutinin of *Bordetella pertussis*. *Cell* 1990;61:1375–1382.

48. Finlay BB, Heffron F, Falkow S: Epithelial cell surfaces induce *Salmonella* proteins required for bacterial adherence and invasion. *Science* 1989;243:940–943.

49. Tsai CL, Schurman DJ, Smith RL: Quantitation of glycocalyx production in coagulase-negative *Staphylococcus*. *J Orthop Res* 1988;6:666–670.

50. Davenport DS, Massanari RM, Pfaller MA, et al: Usefulness of a test for slime production as a marker for clinically significant infections with coagulase-negative *Staphylococci*. *J Infect Dis* 1986;153:332–339.

51. Van Pett K, Schurman DJ, Smith RL: Quantitation and relative distribution of extracellular matrix in *Staphylococcus epidermidis* biofilm. *J Orthop Res* 1990;8:321–327.

52. Sannomiya P, Craig RA, Clewell DB, et al: Characterization of a class of nonformulated *Enterococcus faecalis*-derived neutrophil chemotactic peptides: The sex pheromones. *Proc Natl Acad Sci USA* 1990;87:66–70.

53. Galli D, Wirth R, Wanner G: Identification of aggregation substances of *Enterococcus faecalis* cells after induction by sex pheromones: An immunological and ultrastructural investigation. *Arch Microbiol* 1989;151:486–490.

54. Wanner G, Formanek H, Galli D, et al: Localization of aggregation substances of *Enterococcus faecalis* after induction by sex pheromones: An ultrastructural comparison using immuno labelling, transmission and high resolution scanning electron microscopic techniques. *Arch Microbiol* 1989;151:491–497.

55. Signäs C, Raucci G, Jönsson K, et al: Nucleotide sequence of the gene for a fibronectin-binding protein from *Staphylococcus aureus*: Use of this peptide sequence in the synthesis of biologically active peptides. *Proc Natl Acad Sci USA* 1989;86:699–703.

56. Schmoll T, Ott M, Oudega B, et al: Use of a wild-type gene fusion to determine the influence of environmental conditions on expression of the *S fimbrial* adhesin in an *Escherichia coli* pathogen. *J Bacteriol* 1990;172:5103–5111.

57. Christensen GD, Barker LP, Mawhinney TP, et al: Identification of an antigenic marker of slime production for *Staphylococcus epidermidis*. *Infect Immun* 1990;58:2906–2911.

58. Su CJ, Dallo SF, Baseman JB: Molecular distinctions among clinical isolates of *Mycoplasma pneumoniae*. *J Clin Microbiol* 1990;28:1538–1540.

Future Directions

The preceding sections on microorganisms and microbial adhesion have defined the current state of knowledge about the characteristics and behavior of bacteria in orthopaedic infections. There are important gaps in our knowledge.

Bacterial Adhesins and Host Cell Receptors

Further understanding of bacterial adhesins and host cell receptors is necessary, including immobile receptors in parenchymal tissue and mobile receptors present as macromolecules and on motile cells. The mechanism of bacterial adhesion to biomaterials and human tissue needs to be assessed, including adhesion to viable tissue, to nonviable tissue, and to vascularized and compromised tissue at the site of biomaterial implantation. Specifically, an understanding of the exact bacterial structures that interact with these materials will enhance our ability to prevent infection. Why are certain infections biomaterial specific? There may be a genetic predisposition to musculoskeletal infection. The exact structure of receptor molecules is clearly DNA regulated. The contribution of various receptor structures to bacterial adherence is essentially unknown. The human histocompatibility complex affects the immune system and has been associated with various diseases. The association of the histocompatibility complex system with infection and other orthopaedic disease should be further studied.

Clinically Relevant In Vitro Tests

There is a need for clinically relevant in vitro tests to study the bacterial adhesion process. The goals are to create biomaterials that are better able to resist bacterial colonization and to modulate the adhesion process itself to minimize the risk of infection. In vitro tests, such as the double radioisotope labelling mentioned in this chapter, will facilitate such work.

Prevention of Adherence In Vivo

In addition to understanding the adherence of bacteria in vitro, there is a need to define methods for the prevention of adherence in vivo. Organisms should be studied individually and in polymicrobial infection in the setting of both hematogenous and contiguous spread of infection. Methods to block bacterial adherence to synthetic biomaterials must be pursued. Soluble products, such as antibody against bacterial adhesins and the use of fibronectin and its fragments, may hold future promise. In addition, vaccines should be developed that will offer additional protection for patients with bioimplants. Alterations to host immune function or receptor integrity must be approached cautiously, to avoid harming the host by interfering with a receptor system that is necessary for more than bacterial adherence.

Clinical Microbiology Laboratory

A better assessment of the etiologic agents involved in orthopaedic infections can be achieved by increasing the role of the clinical microbiology laboratory. The coagulase negative staphylococci are ubiquitous and have emerged as a major cause of biomaterial-associated infection. It remains difficult, at times, to determine the role of these bacteria in infection. If the microbiologist is given specific information as to the appearance and site of origin of the clinically obtained culture, input can be offered as to the likelihood that a positive culture actually represents infection rather than skin flora contamination. In addition, the coagulase negative staphylococci are phenotypically variable, and the signs and symptoms of clinical infection are often subtle. The microbiologist must be informed that a biomaterial site is involved to ensure that the coagulase negative staphylococci are appropriately cultured, identified, and evaluated. Communication between the clinical practitioner and the microbiologist must be improved, and the necessary information to be conveyed must be better defined.

Within the microbiology laboratory, better diagnostic aids are needed for the various agents. These tests must be sensitive, specific, and rapid to allow accurate and early intervention. Tests must identify the causative agent and its subtype, in order that appropriate treatment modalities can be selected. A generalized test to distinguish the infected from the noninfected patient would also be of value. A variety of tests should be explored, including blotting and polymerase chain reactions. The development of these procedures should not be limited to sophisticated new tests, but should also focus on improvements for traditional procedures, including staining techniques for light microscopy.

Animal Models

Animal models have provided significant information about infection in the past, and improved models will be necessary for future understanding. Models should be developed that will address the pathogenesis of minor strains of coagulase negative staphylococci, other less common organisms, and polymicrobial infections, and that will permit the evaluation of better antimicrobial treatment modalities. Although the dog remains an important animal model for many orthopaedic infections, especially those involving joint replacement, other models available may offer advantages in addition to lower costs. Animal models should take appropriate care in the use of animals as defined in guidelines established by the National Institutes of Health.

Section Three
Biomaterials

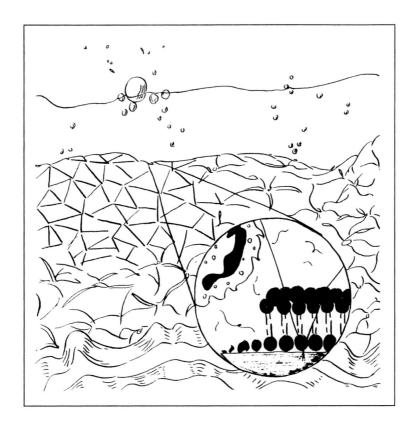

Introduction

John L. Esterhai, Jr., MD
Jeffrey S. Gelb, BS
Anthony G. Gristina, MD

Musculoskeletal infections have been extraordinarily resistant to treatment. The molecular mechanism of pathogenesis and treatment of biomaterial and musculoskeletal sepsis is based in part on the responses of tissue and bacteria to biomaterials.

Many of the advances in orthopaedic surgery in recent years have involved biomaterial implantation. Although these surgical interventions have offered incredible benefits to the patient, the risk of implant failure and infection continues to provide significant concern. Two barriers to the expanded use of devices are the lack of successful tissue integration, or compatibility with biomaterial surfaces, and bacterial adhesion. Biomaterials, devitalized tissue, and bone are physiochemically active and may directly modulate events, such as immunologic responses, tissue integration, and bacterial adhesion, at their surfaces.

The first chapter of this section, by Lemons, presents the requirements and rationale for choosing metals, polymers, and ceramics for surgical implants. Attention is given to the types and constituents of biomaterials, with emphasis on the mechanical, physical, electrical, and biologic properties of the material. Biodegradation, wear products, and material properties are different under static and dynamic conditions. All these variables have been shown to influence local tissue responses.

The second chapter, by Boyan and associates, details the response of bone-forming cells to ceramic surfaces in vivo and in vitro. Materials that stimulate primary bone mineralization are referred to as bone-bonding materials. Nonbonding materials also influence cell differentiation. Failure of bone to bond to a biomaterial may be related to toxic implant materials or a defect in cellular maturation.

The third chapter, by Meyer and Baier, discusses the macromolecular films formed on biomaterial surfaces after implantation. The initial substrate critical surface tension determines the ultimate properties, thickness, and density of the film. In theory, any chemical or biologic treatment of the implant before insertion and the mechanical forces applied during and after insertion can alter the surface energies of the newly formed films. Research on specific marine plants and animals has demonstrated that many possess "antifouling" defense mechanisms against microorganisms. Intensive efforts are under way to isolate and purify the active components of marine exudates that could prove useful in the future as controlled-release "drugs" in biomedical applications.

In the fourth chapter, von Recum demonstrates that the microtexture of an implant surface is essential to a favorable tissue response. Optimal modification of macroporosity, microtexture, and mechanical force transfer should allow better implant integration and a reduced likelihood of infection.

Bone and articular cartilage can also serve as substrata. Bone is a relatively acellular composite structure of calcium hydroxyapatite crystals and collagen matrix. The calcium phosphate crystals are formed in plates between collagen fibrils. The protein matrix is arranged as three noncoaxial helical polypeptides composed principally of proline, hydroxyproline, glycine, and alanine. Proline-rich proteins may act as receptors for bacterial adhesion. Devitalized bone, devoid of normal periosteum, presents a collagen protein matrix and acellular crystal substrate to which bacteria may bind.

The chapter by Rosenberg and Eyre details the structure of the proteoglycans and collagens that compose the extracellular matrix of articular cartilage. New information regarding the structure, behavior, and function of articular cartilage has emerged during the last several years. Specifically, the large aggregating cartilage proteoglycan is accompanied by two interstitial dermatan sulfate proteoglycans. Type II collagen is not the only collagen found in articular cartilage. The details of molecular structure, as well as the arrangement and interactions of these molecules within articular cartilage, are discussed, with emphasis on important biochemical properties and biologic function. The acellular articular cartilage surface (lamina obscurans) offers no resistance to colonization by *Staphylococcus aureus* but rather presents receptors for intra-articular bacterial adhesion.

Extracellular matrix components not only promote bacterial adherence but also allow adherence of host tissues. Recent work has identified "integrins" important in embryonic development, maintenance of tissue architecture, inflammation, wound healing, and tumor metastases.[1] Such cell surface receptors may be critical for bone growth, repair, and remodeling. Rat calvarial bone cells adhere to fibronectin, fibrinogen, laminin, vitronectin, and collagen types I and IV in a dose-response manner. This adherence is blocked by polyclonal rabbit antibody raised against rat integrin complex. Two transmembrane rat bone cell integrins have been identified. These may play a role in connecting the extracellular matrix to the intracellular skeleton as well as influencing cell physiologic response.

The final chapter in this section is important because of the novel approach used to bypass the host immune system in soft-tissue bioimplants. Goddard presents work concerning bioartificial neural prostheses for the treatment of Parkinson's disease. Trans-plantation of dopamine-producing cells directly into the corpus striatum would afford excellent treatment for Parkinson's disease. Procuring adequate tissue for transplantation has met with many problems, often because of limited tissue sources. Several techniques have been developed to expand the number and types of tissues suitable for transplantation. The method discussed in this chapter involves the transplantation of small populations of dopaminergic cells encapsulated in a semipermeable polymer capsule. Small molecules (less than 50,000 in molecular weight), including dopamine, nutrients, oxygen, and water, are exchanged through the capsule membrane while cells, antibodies, and other large molecules are excluded. This system protects the implanted cells from the immune system but allows the transplanted cells to survive and remain localized within the implant. Design of the implant capsule and surgical implantation techniques are discussed. Fibrosis surrounding the implant has been a limiting factor that tends to impede diffusion through the capsule pores. Future success with these implants will require exacting biomaterial design and understanding of the host's soft-tissue reaction. This knowledge would certainly be applicable to bioimplants used in orthopaedic surgery.

Tissue integration may be defined as chemical bonding and compatibility. Lack of tissue integration is a form of incompatibility or host rejection. Even a thin fibroinflammatory response may lead to failure of fixation. Adhesive or integrative events for bacteria and tissue cells are critical, interrelated, and based on similar molecular mechanisms. Because of organic adsorbates and the nature of surfaces, potential colonizing cells first encounter a highly altered, reactive interface. If specific tissue cells receptive to the surface establish a secure chemical bond, subsequent bacterial invaders would be confronted by a living, integrated cellular surface. These chapters lay the groundwork for future research in this area.

Reference

1. Brighton CT, Albelda SM: Identification of cell-substratum adhesion receptors (integrins) on cultured rat bone cells. *Trans Orthop Res Soc* 1991;16:400.

Chapter 11

Metals, Polymers, and Ceramics for Surgical Implant Devices

Jack E. Lemons, PhD

Rationale for Materials Selection

Many of the early decisions related to the selection and use of synthetic materials for the construction of surgical implant devices were based on availability and previous experience with marine and industrial applications.[1,2] Equally important considerations for load-bearing musculoskeletal devices were strength and mechanical durability, inertness in saline environments, and the cost of both the material and the fabrication processes. These criteria dominated much of the selection through the early 1900s. The database of clinical applications and evaluations of longevities that evolved through experience resulted in relatively thorough biocompatibility profiles for most classes of the inert alloys by the early 1950s.

The expansion of material property testing to preclinical studies in laboratory animals significantly influenced the approach to the development process.[3,4] Since 1970, there has been a continuing increase in the types of available materials and in the investigations of surface and bulk properties of these candidate biomaterials for surgical implants.[5] Although a variety of established laboratory and animal studies always precede human clinical evaluations, these studies do not provide complete answers to questions about in vivo biocompatibilities, especially in long-term (more than five years) applications.[6,7]

The rationale for biomaterials selection has remained somewhat the same over time, but biocompatibility is now considered the first priority.[8] This chapter emphasizes the biomaterials used in the construction of surgical devices, their bulk and surface properties, how these properties are correlated with known biodegradation processes, and some associated interactions along tissue interfaces.

Bulk and Surface Characteristics

Material characteristics can be generally classified according to basic physical, mechanical, chemical, and electrical properties.[3] Physical properties include elemental constitution, density, conductivity, and color. Mechanical properties are those associated with externally applied force and include strength, ductility, fatigue and wear resistances, and indentation hardness. Modulus of elasticity can be characterized as a mechanical or a physical property and is normally listed as physical-mechanical. Chemical aspects are those identified with environmental reactions such as corrosion. Electrical properties are involved with the flow of electrons through the material. These properties, which can be determined by laboratory tests, provide basic information about the biomaterial's bulk and surface characteristics that can be used to evaluate basic biocompatibilities. Biocompatibility profiles are determined through the experience gained with similar measurements on existing biomaterials and the established knowledge of biologic host reactions to controlled quantities of foreign substances.[9,10]

Another aspect of biocompatibility assessment is host reactions to chronic applications of mechanical forces and the transfer of these forces across biomaterial-to-tissue interfaces.[11] The microscopic distribution of mechanical strain depends on the relative moduli of the synthetic materials and the immediately adjacent tissues, and this property (modulus) must be evaluated simultaneously with the macroscopic strain distributions. The macroscopic distributions are controlled by the geometric form of the device (for example, size, shape, topology, and topography) and the host's anatomic and functional characteristics.[12] Strain distribution is quite complex and requires analyses of force transfer with three-dimensional models to determine interactive conditions along device-to-tissue interface regions.[13]

Biomaterial-Tissue Interfaces

The interfacial zones between biomaterials and tissues are influenced by a wide range of biomaterial and biomechanical factors. In an attempt to better understand these factors, many investigators have focused on the device's attachment to hard and soft tissues. The type of interfacial attachment can also be classified according to its properties.[14] Physical attachment processes include surface interactions that depend on the relatively weak near-surface charge characteristics of the interfacial phases. Debye- or van der Waals-type bonding is included in this list, along with any other attraction depending on an electromagnetic field. In contrast to this type of attachment or bonding, chemical interactions with ionic- or covalent-type bonds can provide relatively high mechanical strength. Mechanical attachment, however, rather than being physical or chemical, is normally associated with shapes or surface features for mutual interlocking of the biomaterial and biologic components.[15]

Many orthopaedic surgical devices have been fabricated with surface characteristics that provide some type of bonding or attachment to the adjacent tissues. The attachment may be physical, chemical, or mechanical in nature, or a combination of any two or of all three. In each situation, the type of attachment and the attachment stability over time have been shown to influence biocompatibility profiles directly.[3]

Transfers Between Biomaterials and Tissues

All synthetic biomaterials transfer elements or compounds and forces to adjacent tissues.[16,17] These transfers depend on the basic surface and bulk properties of the biomaterial, the design of the devices, and, of course, the host conditions. The critical information to be gained is how much is transferred, at what rate, and for how long.[18] At the interface, the elemental or compound transfers can be described through the chemical properties of the biomaterial and the biochemical responses within the host environment. Under relatively static conditions, biodegradation processes can be further described in terms of the electrochemical corrosion of metals and alloys[3] and the nonelectrochemical degradation characteristics of ceramics and polymers. Elemental compound transfers from ceramics and the preferential leaching of low-molecular-weight forms or the oxidative degradation products from polymers have been described in the literature.[19,20]

When dynamic or motion characteristics exist, interfacial shear stresses are introduced, and biomaterial wear processes can be added to the static biodegradation phenomena.[21] Simultaneously, because functional devices are always subjected to mechanical forces, the necessity exists for the transfer of these forces. These characteristics can be described in terms of the mechanical properties of the biomaterial and the associated biomechanical responses of the tissues. The device's design is a primary consideration related to force transfer and the mechanical stresses evolved within the tissues. Along the interfaces, forces and stresses can be resolved in terms of tensile, compressive, and shear components. Because biomaterials and tissues respond differently in terms of the type of imposed stress (tension, compression, or shear), both the design and material properties are quite important to functional stability.[22] Also, the chemical and mechanical properties of the device contribute to interface stability, while, simultaneously, the biochemical and biomechanical properties provide optimal or suboptimal tissue conditions. Obviously, full descriptions of all interfacial interactions have not been developed, but there is a considerable body of data with regard to interfacial transfer of substances and forces.

Types and Constituents of Biomaterials

The standardized biomaterials available for orthopaedic surgery devices include metals and alloys, polymers, ceramics and carbons, and combinations or composites of these synthetic materials.[5]

The metallic alloys used for most loadbearing structural components include alloys based on iron, cobalt, or titanium. The primary alloying elements that are added during the melting and solidification (casting) process, which constitute more than 4% of the weight, are included to influence basic material properties. Wrought iron alloys (for example, 316L stainless steel) include chromium and nickel. The as-cast and wrought types of cobalt alloys include chromium, molybdenum, nickel, tungsten, and iron. The wrought grade of titanium alloy (Ti-6Al-4V) includes aluminum and vanadium. Other metallic and nonmetallic elements are present in these alloys as deliberate additions to control properties but not to provide major compositional variations. Each of these alloy groups has significantly different properties that have been shown to influence biocompatibility profiles both positively and negatively depending on the conditions of use. In each case, the alloy is selected for certain applications where adverse conditions are to be minimized.

The polymeric biomaterials include a wide range of substances, have a relatively high molecular weight distribution, and contain a minimal amount of secondary constituents. These include ultra-high-molecular-weight (UHMW) polyethylene, polymethylmethacrylate (bone cement), polyethylene terephthalate, polytetrafluoroethylene, polyurethane, dimethylpolysiloxane (silicone), and polysulfone. The most common elements included in the constitution of polymers are carbon, oxygen, fluorine, hydrogen, chlorine, and nitrogen. In some cases, catalytic agents or other substances are added, but only in very dilute quantities. The polymers, in general, have much lower moduli of elasticity than metals and ceramics and are most often used where greater flexibility, compliance, and damping characteristics are indicated.

Ceramics and carbons are more similar to metals in overall properties. Although polymers and ceramics are nonconductors of electricity, carbons are similar to metals with regard to conductivity. The inert ceramics include those based on aluminum and zirconium oxides. The bioactive compounds are based on three groups of compounds: calcium phosphates or aluminates, known as the tricalcium phosphates; glass or glass ceramics, based on silicone dioxide or other more complex compounds; and hydroxyapatites. These substances exhibit a wide range of properties, with many provided in bioactive or biodegradable forms. These forms are intended to induce specific tissue responses such as chemical bonding to bone or temporary fillers that are later replaced by tissues. The carbons and carbon-silicon compounds are also classed as bioinert, and are intended for use as structural components, as coatings on other substrates, or as fibers to reinforce polymeric biomaterials. The primary elements within the ceramics include aluminum, calcium, carbon, fluorine, magnesium, oxygen, phosphorus, silicon, and zirconium.

Biomaterial Properties and Biocompatibility

The properties of biomaterials are correlated with biocompatibility characteristics when they are considered in relation to tissue properties or to a specific application. For example, the strengths and moduli of alloys and inert ceramics are much greater than those of compact bone (1.5 to 20 times). In contrast, polymers are lower in magnitude (0.001 to 0.5 times) than bone. These properties are important because they affect function-associated mechanical fractures (strength) of the device or interfacial shear components (moduli) that could result in dynamic tissue conditions (for example, bone to fibrous tissue to reactive or inflamed granulation tissue over time). The carbons and carbon-silicon compounds were selected previously, in part, because of their relatively high strengths and moduli that are similar to those of compact bone. These types of properties should result in a minimal amount of mechanically induced motion along contiguous interfaces with bone because of similar microscopic strain magnitudes under unit stress conditions. Another key factor is the coefficient of friction along articulating surfaces where motion is intended as a part of normal function.[23] Bearings benefit from lubricants, smooth surfaces, and counterfaces matched to minimize wear phenomena.

The biodegradation and wear properties of biomaterials are sometimes different under static (no motion) and dynamic (motion) conditions. Titanium alloy, with the reactive group metal titanium as the primary constituent, oxidizes along all exposed surfaces on contact with air or normal tissue fluids to form an inert continuous oxide film.[24] With static conditions in bone (such as osteointegration), this oxide film provides an inert barrier against significant transport of substances from the biomaterial to the adjacent tissues.[25] If the oxide film is broken for any reason, it reforms instantaneously. The oxide-based passive film provides advantageous properties for porous materials and areas for bone tissue ingrowth and device attachment through mechanical locking.[15] This same characteristic, however, can create adverse circumstances under conditions of interfacial motion. If the passive film articulates with tissues, polymers, or other alloys, conditions exist for continual film disruption, removal, and reformation, and, thereby, debris accumulation.[26] This is classified as fretting-corrosive wear and can result in a finely divided oxide particulate that can further enhance the breakdown process through third-body abrasive wear mechanisms.[27]

Titanium alloys are surface-treated with secondary ions or compounds to improve surface properties and thereby minimize wear-related degradation processes.[28,29] In some situations, therefore, surface chemical properties, when combined with the relatively low modulus of elasticity, offer advantageous characteristics for bonding or attachment to bone. In contrast, the fretting-corrosion properties, which evolve from a combination of mechanical and chemical properties, can contribute to interface breakdown along regions of interfacial motion.

The hard and inert oxide ceramics (such as alumina and zirconia) and the alloys of cobalt (especially as-cast cobalt-chromium-molybdenum) offer a combination of surface (oxides of aluminum, zirconium, or chromium) and bulk mechanical properties (strength, hardness, and wear resistance) that are much more favorable with regard to minimizing surface breakdown during wear.[21] However, these materials have relatively high moduli of elasticity compared with titanium alloy and bone, and, therefore, require specialized designs to accommodate their basic properties.

This same type of analogy can be applied to the other classes of biomaterials. However, when the possibility of ionic- or covalent-type chemical bonding to bone is introduced, the aspects of interfacial element and force transfer must be reconsidered.[30] For example, if a calcium phosphate compound were chemically bonded to bone, all of the bonded surfaces, whether loaded in compression, tension, or shear, would be capable of transferring mechanical force. This would greatly increase the relative areas available for force transfer and thereby normalize or redistribute the overall mechanical stresses along the various interfacial zones. Simultaneously, the bonded areas could be provided with a relatively protective zone of mineralized tissue that could influence biodegradation phenomena. However, if these surface compounds were subjected to mechanical motion, biomaterial breakdown would be anticipated for current-generation coatings based on calcium phosphate.

It is known that motion along UHMW polyethylene, polymethylmethacrylate, and other polymeric biomaterial surfaces results in wear debris.[23] These are normally particulates of the primary components and in some cases can be a mixed fraction of irregular compositions, sizes, and shapes. For example, metallic and inert ceramic particulates are oxides, whereas polymers are particulates of their primary compositions (UHMW polyethylene or polymethylmethacrylate, for example). With the superimposition of static-condition biodegradation products, simultaneously biodegraded metallic ions or compounds could form a wide range of reactive substances with biologic macromolecular species or ions.

These metallo-products would depend on the valence state of the ion or compound transferred to the host at the time of the environmental interaction. The combined process could, therefore, result in a very complex milieu, with possibilities for acidic or basic conditions introduced by the various chemical species present.[15,18,31,32] Obviously, a multifactorial situation exists with regard to the prediction of biologic reactions. Local environments (acidic or basic), transfer to tissue components or cells, and transport to systemic areas could exist simultaneously. Also, because inflammatory conditions can be introduced by particulates independent of material composition, sorting of definitive, single-source reasons for device-related tissue reactions becomes a difficult task.

Tissue responses to foreign substances have been described qualitatively and quantitatively under somewhat less complex conditions.[8,18,27] Bone has been shown to alter its basic structure to that of fibrous tissue in the presence of foreign substances[16] or of interfacial motions[10] that contain predominantly shear-directed stresses. Specifically, the dimensions and internal structures of this fibrous tissue zone have been said to increase in thickness and to become more acellular with increased quantities of substances or shear stress transfer. However, these general hypotheses have not been fully proven. For example, do these conditions evolve independently or is there a synergism of interactions? Defined cause-and-effect relationships have not been fully established for the various synthetic biomaterials or the biomechanical designs of devices. Although these basic concepts are thought to be correct, it is necessary to establish more quantitative relationships for controlled quantities of known substances under biomechanical stress conditions.

Within this complex series of interactions, it is vital to relate the local or systemic alterations in tissue conditions to the abilities or inabilities of the tissues and interface regions to resist infection. One speculation is that biomaterial-based environmental conditions can introduce either favorable or unfavorable circumstances for the introduction of an infection. This interaction could also depend on the specific foreign substance or substances present, their amount, their reaction products, the biomechanical environment, and the local and systemic condition of the host.[15,18] At this time, most of these questions with regard to tissue interactions remain to be answered. Because of the many complexities associated with biomaterial-to-tissue interactions, especially with total joint replacement devices, assessments of biomaterial product-based infections require many additional investigations under controlled laboratory and laboratory animal environments.

References

1. Ludwigson DC: Today's prosthetic metals. *J Metals* 1964;16:226–231.
2. Crimmins DS: The selection and use of materials for surgical implants. *J Metals* 1969;21:38–42.
3. von Recum AF (ed): *Handbook of Biomaterials Evaluation: Scientific, Technical, and Clinical Testing of Implant Materials*. New York, Macmillan, 1986.
4. Williams DF, Roaf R: *Implants in Surgery*. London, WB Saunders, 1973.
5. *American Sociey for Testing and Materials; Annual Book of ASTM Standards, Vol. 13.01 Medical Devices*. Philadelphia, American Society for Testing and Materials, 1989.
6. Weinstein A, Gibbons D, Brown S, et al (eds): *Implant Retrieval: Material and Biological Analysis*. Washington, DC, U.S. Department of Commerce, National Bureau of Standards, 1981.
7. Retrieval and analysis of surgical implants and biomaterials. *Trans Soc Biomater Spec Symp* 1988;11:1–67.
8. Brown SA (ed): *Cell-Culture Test Methods: A Symposium*. Philadelphia, American Society for Testing and Materials, 1983.
9. Williams DF (ed): *Biocompatibility of Clinical Implant Materials*. Boca Raton, FL, CRC Press, 1981, vol 1.
10. Mears DC: *Materials and Orthopaedic Surgery*. Baltimore, Williams & Wilkins, 1979.
11. Lemons JE: Phase-boundary interactions for surgical implants, in Rubin LR (ed): *Biomaterials in Reconstructive Surgery*. St. Louis, CV Mosby, 1983, pp 662–665.
12. Dieter GE: *Mechanical Metallurgy*. New York, McGraw-Hill, 1961.

13. Huiskies R: Biomechanics of bone and implants. Presented at the Meeting of the Society for Biomechanics, San Diego, CA, September, 1990.

14. Hench LL, Ethridge EC: *Biomaterials: An Interfacial Approach.* New York, Academic Press, 1982.

15. Lemons JE (ed): *Quantitative Characterization and Performance of Porous Implants for Hard Tissue Applications: A Symposium.* Philadelphia, American Society for Testing and Materials, 1987.

16. Lemons JE: Symposium on advanced biomaterials: The future of orthopaedics. *Contemp Orthop* 1989;119:150–185.

17. Ferguson AB Jr, Akahoshi Y, Laing PG, et al: Characteristics of trace ions released from embedded metal implants in the rabbit. *J Bone Joint Surg* 1962;44A:323–336.

18. Lang B, Morris H, Razzoog M (eds): *International Workshop: Biocompatibility, Toxicity and Hypersensitivity to Alloy Systems Used in Dentistry.* Ann Arbor, University of Michigan Press, 1985.

19. Ducheyne P, Lemons JE (eds): *Bioceramics: Material Characteristics Versus In Vivo Behavior* (Annals of the New York Academy of Sciences, vol 523). New York, New York Academy of Sciences, 1988.

20. Li S: Breakdown of polyethylene knee components by oxidation. Presented at the Dartmouth Biomedical Engineering Conference on Techniques and Science of Successful Total Joint Arthroplasty, Burlington, VT, October, 1990.

21. Clark IC, McKellop HA: Wear testing, in von Recum AF (ed): *Handbook of Biomaterials Evaluation: Scientific, Technical, and Clincal Testing of Implant Materials.* New York, Macmillan, 1986, pp 114–130.

22. Brunski JB, Moccia AF Jr, Pollack SR, et al: The influence of functional use of endosseous dental implants on the tissue-implant interface: Part 1. Histological aspects. *J Dent Res* 1979;58:1953–1969.

23. McKellop H, Clarke I, Markolf K, et al: Friction and wear properties of polymer, metal, and ceramic prosthetic joint materials evaluated on a multichannel screening device. *J Biomed Mater Res* 1981;15:619–653.

24. Collings EW: *The Physical Metallurgy of Titanium Alloys.* Metals Park, OH, American Society for Metals, 1984.

25. Brånemark P-I, Zarb GA, Albrektsson T (eds): *Tissue-Integrated Prostheses: Osseointegration in Clinical Dentistry.* Chicago, Quintessence Publishing, 1985.

26. Buchanan RA, Bacon RK, Williams JM, et al: Ion implantation to improve the corrosive wear resistance of surgical Ti-6Al-4V. *Trans Soc Biomater* 1983;6:106.

27. Fraker AC, Griffin CD (eds): *Corrosion and Degradation of Implant Materials: Second Symposium.* Philadelphia, American Society for Testing and Materials, 1985.

28. Sioshansi P: Ion beam modification of materials for industry. *Thin Solid Films* 1984;118:61–71.

29. Lucas L, Lemons J, Lee J: An in vitro corrosion evaluation of surface modified Ti-6Al-4V, in Sauer BW (ed): *Biomaterial Engineering IV.* New York, Pergamon Press, 1985, pp 11–18.

30. Lemons JE: Hydroxyapatite coatings. *Clin Orthop* 1988;235:220–223.

31. Brown GC, Lockshin MD, Salvati EA, et al: Sensitivity to metal as a possible cause of sterile loosening after cobalt-chromium total hip-replacement arthroplasty. *J Bone Joint Surg* 1977;59A:164–168.

32. Lucas LC, Bearden LJ, Lemons JE: Ultrastructural examination of in vitro and in vivo cells exposed to elements from type 316L stainless steel, in Fraker AC, Griffin CD (eds): *Corrosion and Degradation of Implant Materials: Second Symposium.* Philadelphia, American Society for Testing and Materials, 1985, pp 208–222.

Chapter 12

Response of Bone-Forming Cells to Ceramic Surfaces in Vivo and in Vitro

Barbara D. Boyan, PhD
Zvi Schwartz, DMD, PhD
Larry D. Swain, DDS, MS
Aruna Khare, PhD
Tom Marshall, DDS
David Amir, MD
Jona Sela, DMD
Alfred S. Windeler, DDS, PhD
C. Müller-Mai, MD
Ulrich Gross, MD

Introduction

Many studies have shown that ceramic implants differ in their ability to promote close adaptation to the surrounding bone. The relative adherence of the healing bone to the implant surface is referred to as bone bonding,[1-4] a loosely defined term referring to the histologic appearance of the bone-implant interface. In general, the fibrous connective tissue interface between bone and bone-bonding materials is smaller than the interface between bone and nonbonding implants. In many instances, there appears to be a direct intercalation of bone mineral and the bone-bonding implant material; this is particularly true of titanium.[5]

Little is known concerning the behavior of bone-forming cells at this interface. It has been suggested that cells adapt to implant surfaces made of hydroxyapatite in a more physiologic fashion because of its chemical similarity to bone mineral. Gross and associates[6-8] have shown that in tissues adjacent to bone-bonding implants, the cells appear to produce matrix vesicles, which are extracellular organelles associated with the onset of primary hydroxyapatite formation during bone healing.[9-12] In fact, the bioglass implants have been reported to stimulate primary mineral formation, but the mechanism of this is unknown.

To begin to understand the nature of the cell-implant response, we developed two models. To examine primary bone formation in vivo, we adapted the rat tibial marrow ablation model described by Chisin and associates.[13] During normal primary bone formation after tibial marrow ablation, matrix vesicle production is enhanced and the vesicles undergo a maturation process that includes changes in morphology, density, and distance from the mineralization front.[14] Changes in biochemical features associated with hydroxyapatite formation, particularly alkaline phosphatase activity, correlate with the morphologic changes.[15,16] Observation of the transmission electron microscopic appearance of interface tissue during primary bone healing next to bone-bonding and nonbonding implants and analysis of the matrix vesicles isolated from the tissue make it possible to use the model to study cellular response in vivo.

In the second model, we used cell cultures to examine the specific regulation of osteoblastic response to implant materials. The classic surface for cell culture is plastic. Recent attempts to characterize the response of bone cells to implants have used thin disks of the material or bulk-phase extracts in solution with monolayer cells.[17,18] However, with these methods cell culture is difficult because of opacity, and possible observations are limited. Thus, we use culture surfaces sputter-coated with ultrathin films of the material of interest.[19] With these films, the cells can be cultured, cell growth monitored, biochemical characteristics of the cells assessed, and the cytomorphometry of the interface described.

Methods

Intramedullary Bone Implants

With the animals under ketamine anesthesia, marrow was ablated from the tibias of mature Sabra rats as described previously.[13] Bone-bonding and nonbonding ceramic implants, Kg Cera and KGy 213, respectively,[2-3] were inserted into the marrow cavity. On days 0 (primary bone obtained during ablation), 3, 6, 14, and 21, the healing primary bone was removed and frozen at -70 C. Eighteen rats were killed for each treatment regimen (normal healing, bone-bonding implant, and nonbonding implant) at each time and the tissue from three rats pooled for matrix vesicle isolation, resulting in six values for each time point. Matrix vesicles were prepared from thawed, homogenized tissue as described by Hale and associates[20] and modified in our laboratory.[21] The specific activity of alkaline phosphatase was measured as the release of para-nitrophenol from para-nitrophenylphosphate at pH 10.2. We used analysis of variance and Student's t-test to determine statistical significance.

Bone Cell Cultures

Polystyrene culture dishes (35 mm) were sputter-coated with targets composed of implant-quality aluminum oxide (nonbonding) and commercially pure titanium (bone-bonding). Oxygen was introduced during titanium sputtering to produce titanium dioxide. UMR-106 cells, a rat osteoblastic osteosarcoma cell line,[22] were seeded at a density of 10,000 cells/cm^2 and cultured in Dulbecco's modified Eagle's medium containing 10% fetal bovine serum and antibiotics in an atmosphere of 5% carbon dioxide at 37 C. The medium was changed after 24 hours and then at three-day intervals. Cell number was determined at 24 hours (day 1) to assess the number of adherent cells and at day 7 to assess cell proliferation. The specific activity of alkaline phosphatase, the matrix vesicle marker enzyme, was measured in the cell layer.[23] The mRNA levels for alkaline phosphatase were determined and compared with those of actin.[24]

Discussion

Changes in the matrix vesicles isolated from primary bone during normal healing confirmed previous findings of increased matrix vesicle production in the healing primary bone as early as day 3 after marrow ablation.[13–15] After that time, the diameter of the matrix vesicle increased and the mean distance from the calcified front decreased. There was a distinct shift from empty vesicles to vesicles containing amorphous material (day 6) and hydroxyapatite crystals (day 14). Biochemical analyses demonstrated a marked increase in alkaline phosphatase activity at day 6, correlating with the increase in matrix vesicles with amorphous interiors.[16] Alkaline phosphatase activity remained increased at day 14, when hydroxyapatite crystals were being formed, but decreased by day 21, corresponding to the transmission electron microscopic appearance of ruptured vesicles and bulk mineralization of the extracellular matrix.

Exposure to the bone-bonding implant appeared to stimulate an increase in the alkaline phosphatase activity associated with bone healing (Fig. 1). Because specific activity is expressed as a function of matrix vesicle protein content, the increase reflected a real difference in the biochemistry of the matrix vesicles rather than just their increased density on the transmission electron micrographs of the tissue adjacent to the implants.[25] By day 6, alkaline phosphatase specific activity in matrix vesicles isolated from the implanted tissue was identical to that isolated from control animals.

In matrix vesicles isolated from tissue adjacent to nonbonding implants, alkaline phosphatase specific activity was initially identical to that of the normal healing primary bone but no further increase in enzyme activity was detected in the matrix vesicles isolated from adjacent tissue. Similarly, the morphometric characteristics of the matrix vesicles differed significantly from those of normal primary bone healing.[25] This suggests that the matrix vesicles produced by osteoblasts in response to the nonbonding implants were defective or that material leaching from the implants inhibited enzyme activity and matrix vesicle maturation.

The glass-ceramic implants used in the in vivo studies were actually composites of a number of compounds, making it difficult to assess the relative roles of any one of the constituents. Results from the cell culture experiments (Table 1) demonstrated that the expression of the osteoblastic phenotype is sensitive to the type of ceramic present. Cell proliferation was inhibited by all other materials in comparison with plastic, the conventional cell culture surface. This was not the result

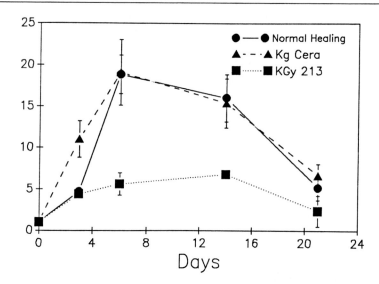

Fig. 1 *Change in matrix vesicle alkaline phosphatase specific activity in healing rat tibial bone following marrow ablation. Matrix vesicles were isolated from the endosteum adjacent to implants of Kg Cera (bone bonding glass ceramic) or KGy 213 (nonbonding glass ceramic) or from unimplanted bone at days 3, 6, 14, and 21 following ablation of the marrow. Alkaline phosphatase specific activity was measured (μmol Pi/mg protein/minute) and the fold increase in activity plotted in comparison with day 0 control bone. Each value represents the mean ± standard error of the mean of 6 samples, where each sample is the combined matrix vesicles isolated from 3 limbs. (Data are taken from Marshall TS, Schwartz Z, Swain LD, et al: Matrix vesicle enzyme activity in endosteal bone following implantation of bonding and non-bonding implant materials.* Clin Oral Implants Res *1991, in press.)*

of cell death because an analysis of cell viability by trypan blue dye exclusion demonstrated no differences among the cultures. Some of the apparent inhibition may have resulted from a decrease in cell attachment because the treatment-control ratio for day 1 was reduced in the experimental cultures. It is more likely that the inhibition in proliferation reflected stimulated cell differentiation, because the treatment-control ratio exhibited a further reduction in the experimental cultures at day 7, and there were distinct differences in expression of alkaline phosphatase activity and mRNA levels as well.

Alkaline phosphatase activity was sensitive to the type of surface to which the osteoblastic UMR 106 cells were exposed. In cultures exposed to aluminum oxide, alkaline phosphatase was comparable to the control cultures at day 1, but at day 7, enzyme activity was more than four times that in the control cultures, the highest increase observed. In contrast, alkaline phosphatase activity in the cells cultured on titanium or titanium dioxide was significantly lower than that in the control cultures at day 1 but was increased over that in the control cultures on day 7. Despite the initial inhibition in alkaline phosphatase activity, the cells cultured on the bone-bonding ceramic surfaces dem-

Table 1 Effect of culture surface on UMR 106 cell proliferation

Culture Surface and Time in Culture	Cells/Dish		Alkaline Phosphatase		mRNA Levels	
	Cells × 10⁵	T-C Ratio*	Activity	T-C Ratio*	AP-Actin Ratio	T-C Ratio*
Plastic						
1 day	0.5 ± 0.07	—	0.03 ± 0.00	—	—	—
7 days	7.1 ± 0.03	—	3.77 ± 0.02	—	1.5	—
Aluminum oxide						
1 day	0.4 ± 0.02	0.78	0.03 ± 0.01	1.24	—	—
7 days	3.2 ± 0.09	0.45	15.80 ± 0.15	4.19	3.0	2.0
Titanium						
1 day	0.3 ± 0.02	0.64	0.01 ± 0.02	0.52	—	—
7 days	3.3 ± 0.50	0.46	10.61 ± 2.86	2.81	1.8	1.2
Titanium dioxide						
1 day	0.3 ± 0.02	0.73	0.01 ± 0.00	0.40	—	—
7 days	3.7 ± 0.02	0.52	9.96 ± 1.10	2.64	1.3	0.9

*T-C ratio, treatment-control ratio.
Activity measured in micromoles of inorganic phosphate released per 10^5 cells/minute.
AP-actin ratio, alkaline phosphatase-actin ratio.

onstrated the greatest stimulation in enzyme activity between day 1 and day 7 (plastic, 151-fold; aluminum oxide, 510-fold; titanium, 816-fold; and titanium dioxide, 996-fold).

Variation in alkaline phosphatase mRNA levels depended on the culture surface, whereas actin mRNA levels were constant. At day 7, mRNA levels for both proteins were comparable in cultures incubated on plastic. In contrast, in cultures incubated on aluminum oxide, alkaline phosphatase mRNA levels were 300% that of actin and 200% that of cells incubated on plastic. Levels in the cells incubated on titanium or titanium dioxide were similar to those in cells incubated on plastic.

It is possible that any surface-dependent differences in alkaline phosphatase mRNA levels may have already been expressed and translated, and the message degraded by day 7. This is likely in the cells cultured on the bone-bonding materials because they exhibited marked increases in enzyme activity. Alkaline phosphatase has been shown to be a marker enzyme in matrix vesicles isolated from bone cell cultures[26] because of its enrichment in this extracellular membrane fraction.

These studies demonstrated that the response of bone-forming cells to implant materials differs with the nature of the material. This differential response to implant materials can be studied both in vivo, using the marrow ablation model, and in vitro, using conventional culture techniques on ceramic-coated surfaces. Bone-bonding materials appear to stimulate matrix vesicle alkaline phosphatase activity, suggesting that they stimulate primary mineralization. Nonbonding materials also influence cell differentiation, as demonstrated by the cell culture experiments on aluminum oxide. Failure of the bone to bond with these materials may be the result of defective maturation of the cells and the matrix vesicles they produce or of toxic effects of the implant materials.

Acknowledgment

This study was supported by grants DE-05937 and DE-08603 from the Public Health Service and from the US-Israeli Binational Foundation. Ruben Gomez, Virginia Ramirez, and Cyndi Tschirhart assisted with cell culture and biochemical analysis.

References

1. Hench LL, Splinter RJ, Allen WC, et al: Bonding mechanisms at the interface of ceramic prosthetic materials. *J Biomed Mater Res* 1971;5:117–141.
2. Gross UM, Strunz V: The anchoring of glass ceramics of different solubility in the femur of the rat. *J Biomed Mater Res* 1980;14:607–618.
3. Gross U, Strunz V: The interface of various glasses and glass ceramics with a bony implantation bed. *J Biomed Mater Res* 1985;19:251–271.
4. Nakamura T, Yamamuro T, Higashi S, et al: A new glass-ceramic for bone replacement: Evaluation of its bonding to bone tissue. *J Biomed Mater Res* 1985;19:685–698.
5. Gross U, Strunz V: Bone connection, a principle for biomaterials engineering in bone and tooth replacement, in Lee AJC, Albrektsson T, Brånemark P-I (eds): *Clinical Applications of Biomaterials*. New York, John Wiley & Sons, 1982, pp 237–244.
6. Gross U, Brandes J, Strunz V, et al: The ultrastructure of the interface between a glass ceramic and bone. *J Biomed Mater Res* 1981;15:291–305.
7. Gross U, Muller-Mai C, Voigt C, et al: Morphology of early host and material response after implantation of surface reactive ceramics in the rat femur, in Oonishi H, Aoki H, Sawai K (eds): *Bioceramics*. Tokyo, Ishiyaky EuroAmerica, 1989, pp 163–168.
8. Gross U, Kinne R, Schmitz H-J, et al: The response of bone to surface-active glasses/glass-ceramics. *CRC Crit Rev Biocompat* 1988;4:155–179.
9. Sela J, Brandes J, Strunz V, et al: Primary mineralization and extracellular matrix vesicles in rat bone after administration of glass-ceramic implants. *Arch Orthop Trauma Surg* 1981;98:237–240.
10. Anderson HC: Electron microscopic studies of induced cartilage development and calcification. *J Cell Biol* 1967;35:81–101.
11. Bonucci E: Fine structure of early cartilage calcification. *J Ultrastr Res* 1967;20:33–50.
12. Anderson HC: Matrix vesicles of cartilage and bone, in Bourne HG (ed): *The Biochemistry and Physiology of Bone*. New York, Academic Press, 1976, vol 4, pp 136–157.
13. Chisin R, Gazit D, Ulmansky M, et al: 99mTC-MDP uptake and histological changes during rat bone marrow regeneration. *Int J Rad Appl Instrum* 1988;15B:469–476.
14. Sela J, Amir D, Schwartz Z, et al: Changes in the distribution of extracellular matrix vesicles during healing of rat tibial bone (computerized morphometry and electron microscopy). *Bone* 1987;8:245–250.
15. Bab I, Deutsch D, Schwartz Z, et al: Correlative morphometric and biochemical analysis of purified extracellular matrix vesicles from rat alveolar bone. *Calcif Tissue Int* 1983;35:320–326.
16. Schwartz Z, Sela J, Ramirez V, et al: Changes in extracellular matrix vesicles during healing of rat tibial bone: A morphometric and biochemical study. *Bone* 1989;10:53–60.
17. Styles JA: Tissue culture methods for evaluating biocompatibility of polymers, in Williams DF (ed): *Fundamental Aspects of Biocompatibility*. Boca Raton, FL, CRC Press, 1981, vol 2, pp 219–231.

18. Pizzoferrato A, Vespucci A, Ciapetti G, et al: Biocompatibility testing of prosthetic implant materials by cell cultures. *Biomaterials* 1985;6:346–351.

19. Windler S, Boyan B, Norling D, et al: Applications of RF sputter coating to implant technology. *Trans Soc Biomat* 1987;46:194.

20. Hale LV, Kemick ML, Wuthier RE: Effect of vitamin D metabolites on the expression of alkaline phosphatase activity by epiphyseal hypertrophic chondrocytes in primary cell culture. *J Bone Min Res* 1986;1:489–495.

21. Schwartz Z, Boyan B: The effects of vitamin D metabolites on phospholipase A_2 activity of growth zone and resting zone cartilage cells in vitro. *Endocrinology* 1988;122:2191–2198.

22. Partridge MC, Alcorn D, Michelangeli VP, et al: Morphological and biochemical characterization of four clonal osteogenic sarcoma cell lines of rat origin. *Cancer Res* 1983;43:4308–4314.

23. Majeska RJ, Rodan GA: Alkaline phosphatase inhibition by parathryoid hormone and isoproterenol in a clonal rat osteosarcoma cell line: Possible mediation by cyclic AMP. *Calcif Tissue Int* 1982;34:59–66.

24. Davis LG, Dibner MD, Battery JF: *Basic Methods in Molecular Biology.* New York, Elsevier, 1986, pp 136–138.

25. Schwartz Z, Amir D, Boyan BD, et al: Effect of glass ceramic and titanium implants on primary calcification during rat tibial bone healing. *Calcif Tissue Int*, 1991;49, in press.

26. Boyan BD, Schwartz Z, Bonewald LF, et al: Localization of 1,25–$(OH)_2D_3$-responsive alkaline phosphatase in osteoblast-like cells (ROS 17/2.8, MG 63, and MC 3T3) and growth cartilage cells in culture. *J Biol Chem* 1989;264:11879–11886.

Chapter 13

Dynamic Control of Interfacial Infections: The Effect of Surface Properties on Biologic Adhesion

Anne E. Meyer, PhD
Robert E. Baier, PhD

Introduction

Figure 1 depicts the ways in which biologic interactions with artificial substrata can be viewed, be they orthopaedic, vascular, and ophthalmologic implants, or even the sides of ocean-going vessels. Depending on the level of analysis used, the interfacial events can be described in macroscopic or microscopic terms; for the latter, the focus is on the deposition and retention of biologic macromolecules (such as proteins and lipids) and cells on the material. Work conducted in the 1960s proved that, when a biomaterial is introduced into a biologic system, an important initial event is the spontaneous biologic coating of that material with a macromolecular film. The films typically observed are very thin and composed primarily of similar glycoproteins that arrange themselves differently at each surface in response to the unique properties of that surface and its environment.[1-7] It is not that cells cannot deposit and attach to a bare biomaterial,[8-10] but that in a real situation, the macromolecular films always form on the surface first, and only then do the cells deposit and remain attached.

Methods Used To Characterize Biomaterials and Biologic Films

Many analytical techniques can be used to clarify interfacial events.[11-13] Comprehensive contact-angle measurements can determine the following useful characteristics of the substratum and its acquired biologic film: critical surface tension,[14] composite surface free energy, and relative polarity and apolarity of that material.[15-17] Infrared spectroscopy of the materials and the acquired biologic films, specifically internal-reflection infrared spectroscopy,[18] provides an analysis of the chemistry of both the outermost surface zone of the materials and their very thin films (less than 10 nm) of acquired macromolecules. Another important tool in characterizing macromolecules on prosthetic materials is thin-film ellipsometry; this technique is particularly

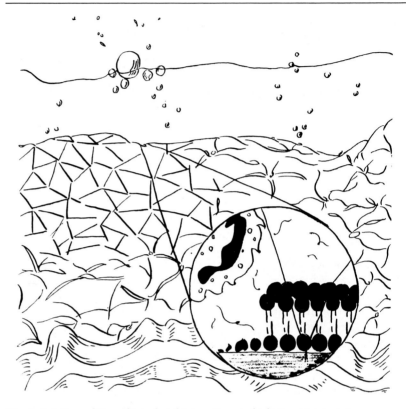

Fig. 1 *Artist's rendition of interfacial interactions in biologic environments.*

useful with highly polished and reflective substrata such as metals.[19-21] The data obtained from ellipsometric measurements allow precise calculations of film thickness. The technique is most suitable for thicknesses between 0.5 and 100 nm, a range that other techniques cannot easily measure. It is especially suited to the analysis of the proteinaceous "conditioning" film, which typically is 10 to 30 nm thick. Scanning electron microscopy (for surface texture and visual analysis of the material), energy-dispersive X-ray analysis (for a general elemental analysis), and classic cross-sectional techniques (histochemical or ultrastructural) also provide important information.

Comprehensive contact-angle methods are sensitive to the outermost atomic layer of the surface; for a perfect monolayer, this translates to a "sampling depth" of approximately 0.5 nm.[22] Internal-reflection infrared spectroscopic analysis is useful for characterizing the outermost portion of the sample, about 1.5 to 200 nm thick. Energy-dispersive X-ray analysis generally characterizes a depth between 50 and 1,000 nm (1 μ). Most of these techniques are performed under ambient conditions or moderate vacuum conditions. Relatively new analyses use high and ultra-high vacuum techniques[23-26]; these include secondary ion mass spectrometry, scanning Auger microscopy, and electron spectroscopy for chemical analysis, also called X-ray photoelectron spectroscopy. Secondary ion mass spectrometry produces a chemical analysis of components in the outermost 0.5 to 2 nm of the sample. Scanning Auger microscopy is most useful in the outermost 1 to 5 nm, but can sputter deeper into the surface zone and provide information on a cross-sectional basis. Electron spectroscopy probes between 1 and 10 nm of the sample surface.

Many biomedical materials are in use today.[13] Each material has a set of physicochemical characteristics that must be identified and confirmed so that subsequent interfacial interactions in vitro and in vivo can be evaluated. The critical surface tensions and general surface energy, as well as the overall chemistry of biomaterials, must be known in order to study the initial events of biologic deposition and adhesion.[27,28] Polymeric materials used as implants include fluorocarbons, silicones (polydimethylsiloxane), polyethylenes, polyacrylates, polyamides, polyesters, polyurethanes, and others. The critical surface tensions of the polymers range from very low (< 20 mN/m) for Teflon to moderately high (> 30 mN/m) for such polymers as polyurethane to quite high (> 40 mN/m) for nylon 6. Medical-grade silicones have critical surface tensions between 20 and 30 mN/m. Clean metals, alloys, glasses, and ceramics theoretically have surface tensions in excess of 100 mN/m, but in practice have only medium to relatively high critical surface tensions (> 30 mN/m) because their actual surfaces are covered with tightly bound layers of adsorbed moisture. When freshly cleaned,[29] these materials display their intrinsically higher critical surface tensions, well above 50 mN/m, and are extremely polar.[27]

Biomaterials and Adhesion

In the absence of antibiotics, the infection of orthopaedic sites can be viewed as the result of the higher relative strength of adhesion of the infecting bacteria to the implant material (and/or surrounding tissue) compared with the removing forces. The relative strengths of adhesion of other cells present at the site, whether osteocytes, osteoblasts, osteoclasts, macrophages, or fibroblasts, must also be considered. More than 20 years of research has shown that there is a useful correlation between the strength of biologic adhesion and the critical surface tension of the biomaterial in its preimplant condition.[4,30,31] It has been observed that there is a zone of minimal biologic adhesion (macromolecular, bacterial, or cellular) for materials with critical surface tensions between approximately 20 and 30 mN/m, including materials such as methyl-silicones. It is not necessary to use a bulk medical-grade silicone material to achieve this minimal biologic adhesion; another material that can be coated with a thin methyl-group-dominated film that produces properties similar to those of medical silicone can be considered. Teflon materials, having critical surface tensions even lower than those of the silicones, surprisingly tend to maintain

173

higher strengths of biologic adhesion than do the methyl-silicones[31-33]; this has been attributed to a greater unbalanced surface energy for Teflon-type materials in underwater environments.[34] Other common polymers, metals, and ceramics are also retentive of biologic macromolecules and cells because they have critical surface tensions greater than 30 mN/m.

Preparation of Materials and Implant Failure

It is important to note that the materials discussed are generally "clean," that is, the substrata are not covered, partially or completely, by surface contaminants that significantly alter their physicochemical character. There are, however, several potential sources and types of surface contamination of implants.[35] Unspecified trace components in the raw materials used for the implant production may cause contamination. Machining or shaping with tools of different composition may leave foreign materials on the surface. Polishing residues, which generally result in low-energy films or small particles of different composition on the surface of the material, must also be considered; this is especially true for implants made from metals or alloys. Cleaning procedures may leave detergent residues or other types of surfactants or organic material on implant surfaces. Sterilization procedures tend to leave residues on biomedical implants and devices, including materials that can lower surface energy.[29,35-37] Packaging and storage conditions may also affect surface properties. Not to be overlooked is surgical handling of the implant or material, and the many possibilities during surgery for modification of its surface properties. Further, during placement of the implant into the surgical site, it is almost impossible to avoid coating the implant with blood; this particular "contamination" of the implant may be beneficial, because the deposited plasma components may contribute the initial macromolecular conditioning film.

The new technical fields of biomaterials and biomedical devices require scientists and physicians to address the solution of chronic problems from many points of view; the prevention and treatment of implant infection is one such problem, and implant failure because of suboptimal tissue response is another. When scientists approach these problems, observations of relative success or failure tend to be based on whether adhesive or cohesive failure was at work. True adhesive failure occurs cleanly between two dissimilar materials at their interface, whereas cohesive failure occurs within one of the materials making that bond. Almost all material failures are cohesive in character. For instance, even if infecting bacteria are removed from the biologic film on a surface, it is unlikely that all the underlying macromolecular conditioning film will be removed. In the case of strong adhesion of bacteria and other types of cells, cohesive failure of the cellular layers may result in torn cellular fragments remaining on the surface.

Both sides of the "plane of failure" are rich sources of information for the biomaterials scientist and the pathologist, especially as more reliable techniques are being developed for ultrastructural analysis of unperturbed interfaces.[38]

Remodeling of Surfaces by the Biofilm

Implants   The common sequence of events, formation of the macromolecular conditioning film and then cellular deposition and retention, allows a number of different systems to be used to examine the effects of the physicochemical properties of the preimplant materials on the biologic strength of adhesion. One in vivo test system that has proved to be fruitful is placing the material into the subdermal fascial plane of the back of the New Zealand white rabbit.[39,40] This is a soft-tissue site, but has also been predictive of the general sequence and degree of initial interactions within hard-tissue sites.[41] Materials with low critical surface tensions (20 to 30 mN/m) most often maintain these apparent surface properties, despite having adsorbed thin macromolecular and cellular films, after more than 20 days of implantation.

Materials with medium initial critical surface tensions acquire biologic films with adhesive properties generally similar to those of films on materials with high critical surface tensions. The mean apparent volume fraction of fibroblasts around high-energy implants in the soft-tissue site did exceed that around the medium-energy materials in one study,[42] and this seems to be a general feature of the higher-energy materials.

After a ten-day period in the fascial plane of the rabbit back, biologic matter retained on the low-energy implants ranges from acellular macromolecular film patches to a few small patches of rounded cells. At 20 days, the low-energy implants still retain only a patchy macromolecular film with a few rounded fibroblasts. On the medium-energy materials, some flattened cells, as well as the macromolecular film, are usually observed at ten days. By 20 days, many more flattened cells and several extensive tissue patches can be observed on these implants. On the high-energy materials, cellular patches are regularly strongly adhesive to the implants by ten days; disrupted, torn cells can be noted when the implants are taken from the sites. This observation is confirmed at 20 days. The cohesive failure occurs through the tissues that grow around the medium- and high-energy implants. When low-energy

Table 1 General appearance of plane of parting in a rabbit model at 21 days

Implant Type	Film Retained on Implant	Cells Remaining With Bulk Tissue	
		Appearance	Average Capsule Thickness (No. of Cell Layers)
Cobalt-chromium-molybdenum	Not all cellular; thick film	Flat	8
Titanium alloy	Tissue/cellular patches	Flat	15
Calcium hydroxyapatite	Variable response	Mostly flat	12
Low-density polyethylene	Flat and disrupted cells	Flat	6

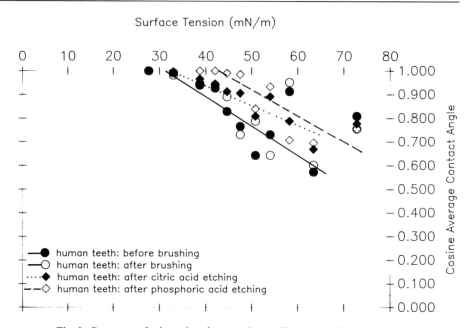

Fig. 2 *Contact-angle data plots from analyses of human teeth in situ, before and after brushing and after acid etching. Each data point represents multiple measurements with a particular pure diagnostic liquid; several different liquids are used in the analysis, and each liquid has a different liquid-vapor surface tension. The smaller the angle of contact between the liquid and the tooth surface, the greater the cosine of the contact angle. The "critical surface tension" is defined as the intercept of the plotted line with the surface tension axis.*

materials are implanted, cohesive failure occurs within the macromolecular films that form on the surfaces.

In a cross-sectional analysis of the tissue side of the plane of failure around medium-energy materials (metals, dense hydroxyapatite, and low-density polyethylene), the surface-contacting cells are flat in almost every sample. The average tissue-capsule thickness, however, can differ from material to material (Table 1). In one study, more layers of cells apparently formed around titanium alloy (titanium, aluminum, and vanadium) and dense calcium hydroxyapatite implants; in this study, these two materials were more textured than the other implants.[43] The thinnest tissue capsule observed, including the tissue retained on the implant, was formed around relatively apolar, low-density polyethylene. Again, flattened and disrupted cells indicated strong tissue adhesion to all of these medium-energy materials.

The general chemical composition of the biologic film that forms around these implants and that remains on the implant materials after the implant has been removed from the tissue is similar for almost every implant type: glycoprotein. The same type of chemistry is detected for biologic films on dental implants, orthopaedic implants,

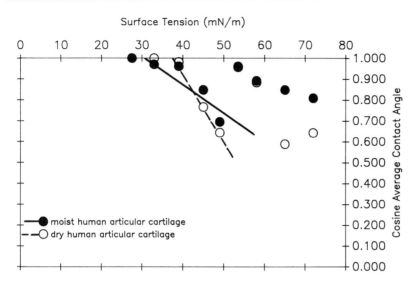

Fig. 3 *Contact-angle data plots for human articular cartilage in different states of hydration. The more polar diagnostic liquids used in the analysis have liquid-vapor surface tensions above 50 mN/m. Note the increase in critical surface tension, but decrease in polarity, as a result of drying.*

ophthalmologic materials (intraocular lenses and contact lenses), and cardiovascular implants. The salivary pellicles that form on dental prosthetic materials and teeth are also glycoproteinaceous.

Natural Tissue Surfaces   Again, the similarity of the physicochemical properties of natural biologic surfaces can be demonstrated by several techniques, including comprehensive contact-angle analyses. The critical surface tension and polar properties of human teeth, determined in situ, do not change significantly as a result of brushing (Fig. 2), indicating that the binding strength of the acquired pellicle is quite high. The brushed tooth enamel is not clean mineral; there is a great deal of organic macromolecular material present. After citric acid etching, which temporarily removes the salivary macromolecular components from the enamel, a modest increase in critical surface tension and polarity of the surface is observed.[4,44] The surface properties of the etched tooth are similar to those of synthetic ceramics. Phosphoric acid etching, which also uncovers a significant depth of tooth mineral, further increases the apparent surface energy as an artifact of the roughness induced.[4]

Contact-angle data plots from preliminary studies of human articular cartilage are shown in Figure 3. The moist cartilage is similar to the teeth in that the critical surface tensions are between 30 and 33 mN/m and both surfaces are polar. When the articular cartilage is air-dried, there is an increase in the critical surface tension, as well as a

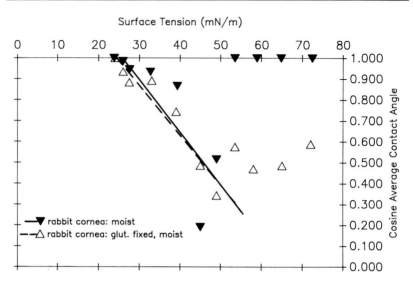

Fig. 4 *Contact-angle data plots for moist rabbit corneal surfaces. Fixation by dilute glutaraldehyde does not significantly alter the critical surface tension of the tissue, but causes a large decrease in surface polarity.*

loss of some polarity. Fixation of similar tissue (retrieved from a rabbit hip) in 2% glutaraldehyde resulted in the critical surface tension being maintained between 30 and 40 mN/m, but the polarity of the surface was significantly lower than for an unfixed control, indicating partial "quenching" of the material's surface energy by glutaraldehyde's primary cross-linking across the terminal amino groups of lysine residues.

Figure 4 summarizes contact-angle analyses of rabbit corneal surfaces, and Figure 5 provides a similar characterization of oral mucosa in human volunteers. These latter two surfaces exhibit practical "fouling release" qualities not obviously shared by the tooth or cartilaginous surfaces, despite their similar polar (or water-loving) qualities. Thus, it must be the differences in surface energy qualities that correlate with the lower bioadhesive strength.

The blood-contacting surfaces of natural blood vessels can be represented by contact-angle data plots like the one given in Figure 6 for the inner surface of a human saphenous vein. The critical surface tension of the luminal surfaces of natural blood vessels is between 20 and 30 mN/m; again, the surfaces also are quite polar, as expected for substances in direct contact with aqueous fluids, whether or not the polar groups participate in bioadhesive events. A data plot for the luminal surface of a nonthrombogenic arterial graft (umbilical cord vein) is also given in Figure 6; note that the surface properties of the natural blood vessel have been reproduced in the artificial graft, which has no living endothelial cells on its surface.[45]

The natural surfaces described above, which generally remain free

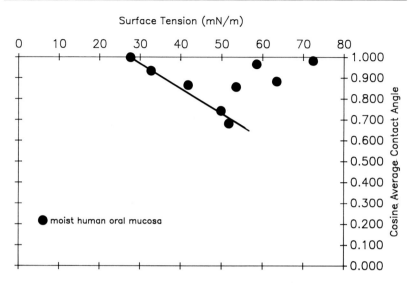

Fig. 5 *Contact-angle data plot for moist human oral mucosa (in situ). Note the similarity in critical surface tensions among the mucosal, corneal (Fig. 4), and vascular (Fig. 6) surfaces. Note the difference between the critical surface tension of the mucosa and those of teeth (Fig. 2) and articular cartilage (Fig. 3).*

of biologic film buildup and display weak bioadhesion, all have low critical surface tensions. In contrast, tooth and articular cartilage surfaces are both very retentive of their acquired macromolecular overlayers, which serve the important function of boundary lubrication under repetitive and often severe mechanical challenges. It is the bioretentive quality indicated by the higher (about 34 to 36 mN/m) critical surface tensions of these two wear-protected materials that also renders them susceptible to undesirable biodeposits such as dental plaque or infective lesions.

Mechanical Shear Challenge

Investigators must determine how mechanical forces, such as interfacial shear, alter the composition or structure of the biologic films. Shear may play an unexpected role in the maintenance of corneal, cartilage, and cardiovascular surfaces. Application of shear stress certainly is one way to create cohesive failure within a biologic film, but it may produce planes of failure by removing material nearer the implant or nearer natural tissue surfaces. Application of shear forces also presents opportunities for the delivery of additional film components to the site, or "turnover" of molecules already in the vicinity.

One helpful method of elucidating the effects of shear in vitro uses parallel plates in a flow-cell arrangement. Flat specimens of sample substrata can be exposed to a liquid pumping system through which the operational fluid dynamics (such as velocity and shear rate) can

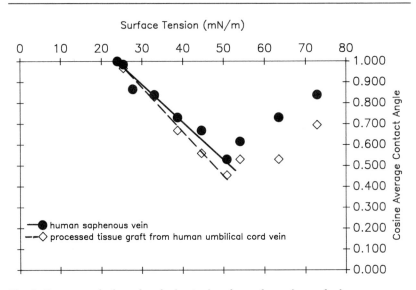

Fig. 6 *Contact-angle data plots for luminal surfaces of vascular grafts: human saphenous vein and processed human umbilical cord vein. The processing for the umbilical cord vein included treatment with dilute glutaraldehyde.*

be controlled.[7,46,47] In addition to its use in the study of macromolecular film formation, this method has been applied to research on processes of bacterial retention on materials with different initial surface properties.[48-52] Recent work with *Escherichia coli* confirmed that the attachment rate of macromolecular and cellular species is not predictive of the ultimate strength of adhesion.[52] Other investigators who simply counted the organisms often drew the conclusion that materials with larger numbers of quickly attaching organisms are more adhesive than materials with fewer organisms attaching during short exposures. It is difficult to estimate such relative strengths of adhesion when experiments are conducted under static conditions, in which the mechanical detaching forces are too weak to discriminate among materials that may actually bind microbes with vastly different strengths. This problem is compounded by the fact that much of the published literature on biologic adhesion fails to define exposure conditions (sample rinsing conditions are the most poorly defined) in the discussion of results. Adhesive strength can only be elucidated by challenges that are sufficient to separate microorganisms or other test particles from some, but not all, substances. Rapidly attaching organisms, for instance, exposed to shear forces by controlled rinsing or increased flow rate of the original test fluid may readily slough from some surfaces while being retained on others.

An interesting related observation by Rittle and associates[52] was the demonstration that rates of attachment can also change as a function of exposure time. "Hydrophobic" surfaces (such as medical silicones) acquired bacterial cells from the flowing stream at a high rate in the early stages of exposure. Subsequent challenge by increased shear rate, however, removed most of the cells from the surface. Medium- and high-energy substrata tended to acquire cells at a lower rate during the early exposure period, but the numbers of attached cells increased with time as the surface-bound water layers of these intrinsically more hydrophilic substrata were eventually penetrated by the biofilm-forming macromolecules and cells. The long-term strength of adhesion of the cells to the higher-energy substrata was significantly greater than that to the lower-energy materials. This observation parallels the findings for soiled rigid, gas-permeable contact lenses, for example,[53] unlike soiled soft contact lenses, which collect material more slowly but are more difficult to clean.

In flow cell studies of whole saliva exposed to medium-energy materials, it was noted that shear rate altered both the formation rate and the organization of the deposited salivary films.[54] Fluid shear rate affected many important film properties, including critical surface tension, polarity, thickness, density, and film mass. Increased shear stress decreased the critical surface tensions of the macromolecular films, perhaps as a result of a type of surface "polishing" to the weakest (least adhesive) plane of parting. Conditions of increasing flow rate seem capable of producing different planes of failure in the films once they exceed the so-called critical shear stress and remove the bulk of the film from regions not immediately adjacent to the substratum.[55]

The flow cell experiments with whole saliva demonstrated that the polarities of the retained biologic films can increase with increased shear, and the critical surface tension can indicate decreased bioadhesive tendencies at the same time. In addition, the densities of the films were much greater with increased shear stresses, indicating compaction of the films and perhaps delivery of more material to the interface (rather than simple stripping and removal of initially deposited material). These effects of shear stress on the properties of the biologic films retained on various materials were reproduced, although at different kinetics, in flow cell experiments with natural seawater.[54]

Studies of the interfacial properties of the biologic adhesive produced by the New England blue mussel in seawater conditions indicate that a particular range of polarity of the macromolecular conditioning film, in addition to critical surface-tension criteria, may be important in the support of optimal cellular adhesion.[56] Figure 7 shows values of the polar components of films of the adhesive as a function of applied concentration and effective cellular adhesion.

These observations should be factored into the evaluation of infected wound sites. Shear forces produced in a joint area may compact the biologic film on the surface, resulting in even more reclusive conditions for pathogens. Conversely, increased shear may affect the removal of the bacteria from the site, rendering them more, or less, vulnerable to external treatment. Shear forces produced by irrigating the infected site may have similar advantages and disadvantages.

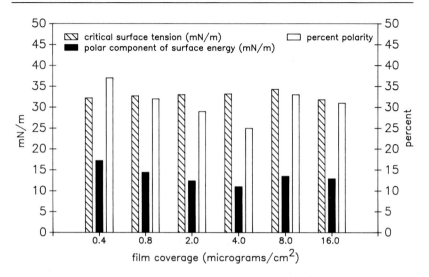

Fig. 7 *Surface-energy properties of prepared films of mussel adhesive protein isolated from* Mytilus edulis. *Film dimensions were greater than a single macromolecular layer. Several studies demonstrated that a surface concentration of 2 μg/cm² of the protein provides optimal conditions for cellular adhesion. Graph plotted from data in Olivieri and associates.*[56]

Surface Properties of Pathogenic Bacteria

The special challenges of infection and infection control also require more understanding of the physicochemical characteristics of the organisms themselves. A limited study of a variety of microorganisms of varying pathogenicities concluded that the more pathogenic bacteria were more adept at modifying their own surfaces and the environment immediately surrounding them (A.E. Meyer, R.E. Baier, M.S. Vejins, and associates, unpublished data). The pathogens modify the surface energetics of their local microenvironment through the elution of surface-active amphipathic substances. Simple expression, with no frank elution, of these substances on the cell surface may allow the organisms to adapt to different external conditions, including different types of substrata, successfully. These features may contribute to the difficulty of eradicating the pathogens by physiologic or biochemical means, but do not free the organisms from the fundamental rules of physical chemistry.

Pathogenic microorganisms, like other particles, are less likely to adhere strongly to materials with initially low critical surface tensions. Figure 8 summarizes the results of flow cell studies of bacterial retention to two types of substrata (one with low and one with medium critical surface tension). Although different species were retained in different numbers, possibly indicating some degree of adaptive substratum specificity after their initial deposition, all species were less

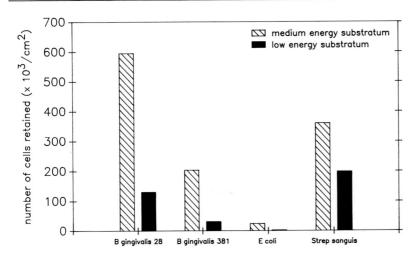

Fig. 8 *Numbers of the bacteria retained on medium- and low-energy substrata after identical exposure times and challenge by shear forces.* B gingivalis *28 is, in the human oral cavity, more pathogenic than* B gingivalis *381.*

likely to adhere strongly to the low-energy substrata (Christersson and associates[51] and Meyer and associates, unpublished data).

Specific reactions and interactions of particular peptides and cell receptors may occur over longer periods, but the initial events so important to determining the success or failure of a material are clearly more strongly related to fundamental physicochemical processes than they are to slower-acting factors such as receptor-lectin recognition, for example.

Prevention and Treatment of Infection

Thus, from a physicochemical point of view, the relative retention of biologic macromolecules and cells can be controlled by the interfacial properties of the implant materials before their placement and/ or the forces they experience afterward, such as mechanical shear. Development of more effective treatments or methods for prevention of biomaterials-centered infection is likely to require a combination of physiologic, biochemical, and physicochemical approaches and depends on productive collaboration among basic and clinical research teams.

Approaches may include removal of bacteria, removal of protective macromolecular constituents, and killing the infective organisms; the last has been almost the sole focus of treatments in wide use today. Serious consideration also should be given to the prevention of bacterial attachment and colonization via the control of substratum properties and biologic film formation.

Competition for the Interface

It is clear that minimization of bacterial retention through the use of materials with low critical surface tensions will be disadvantageous in regard to strong tissue adhesion to the implant. A better technique may be enhanced tissue adhesion to substrata of optimized high-energy surface properties, because local healthy tissue growth and adhesion will put invading bacteria at a significant disadvantage with regard to "lodgement" at that interface. Gristina[57] described this competition as the "race for the surface."

Learning From the Natural Defense Mechanisms of Plants and Animals

In studying the control of bacterial attachment and retention mechanisms, biomedical research may find some interesting clues in the field of marine biology. As discussed earlier, there is still much to learn about specialized underwater adhesives produced by aquatic animals such as mussels and barnacles.[56,58] Research on specific marine plants (such as eel grass) and animals (such as sea fans, or gorgonian corals) has demonstrated that many of them possess "antifouling" defense mechanisms against microorganisms. The defense mechanisms include (1) passive features, including low-energy surfaces and mechanical processes such as weak boundary layers, and (2) active chemical processes, such as the production of diffusible adhesion-inhibiting metabolites.[59-63]

Figure 9 presents contact-angle data plots of eel grass leaves at different stages of maturation and environmental exposure. When the eel grass leaves are relatively young, very few bacteria are retained on their surfaces; the critical surface tensions of the plant's new leaf surfaces are between 20 and 30 mN/m, the zone identified earlier as defining conditions for minimal biologic adhesion. As the leaves age, more bacteria are retained on their surfaces; the critical surface tensions of the older leaves are greater than those of the new leaves. The reasons for the change in the surface properties of the eel grass leaves are not known, but probably include the deterioration of the initial surface-energy-lowering coating that protects the leaves from easy colonization by arriving microorganisms. Research on sea fans demonstrates that, while incorporation of both passive and active mechanisms can effectively control microbial adhesion over the lifetime of the coral, some fouling-resistant species may possess only the passive mode of control.[61]

Nevertheless, there are now intensive efforts to isolate and purify the active components of marine exudates that can prevent bacterial adhesion and colonization (R.E. Baier, unpublished data). If these components prove to be nontoxic, they may indeed be useful as controlled-release "drugs" for both environmental and biomedical applications.

Disruption of Protective Films

Closer to fruition for biomedical applications is development of powerful, but biologically safe, matrix-disruption agents that might be

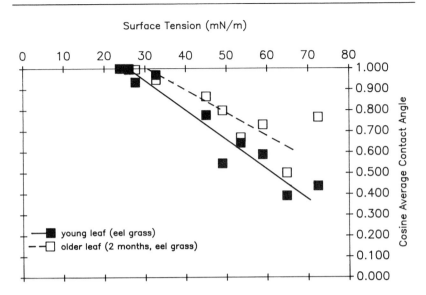

Fig. 9 *Contact-angle data plots of eel grass* (Zostera marina) *leaves of different ages. The younger leaves retain very few microorganisms on their surfaces, whereas the older leaves become increasingly retentive of deposited bacteria. Note the change in critical surface tension of the surface as the leaves age.*

used in topical treatment of infected sites. Currently under development for dental plaque removal and prevention are compounds that dramatically congeal the "glycocalyx" (extracellular matrix, slime films) around the bacteria, destroying the architecture and mechanical strengths of the entire plaque film.[64,65] Use of such a disrupting agent at an infected site also can render the bacteria much more susceptible to treatment by antibiotics and other types of antimicrobials.

Photodynamic Therapy

Another new approach being studied for its potential application to control of infection is photodynamic therapy, which has been employed, so far, primarily for the treatment of carcinomas.[66,67] The treatment works via the activation of a photosensitive organic molecule (from the class of porphyrin compounds) by visible light; certain wavelengths are more efficient than others. Although details are lacking, it is surmised that the activated porphyrin produces reactive species, such as oxygen radicals, leading to local necrosis. It is not yet known if it is necessary for the photosensitive molecules to be taken up into the interiors of the cells to achieve cell death. Recent research has shown photodynamic therapy to be useful for the destruction of gram-positive bacteria, *Mycoplasma* organisms, and yeasts.[68] The technique has not so far been effective against gram-negative bacteria.

Photodynamic therapy is a technique worth exploring in much

greater depth. As practiced in clinical trials for cancer therapy, the activating light is directed to the site by thin fiberoptics for precision and minimization of damage to surrounding healthy tissue. Eventual goals include noninvasive treatment, which may be possible if activating light wavelengths and intensities of light can be identified that can penetrate the skin and other tissues harmlessly.

References

1. Baier RE, Dutton RC: Initial events in interactions of blood with a foreign surface. *J Biomed Mater Res* 1969;3:191–206.
2. Vroman L, Adams AL: Possible involvement of fibrinogen and proteolysis in surface activation: A study with the recording ellipsometer. *Thromb Diath Haemorrh* 1967;18:510–524.
3. Glantz P-O: On wettability and adhesiveness. *Odontol Rev* 1969;20(suppl 17):1–132.
4. Baier RE: Occurrence, nature, and extent of cohesive and adhesive forces in dental integuments, in Lasslo A, Quintana RP (eds): *Surface Chemistry and Dental Integuments*. Springfield, IL, Charles C Thomas, 1973, pp 337–391.
5. Sönju T, Rölla G: Chemical analysis of the acquired pellicle formed in two hours on cleaned human teeth in vivo: Rate of formation and amino acid analysis. *Caries Res* 1973;7:30–38.
6. Baier RE: Influence of the initial surface conditions of materials on bioadhesion, in *Proceedings: Third International Congress on Marine Corrosion and Fouling*. Evanston, IL, Northwestern University Press, 1973, pp 633–639.
7. Meyer AE, Baier RE, King RW: Fouling of nontoxic coatings in fresh, brackish, and sea water. *Can J Chem Eng* 1988;66:55–62.
8. Schakenraad JM, Arends J, Busscher HJ, et al: Kinetics of cell spreading on protein precoated substrata: A study of interfacial aspects. *Biomaterials* 1989;10:43–50.
9. Steinberg J, Neumann AW, Absolom DR, et al: Human erythrocyte adhesion and spreading on protein-coated polymer surfaces. *J Biomed Mater Res* 1989;23:591–610.
10. Borenstein N, Brash JL: Red blood cells deposit membrane components on contacting surfaces. *J Biomed Mater Res* 1986;20:723–730.
11. Baier RE, Meyer AE: Surface analysis, in von Recum AF (ed): *Handbook of Biomaterials Evaluation: Scientific, Technical, and Clinical Testing of Implant Materials*. New York, Macmillan, 1986, pp 97–108.
12. Meyer AE: Reference materials, in von Recum AF (ed): *Handbook of Biomaterials Evaluation: Scientific, Technical, and Clinical Testing of Implant Materials*. New York, Macmillan, 1986, pp 131–139.
13. Meyer AE, Baier RE, Glantz P-OJ, et al: Biomaterials: Selection, evaluation, and preparation, in Babbush CA (ed): *Oral Implants*. Philadelphia, WB Saunders, 1991.
14. Zisman WA: Relation of the equilibrium contact angle to liquid and solid constitution. *Adv Chem* 1964;43:1–51.
15. Fowkes FM: Role of acid-base interfacial bonding in adhesion. *J Adhesion Sci* 1987;1:7–27.
16. Kaelble DH: Dispersion-polar surface tension properties of organic solids. *J Adhesion* 1970;2:66–81.
17. van Oss CJ, Good RJ, Chaudhury MK: Additive and nonadditive surface tension components and the interpretation of contact angles. *Langmuir* 1988;4:884–891.

18. Harrick NJ: Surface chemistry from special analysis of totally internal reflected radiation. *J Phys Chem* 1960;64:1110–1114.

19. McCrackin FL, Passaglia E, Stromberg RR, et al: Measurement of the thickness and refractive index of very thin films and the optical properties of surfaces by ellipsometry. *J Res Natl Bur Standards Appl Phys Chem* 1963;67A:363–377.

20. Cuypers PA: *Dynamic Ellipsometry: Biochemical and Biomedical Applications,* thesis. The Netherlands, Rijksuniversiteit Limburg, 1976.

21. Arnebrant T, Ivarsson B, Larsson K, et al: Bilayer formation at adsorption of proteins from aqueous solutions on metal surfaces. *Progr Colloid Polymer Sci* 1985;70:62–66.

22. Troughton EB, Bain CD, Whitesides GM, et al: Monolayer films prepared by the spontaneous self-assembly of symmetrical and unsymmetrical dialkyl sulfides from solution onto gold substrates: Structure, properties, and reactivity of constituent functional groups. *Langmuir* 1988;4:365–385.

23. Feldman LC, Mayer JW: *Fundamentals of Surface and Thin Film Analysis.* New York, Elsevier, 1986.

24. Reed SJB: *Electron Microprobe Analysis.* Cambridge, Cambridge University Press, 1975.

25. Gardella JA Jr, Pireaux JJ: Analysis of polymer surfaces using electron and ion beams. *Anal Chem* 1990;62:645A.

26. Ratner BD (ed): *Surface Characterization of Biomaterials: Progress in Biomedical Engineering, Vol 6.* New York, Elsevier, 1988.

27. Baier RE, Meyer AE: Implant surface preparation. *Int J Oral Maxillofac Implants* 1988;52:788–791.

28. Baier RE: Conditioning surfaces to suit the biomedical environment: Recent progress. *J Biomech Eng* 1982;104:257–271.

29. Meyer AE: Gas plasma treatments, in *Sterilization in the 1990s: Proceedings of the HIMA Educational Seminar.* Washington, DC, Health Industry Manufacturers Association, 1989, pp 75–82.

30. Baier RE: Substrata influences on the adhesion of microorganisms and their resultant new surface properties, in Bitton G, Marshall KC (eds): *Adsorption of Microorganisms to Surfaces.* New York, Wiley, 1980, pp 59–104.

31. Baier RE, Meyer AE: Surface energetics and biological adhesion, in Mittal KL (ed): *Physicochemical Aspects of Polymer Surfaces.* New York, Plenum Press, 1983, vol 2, pp 895–909.

32. Grinnell F: Cellular adhesiveness and extracellular substrata. *Int Rev Cytol* 1978;53:65–144.

33. Dexter SC: Influence of substratum critical surface tension on bacterial adhesion: In situ studies. *J Colloid Interface Sci* 1979;70:346–354.

34. Schrader ME: On adhesion of biological substances to low energy solid surfaces. *J Colloid Interface Sci* 1982;88:296–297.

35. Baier RE, Meyer AE: Future directions in surface preparation of dental implants. *J Dent Educ* 1988;52:788–791.

36. Baier RE, Meyer AE, Akers CK, et al: Degradative effects of conventional steam sterilization on biomaterial surfaces. *Biomaterials* 1982;3:241–245.

37. Keller JC, Draughn RA, Wightman JP, et al: Characterization of sterilized CP titanium implant surfaces. *Int J Oral Maxillofac Implants* 1990;5:360–367.

38. Bjursten LM, Emanuelsson L, Ericson LE, et al: Method for ultrastructural studies of the intact tissue-metal interface. *Biomaterials* 1990;11:596–601.

39. Baier RE, Meyer AE, Natiella JR, et al: Surface properties determine bioadhesive outcomes: Methods and results. *J Biomed Mater Res* 1984;18:327–355.

40. Meyer AE, Baier RE, Natiella JR, et al: Investigation of tissue/implant interactions during the first two hours of implantation. *J Oral Implant* 1989;14:363–379.

41. Stachowski MJ: *Mechanical Properties of the Bone Titanium Interface With Implants of Various Surface Treatments in Vivo*, thesis. State University of New York at Buffalo, 1991.

42. Carter JM, Natiella JR, Baier RE, et al: Fibroblastic activities post implantation of cobalt chromium alloy and pure germanium in rabbits. *Artif Organs* 1984;8:102–104.

43. Meyer AE, Baier RE, Natiella JR: An experimental model to predict tissue implant adhesion. *Trans Soc Biomater* 1990;13:296.

44. Glantz P-O, Jendresen M, Baier RE: A clinical method for the study of in vivo adhesiveness of teeth. *Acta Odontol Scand* 1980;38:371–378.

45. Baier RE, Akers CK, Perlmutter S, et al: Processed human umbilical cord veins for vascular reconstructive surgery. *ASAIO Trans* 1976;22:514–524.

46. DePalma VA: Apparatus for zeta potential measurement of rectangular flow cells. *Rev Sci Instrum* 1980;51:1390–1395.

47. King RW, Meyer AE, Ziegler RC, et al: New flow cell technology for assessing primary biofouling in oceanic heat exchangers, in Proceedings of the Eighth Ocean Energy Conference. Washington, DC, The Marine Technology Society, 1981, p 431.

48. Meyer AE, Fornalik MS, Baier RE, et al: Microfouling survey of Atlantic ocean waters, in Proceedings of the Sixth International Congress on Marine Corrosion and Fouling. Athens, Greece, 1984, pp 605–621.

49. Meyer AE, DePalma VA, Goupil DW, et al: Human fibrinogen adsorption onto surface-energy-controlled substrata. *J Electroanal Chem* 1986;212:27–41.

50. Christersson CE, Glantz P-OJ, Baier RE: Role of temperature and shear forces on microbial detachment. *Scand J Dent Res* 1988;96:91–98.

51. Christersson CE, Dunford RG, Glantz P-O, et al: Effect of critical surface tension on retention of oral microorganisms. *Scand J Dent Res* 1989;97:247–256.

52. Rittle KH, Helmstetter CE, Meyer AE, et al: *Escherichia coli* retention on solid surfaces as functions of substratum surface energy and cell growth phase. *Biofouling* 1990;2:121–130.

53. Meyer AE, Palmer GR, Sabers SL, et al: Initial deposits on contact lenses: Subject and material variations. *Trans Soc Biomater*, 1991;14:135.

54. Meyer AE: *Dynamics of "Conditioning" Film Formation on Biomaterials*, thesis. Lund University, Sweden, 1990.

55. Powell MS, Slater NKH: Removal rates of bacterial cells from glass surfaces by fluid shear. *Biotech Bioeng* 1982;24:2527–2537.

56. Olivieri MP, Loomis RE, Meyer AE, et al: Surface characterization of mussel adhesive protein films. *J Adhes Sci Technol* 1990;4:197–204.

57. Gristina AG: Biomaterial-centered infection: Microbial adhesion versus tissue integration. *Science* 1987;237:1588–1595.

58. Waite JH, Tanzer ML: The bioadhesive of *Mytilus byssus*: A protein containing L-dopa. *Biochem Biophys Res Commun* 1980;96:1554–1561.

59. Kirchman DL, Mazzella L, Alberte RS, et al: Bacterial epiphytes on *Zostera marina*. *Mar Ecol Progr Ser* 1984;15:117–123.

60. Baier RE, Zimmerman RC, Meyer AE: Eel grass (*Zostera marina*) leaves as models for natural resistance to biofouling. *Trans Soc Biomater* 1990;13:20.

61. Vrolijk NH, Targett NM, Baier RE, et al: Surface characterisation of two gorgonian coral species: Implications for a natural antifouling defence. *Biofouling* 1990;2:39–54.

62. Davis AR, Targett NM, McConnell OJ, et al: Epibiosis of marine algae and benthic invertebrates: Natural products chemistry and other mechanisms inhibiting settlement and overgrowth, in *Bioorganic Marine Chemistry*. Berlin, Springer-Verlag, 1989, vol 3, pp 85–114.

63. Baier RE, Meyer AE: Biosurface chemistry or fun and profit. *Chemtech* 1986;16:178–185.

64. Attström R, Matsson L, Edwardsson S, et al: The effect of Octapinol on dentogingival plaque and development of gingivitis: III. Short-term studies in humans. *J Periodont Res* 1983;18:445–451.

65. Baier RE, Meyer AE, Akers CK: Safe and effective decontamination of delicate surfaces, in Hall CW (ed): *Biomedical Engineering II: Recent Developments*. New York, Pergamon Press, 1983, pp 293–296.

66. Dougherty TJ: Photosensitizers: Therapy and detection of malignant tumors. *Photochem Photobiol* 1987;45:879–889.

67. Henderson BW, Waldow SM, Mang TS, et al: Tumor destruction and kinetics of tumor cell death in two experimental mouse tumors following photodynamic therapy. *Cancer Res* 1985;45:572–576.

68. Malik Z, Hanania J, Nitzan Y: Bactericidal effects of photoactivated porphyrins—an alternative approach to antimicrobial drugs. *J Photochem Photobiol* 1990;5B:281–293.

Chapter 14

Soft-Tissue Adhesion to Implant Materials

Andreas F. von Recum, DVM, PhD

Introduction

The standard histological response to soft-tissue implants is inflammatory encapsulation. Tissue adhesion to the implant surface is generally not observed. Macroporous implants may allow tissue ingrowth but do not reduce chronic inflammation and do not promote cellular adhesion to the material surface.

Microtextured surfaces, however, within a small range, allow cellular and collagen apposition and reduce chronic inflammation and capsule formation to a minimum.

Mechanical interfacial forces are the apparent modifiers of tissue response. The interrelationship among tissue, bacteria, and microtextured surfaces is an important criterion for implant design.

The Histological Response to Soft-Tissue Implants

Histological sections of the tissue surrounding prosthetic implants show a characteristic inflammatory reaction termed (foreign body) granuloma. Assuming that the implant material is nontoxic, the inflammatory response usually remains localized to the implantation bed. The severity and extent of this tissue response depend on the biocompatibility of the material, the configuration of the implant, and the severity of the surgical insult. Biocompatibility is widely accepted as the degree to which the implant is accepted by the tissue bed, and it is modified by the bulk and surface chemistry and electrochemistry of the implant material.

If an injured site is free or has been free of foreign materials (contaminants, including implants), then the inflammation persists only for a few days and tissue repair results in a fibrous and stable scar within about six weeks. When sterile foreign materials, including implants, remain in the injured site, the initial acute inflammation turns into a chronic one, resulting in tissue encapsulation. This capsule and the inflammatory condition, the foreign body granuloma, can persist for long periods, often worsening gradually with time.

Implants With Smooth Surfaces

Histologically, a granuloma capsule consists of layered tissue that is an accumulation of capillaries, inflammatory cells (specifically of monocytic lineage), a few other white cells (including lymphocytes and plasma cells), and fibroblasts. Inflammatory cells are predominantly concentrated in layers closer to the implant surface, and the percentage of fibroblasts increases in the direction away from the implant. Usually the tissue is not firmly attached to the surface of the implant. Instead, the interface is filled with extracellular fluid and layers of macrophages and their senile conglomerates, the giant cells. A typical example can be seen in Figure 1. A Silastic catheter had been implanted percutaneously in the back of a dog for several months. The thick tissue capsule was densely packed with metabolically active cells. The capsule surface adjacent to the catheter consisted predominantly of macrophages. This tissue response, which is seen around all smooth-surfaced soft-tissue implants, can be responsible for a number of significant clinical problems. The chronic inflammation persists. Often the granulous tissue capsule contracts, leading to unacceptable functional and cosmetic results, as happens in breast implants. The lack of tissue attachment allows widening of the tissue-implant interface, migration of the implant, and eventually bacterial immigration with resulting infection that leads to implant failure.

Porous Implants

In the early 1960s, this lack of tissue attachment led to the concept that a porous implant would allow tissue migration into the implant pores, thereby anchoring the implant firmly in its bed and reducing capsule thickening and contracture. Consequently, a number of polymeric fiber textiles were developed and used for vascular replacement; closing of large tissue gaps; replacement of disks, tendons, and ligaments; and tissue-anchoring cuffs for percutaneous, long-term catheters. Figures 2 and 3 show two different prosthetic blood vessels commonly used in cardiovascular practice. A granulation tissue capsule enveloped the entire implant (not shown here) and tissue processes reached into the implant porosity and filled the spaces. As with smooth implants, all the surfaces were covered with giant cells and macrophages. Peripheral to those, fibroblasts and their extracellular matrix products appeared wherever there was enough physical space between the polymeric fibers and their giant cell sleeves (Fig. 3). Actual attachment of connective tissue to the polymeric surface was usually not achieved.[1-3]

Although these porous implants provided significant functional improvements because of the achieved tissue anchorage to the implant, the persisting inflammation and propensity for infection at the material-tissue interface still represent significant problems.

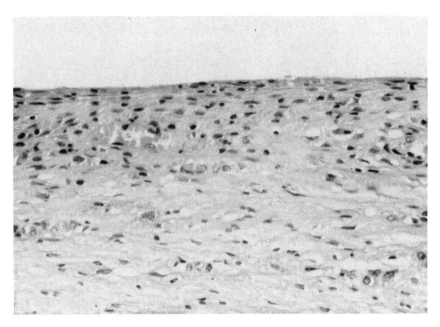

Fig. 1 *Tissue capsule adjacent to a Silastic catheter. The catheter (at top) has been removed for ease of sectioning. The granulous tissue capsule is thick and dense. The content of macrophages increases in the direction of the implant surface (hematoxylin-eosin, ✕ 100).*

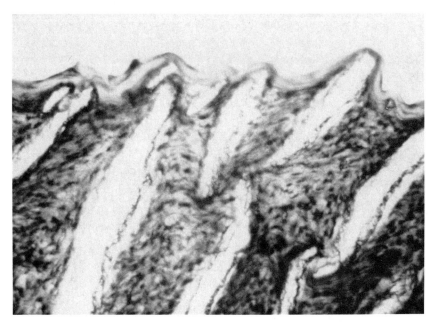

Fig. 2 *Tissue with polytetrafluoroethylene vascular prosthesis implanted in a goat for six weeks. The blood-contacting surface (at top) is lined with a monolayer of cells and a thin film of collagen. The spaces between the Teflon septi are filled with granulation tissue, predominantly macrophages. This general response is observed to be stable and persists throughout the implantation period of this graft.*

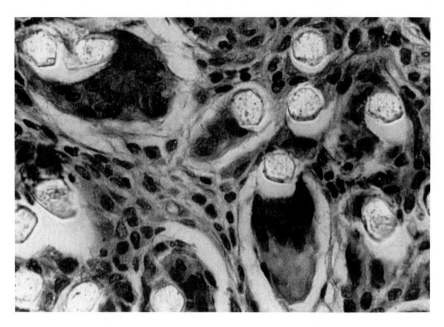

Fig. 3 *Tissue within a polyester terephthalate vascular graft removed from the subcutaneous space of the back of a rabbit after 20 days of implantation. Each polymer fiber is surrounded by a sleeve of macrophages and giant cells. There is little evidence of connective tissue formation (hematoxylin-eosin, × 300).*

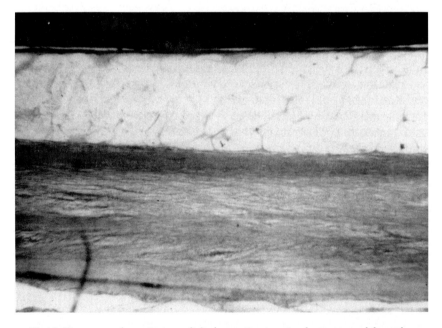

Fig. 4 *Tissue capsule against a polished pure titanium implant, removed from the subcutaneous tissue of the back of a goat after three months of implantation. A thick and dense fibrous capsule has formed around the implant (at top). The capsule does not adhere to the implant. A serum-filled cavity separates the titanium polished surface from the capsule.*

Modification of Tissue Response by Surface Microtexture

Recent histopathologic observations with various implants have suggested that bulk chemistry and surface electrochemistry cannot be the only determinants of biocompatibility and that there must be other strong modifiers of cellular response at the interface. Figures 4 and 5 indicate that the subcutaneous tissue response to commercially pure titanium can vary significantly. In Figure 4 the titanium surface was highly polished. A thick and dense fibrous capsule had developed that did not adhere to the titanium surface; this was demonstrated by the serum- and fibrin-filled space between the implant and the fibrous capsule. In Figure 5 the tympanic membrane implant removed from a cat was made from sandblasted pure titanium. Epidermal cells adhere tightly and there was no evidence of a gap or of inflammatory cells at the interface.[4] We decided, therefore, to investigate the connection between the microtexture of the implant surface and the tissue response.[5]

Experimental Observations

Micropore Dimensions and Connective-Tissue Response

A commercially available filter material (a nylon fiber mesh coated with a copolymer foam) was selected as the test model because it was available in various average micropore sizes from 0.4 to 10 µ without changes of the bulk and surface chemistry. After two- and 12–week implantation periods the implants were studied by light microscopy in an attempt to correlate tissue response with average pore size.

Filters with average pore sizes of less than 1 µ showed histologic responses similar to those of smooth-surfaced implants: Several layers of macrophages floating at the interface were surrounded by a thick capsule of granulous tissue (Fig. 6). The micropore range of 1 to 3 µ stimulated an extremely thin connective tissue capsule that was attached directly to the copolymer foam. There were only occasional macrophage accumulations at the interface (Fig. 7). Filters with average micropore sizes of more than 3 µ showed masses of macrophages filling all pores and coating the implant (Fig. 8).

Within the micropore range tested, those between 1 and 3 µ seemed to have an optimally benign tissue response. All micropore sizes outside this range produced significantly different tissue reactions although the chemical bulk and surface properties of all implants were the same. Among the differences were the following: (1) In the optimal micropore range, fibrocytes were the predominant cell type; in all other micropore sizes, macrophages outnumbered all other cell types. (2) In the optimal micropore range, collagen was deposited directly onto and into the copolymer foam. In the other micropore sizes, collagen could not be stained in the vicinity of the surface. (3) In the optimal micropore

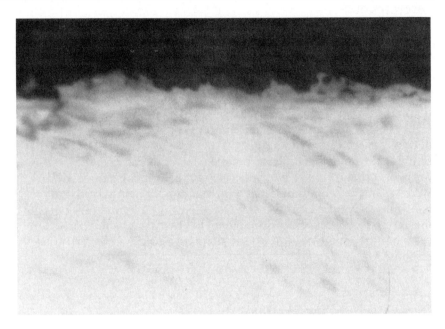

Fig. 5 *Tissue capsule against a sandblasted pure titanium implant in the tympanic membrane of a human patient. Epidermal cells can be seen adhering tightly to the roughened surface without interposed inflammatory cells (hematoxylin-eosin, × 300).*

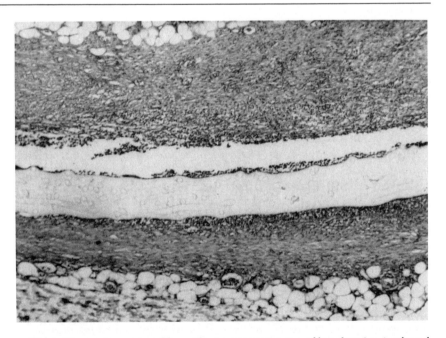

Fig. 6 *Tissue response to a filter with an average pore size of less than 1 μ, implanted in the subcutaneous space of the back of a dog for 20 days. A very inflammatory response characterizes this surface texture, with masses of macrophages flooding the implant surface (hematoxylin-eosin, × 80).*

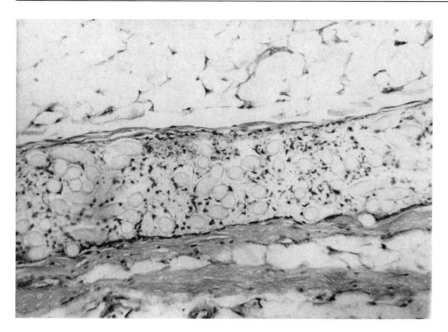

Fig. 7 *Tissue response to a filter with an average pore size of 2 μ, implanted in the subcutaneous space of the back of a dog for 20 days. A monolayer of fibrocytes and collagen line the surface of the implant. No other reactions are evident (trichrome, × 80).*

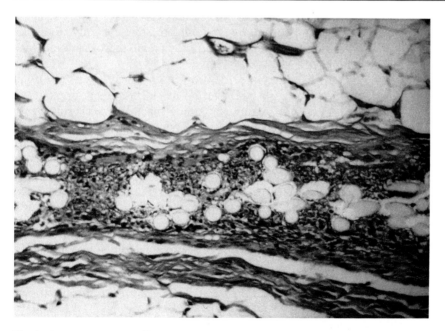

Fig. 8 *Tissue response to a filter with an average pore size of more than 5 μ, implanted in the subcutaneous space of the back of a dog for 20 days. The implant pores are filled with macrophages, and a granulation tissue capsule surrounds the implant (hematoxylin-eosin, × 200).*

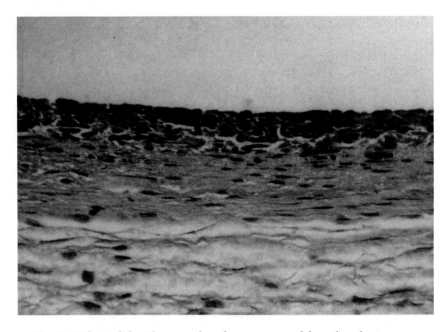

Fig. 9 *A Silastic disk with a smooth surface was removed from the subcutaneous space of the back of a rabbit after six weeks of implantation. A typical granulation tissue capsule is apparent (hematoxylin-eosin, × 300).*

range, fibrocytes and collagen were found to adhere tightly to the co-polymer surface. No tissue adhesion to the copolymer was found with the other micropore sizes.

When Silastic disk implants, identical in chemical composition but different in surface texture, were tested as subcutaneous implants in rabbits, the influence of texture on tissue reaction was verified with nonporous implants (Figs. 9 and 10) (E. Wu, J. Schmidt, and A.F. von Recum, unpublished data).

When human gingival or dermal fibroblasts were cultured on silicone (99.9% pure) disks with grooves etched into the surface (1 μ wide, 1 μ deep, and 1 μ apart), the cells spread over the entire surface and filled the grooves, achieving maximal surface contact and mechanical interlocking (Fig. 11).[6]

Mechanical Forces and Connective-Tissue Formation

Our observations of these and other implants strongly implied that mechanical forces are additional modifiers of connective-tissue formation.

Stiff, porous implants do not produce significant connective-tissue formation within the implant pores regardless of pore size (Fig. 12),

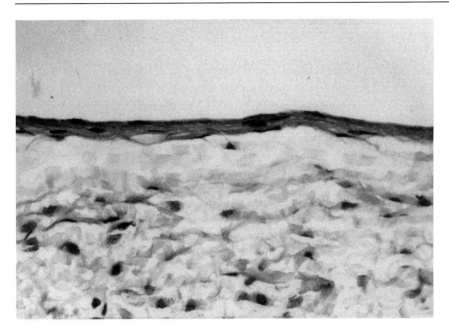

Fig. 10 *A Silastic disk with surface microtexture. A monolayer of fibrocytes coating the implant surface is the only histologically identifiable reaction (hematoxylin-eosin, × 300).*

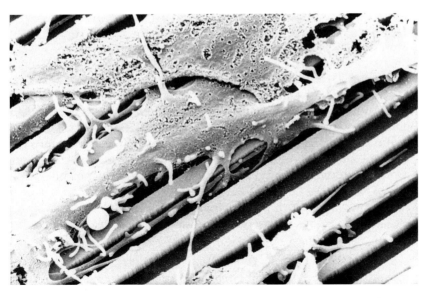

Fig. 11 *Surface electron micrograph of fibroblasts cultured on silicone disks with etched grooves, 1 μ deep and 1 μ apart. The cells conform to all surface changes within these dimensions. (Reproduced with permission from Meyle J, von Recum AF, Gibbesch B, et al: Fibroblast conformation to surface micromorphology.* Appl Biomater, *in press.)*

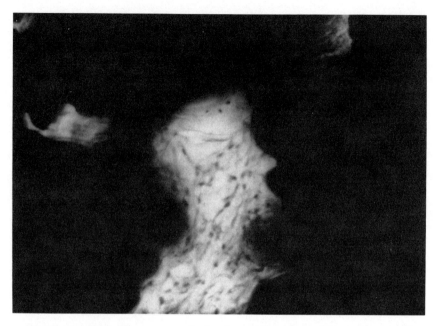

Fig. 12 *Connective-tissue response in the absence of mechanical forces. A very stiff, porous pure titanium implant was implanted for three months in the subcutaneous space of the back of a pig. A young-appearing loose granulation tissue can be seen with few, if any, macrophages. There is little evidence of fibrous tissue (hematoxylin-eosin, × 100).*

especially within the deeper pores, whereas very elastic porous implants allow connective-tissue formation if the pores are sufficiently large (Fig. 13).

Connective tissue cells appear not to cope well with interfacial micromotion.[7] In the absence of tissue attachment to the implant, micromotion appears to be responsible for tissue damage and, as a consequence, macrophages move onto and cover the material surface (see Fig. 1). Where cells attach firmly to the surface, collagen is manufactured right onto and even into the micropores of the implant surface (Fig. 14).

Consequences for Implant Development

The first goal is to provide a functional implant. The second goal must be to provide a safe implant that keeps undesirable side effects, including chronic inflammation, pressure necrosis, capsule contraction, and propensity for infection, to a minimum.

Macroporosity Clinical and experimental experience with macroporous soft-tissue implants have shown that macroporosity maintains chronic inflammation and may harbor bacteria for prolonged periods.

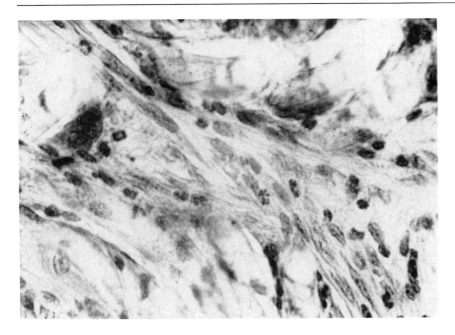

Fig. 13 *Connective-tissue response in the presence of mechanical forces. A very flexible polyester textile implant in the subcutaneous space of the back of the rabbit shows some connective tissue formation between the macrophage-lined polymer fibers (hematoxylin-eosin, × 300).*

Consequently, implant pore sizes of more than 5 μ should be avoided in nonresorbable implants.

Microtexture   Surface microtexture within an optimal range improves the quality and reduces the quantity of the tissue response, possibly because it prevents or significantly reduces micromotion at the implant-tissue interface (Fig. 14).

Mechanical Force Transfer   Tissue necrosis and resultant fibrosis of the tissue capsule can be generated by focal force concentrations. The implant should, therefore, be designed to avoid stress risers, and the implant's elastic modulus should be adjusted to the surrounding tissue whenever possible. Microtexture will then serve to distribute the stress over the entire tissue-implant interface equally and reduce the likelihood of pressure necrosis.

Competition With Bacterial Contaminants at the Interface   It has been observed that microtexture, including surface scratches, promotes cellular attachment of a variety of tissue cells,[8] but also attracts bacterial settlement. Fibroblasts and bacteria may, therefore, compete for attachment sites immediately after implantation. Conversely, once tissue attachment has been achieved, it effectively retards bacterial pro-

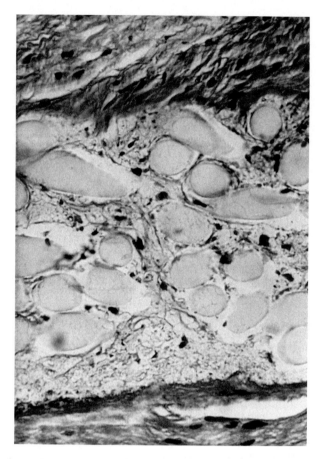

Fig. 14 *Filter with an average pore size of 2 μ, implanted into the subcutaneous space of the back of a dog for two weeks. Collagen is manufactured directly onto and even into the microporous copolymer surface (trichrome, × 300).*

gression on prosthetic surfaces.[9] This could mean that a microtextured surface can retard if not prevent interfacial bacterial contamination or the onset of infection.

Acknowledgments

Most of this review is based on the dissertations of the following graduate students to whose significant contributions the author is indebted: T. Gangjee, 1983; P.D. Schrenders, 1987; J.Y.J. Yan, 1986; C.E. Campbell, 1988; E. Wu, in progress; and J. Schmidt, in progress.

References

1. Gangjee T, Colaizzo R, von Recum AF: Species-related differences in percutaneous wound healing. *Ann Biomed Eng* 1985;13:451–467.
2. Schreuders PD, Salthouse TN, von Recum AF: Normal wound healing compared to healing within porous Dacron implants. *J Biomed Mater Res* 1988;22:121–135.
3. Yan JYJ, Cooke FW, Vaskelis PS, et al: Titanium-coated Dacron velour: A study of interfacial connective tissue formation. *J Biomed Mater Res* 1988;23:171–189.
4. Powers DL, Henricks ML, von Recum AF: Percutaneous healing of clinical tympanic membrane implants. *J Biomed Mater Res* 1986;20:143–151.
5. Campbell CE, von Recum AF: Microtopography and soft tissue response. *J Invest Surg* 1989;2:51–74.
6. Meyle J, von Recum AF, Gibbesch B, et al: Fibroblast conformation to surface micromorphology. *J Appl Biomater*, in press.
7. Kupp T, Hochman P, Hale J, et al: Effect of motion on polymer implant capsule formation in muscle, in Winter GD, Gibbons DF, Plenck H Jr (eds): *Biomaterials 1980*. New York, John Wiley & Sons, 1982, pp 787–797.
8. Burnett DM: Fibroblasts on micromachined substrata orient hierarchically to grooves of different dimensions. *Exp Cell Res* 1986;164:11–26.
9. Myojin K, von Recum AF: Experimental infections along subcutaneous conduits. *J Biomed Mater Res* 1978;12:557–570.

Chapter 15

The Relevance of Proteoglycans and Collagens of the Extracellular Matrix of Articular Cartilage in the Pathogenesis of Bacterial Arthritis

Lawrence C. Rosenberg, MD
David Eyre, PhD

Introduction

In the formation of articular cartilage, chondrocytes synthesize and secrete into the extracellular matrix a variety of macromolecules with elaborate structures. A tissue is formed that consists of relatively few cells distributed throughout an abundant extracellular matrix. The extracellular matrix gives articular cartilage special mechanical properties that are essential for the normal function of diarthrodial joints. These mechanical properties, in turn, are directly related to the structure and properties of the individual extracellular matrix macromolecules and to their interactions with one another.

The extracellular matrix is composed of proteoglycans, collagens, noncollagenous proteins, and water. Until recently, it was believed that the extracellular matrix of articular cartilage was composed primarily of large, aggregating cartilage proteoglycans (Fig. 1) and type II collagen. Type II collagen is an insoluble fibrous protein with tensile strength. The large aggregating cartilage proteoglycan is an elastic molecule that tends to expand in solution and resist compression into a smaller volume of solution. It was believed that the mechanical properties of normal articular cartilage depend on the properties of the fibrous composite formed when the large aggregating proteoglycan at high concentration is enmeshed in and constrained by a dense network of collagen fibers.

However, our understanding of the structure of articular cartilage is now rapidly changing. In the last several years, it has been learned that articular cartilage contains not only the large aggregating proteoglycan, but also two forms of small interstitial dermatan sulfate proteoglycans, which have important biochemical properties and biologic functions. In addition to type II collagen, articular cartilage also contains several other collagen types with quite different structures. Moreover, it is rapidly becoming apparent that there are a variety of interactions between these individual macromolecules, which include both noncovalent associations and the formation of covalent bonds between different collagen species.

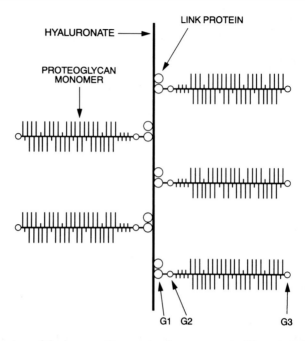

Fig. 1 *Structure of the large cartilage proteoglycan aggregate. The aggregate is formed by the noncovalent association of proteoglycan monomers, link protein, and hyaluronate. Many proteoglycan monomers bind to a single central filament of hyaluronate (central vertical line). The binding of a proteoglycan monomer to hyaluronate is mediated by the G1 globular domain of proteoglycan monomer core protein. Link protein binds simultaneously to G1 and hyaluronate and stabilizes the aggregate against dissociation.*

In the development of a bacterial infection, the attachment and adhesion of bacteria to a substratum is directly involved in the colonization and growth of the bacteria. *Staphylococcus aureus* and other bacteria possess receptors that mediate their adhesion to fibronectin,[1,2] collagens,[2,3] and other extracellular matrix macromolecules. The questions concerning which collagen types in articular cartilage provide substrata for bacterial adhesion, and what domains and amino acid sequences within these domains mediate the binding of bacterial cell-wall receptors, are of basic importance to an understanding of the biochemical mechanisms involved in the development of bacterial arthritis.

In bacterial arthritis, proteoglycans that contribute to the elastic properties of articular cartilage are degraded by proteolytic enzymes and lost from the cartilage extracellular matrix. This degradation of proteoglycans is a central event in the pathogenesis of bacterial arthritis.[4]

This chapter describes the structures of the collagens and proteoglycans in articular cartilage, the interactions between these macromolecules, and their biologic functions.

The Large, Aggregating Cartilage Proteoglycan

Large proteoglycan aggregates are major components of the extracellular matrix of articular cartilage.[5-8] The aggregates are formed by the noncovalent association of proteoglycan monomers, link protein, and hyaluronate.[9-11] In an aggregate, many proteoglycan monomers bind at regular intervals to a single central filament of hyaluronic acid, as shown in Figure 1. Link protein strongly stabilizes the binding of each proteoglycan monomer by binding simultaneously to proteoglycan monomer and hyaluronate.[12-16]

The large, aggregating cartilage proteoglycan monomer, which is initially synthesized and secreted into extracellular matrix, contains a core protein with a molecular weight of approximately 200,000 to which are attached many chondroitin sulfate and keratan sulfate chains. The molecular weight of the proteoglycan monomer initially synthesized and secreted into the extracellular matrix of articular cartilage is approximately 2.5×10^6. When proteoglycan aggregates are formed in extracellular matrix by the noncovalent association of proteoglycan monomers, link protein, and hyaluronate, the size of an individual aggregate is determined primarily by the length and molecular weight of the hyaluronate chain, which in turn determines the numbers of proteoglycan monomers that become bound to hyaluronate in a particular aggregate. However, a typical representative proteoglycan aggregate in articular cartilage has 20 proteoglycan monomers bound at 25-nm intervals to a hyaluronate chain 500 nm in length, and a molecular weight of approximately 50×10^6.[7,8]

Because of the repelling forces of the closely spaced sulfate and carboxylate groups on chondroitin sulfate and keratan sulfate chains, proteoglycans tend to occupy a relatively large volume of solution, and they expand in solution until they are constrained by the surrounding dense network of collagen fibrils. It is this swelling pressure of the proteoglycan aggregates and the constraining influence of the collagen network that give articular cartilage its elastic properties.[17-19] In pyogenic arthritis, bacterial proteases cleave proteoglycan monomer core protein and shatter the proteoglycan aggregate into fragments; when this happens, articular cartilage loses its normal elastic properties.

In recent years, studies of the large, aggregating proteoglycan monomer have focused particularly on the structure of the proteoglycan monomer core protein and its globular domains, which mediate the binding of proteoglycan monomer to hyaluronate and link protein and also serve other functions.

The complete amino acid sequence of proteoglycan monomer core protein of Swarm rat chondrosarcoma has been deduced from cDNA sequences by Doege and associates.[20] The name given to the large, aggregating cartilage proteoglycan monomer was aggrecan.

Aggrecan contains three globular domains, G1, G2, and G3 (Fig. 2). G1 is located at the NH_2-terminus, consists of 331 amino acids (molecular weight, 37,000), and mediates the binding of the proteoglycan monomer to hyaluronate and link protein. G1 is separated from G2

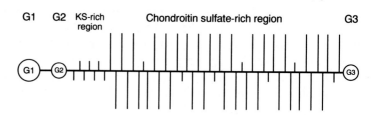

Fig. 2 *Structure of the large aggregating cartilage proteoglycan monomer, which has been called aggrecan.*

by an interglobular domain, which consists of 135 amino acids (molecular weight, 14,000). G2 consists of 200 amino acids (molecular weight, 22,000). G2 apparently does not bind to hyaluronic acid or link protein. The function of G2 is not known.

The third globular domain, G3, is located at the COOH-terminus of the proteoglycan monomer core protein, consists of 222 amino acids (molecular weight, 26,000), and is homologous with a hepatic lectin that binds nonreducing terminal N-acetylglucosamine residues.[21] The function of G3 in articular cartilage is not known.

As shown in Figure 2, the regions rich in keratan sulfate and chondroitin sulfate are located between the G2 and G3 globular domains. The region rich in keratan sulfate contains a short peptide that consists of 113 amino acids (molecular weight, 12,000). The region rich in chondroitin sulfate consists of 1,104 amino acids and contains 117 sequences containing serine-glycine that provide attachment sites for chondroitin sulfate and keratan sulfate chains.

Since the G1 globular domain of proteoglycan monomer core protein mediates the binding of proteoglycan monomer to hyaluronate and link protein, it is clear that G1 is directly involved in the assembly of the cartilage proteoglycan aggregate. To study the binding function of G1, investigators have isolated fragments containing the 37-kd G1 peptide after trypsin degradation of proteoglycan aggregates. Proteolytic enzymes such as trypsin cleave most of proteoglycan monomer core protein, particularly the region rich in chondroitin sulfate, into small fragments,[22] but the G1 domain and link protein, which are bound to each other and to hyaluronate (Fig. 1), are not degraded and are left essentially intact. G1 isolated after the trypsin digestion of proteoglycan aggregates contains both N-linked oligosaccharides and keratan sulfate chains, and is frequently isolated as a glycopeptide with a molecular weight of approximately 65,000. Until recently, glycosylated G1 fragments of this kind were called the hyaluronic-acid-binding region of proteoglycan monomer core protein.[22–24]

As noted, link protein stabilizes the proteoglycan aggregate against dissociation by binding simultaneously to hyaluronate and to the G1 globular domain of proteoglycan monomer core protein.[12–16] Because

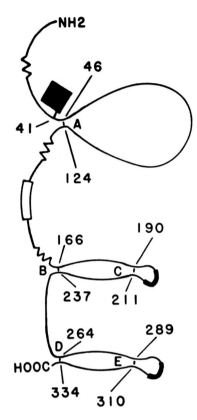

Fig. 3 *Locations of the disulfide bonds, tandem repeats, and immunoglobulin fold in link protein. The numbers refer to the positions of cysteine residues. (Reproduced with permission from Neame PJ, Christner JE, Balker JR: The primary structure of link protein from rat chondrosarcoma proteoglycan aggregate.* J Biol Chem *1986;261:3519–3535.)*

G1 and link protein each bind to hyaluronate in the formation of a proteoglycan aggregate, some degree of similarity or homology in the amino acid sequences of G1 and link protein might be expected, and indeed this is the case.

The complete amino acid sequence of link protein has to be determined.[25–28] Neame and associates[25] have shown that link protein from Swarm rat chondrosarcoma is a single peptide (molecular weight, 38,564) of 339 amino acids. Five disulfide bonds result in the formation of three loops or domains (Fig. 3). The loop nearest the NH$_2$-terminus between Cys[46] and Cys[124] forms a domain which contains the peptide that mediates the binding of link protein to G1. Two loops toward the COOH-terminus between Cys[166] and Cys[334] form domains that mediate the binding of link protein to hyaluronate. These two loops are highly homologous and have been called the link protein tandem repeats. The amino acid sequence of the G1 globular domain of proteoglycan monomer core protein is very similar to that of link protein. G1 contains two tandem repeats that show extensive homology with those of link protein.[29] These are the domains within G1 that mediate the binding of G1 to hyaluronate. The NH_2-terminus of G1 contains an immunoglobulin fold domain similar to that in link protein.[30,31] However, the degree of homology of this NH_2-terminal in G1 and link protein is much less extensive. The immunoglobulin fold domains of G1 and link protein must contain the peptides that mediate the binding of link protein and G1 to one another.

As noted, when the proteoglycan aggregate is degraded by proteolytic enzymes, the region rich in chondroitin sulfate of the proteoglycan monomer is shattered into fragments, but the central portion of the aggregate (Fig. 1), which consists of G1, link protein, and hyaluronate noncovalently associated with one another, is resistant to proteolytic degradation. Whether proteoglycan aggregates are degraded in this fashion in bacterial arthritis, and whether the central complex consisting of G1, link protein, and hyaluronate provides a substratum for bacterial adhesion that facilitates colonization and growth remain to be determined.

The Small, Interstitial Dermatan Sulfate Proteoglycans

Articular cartilage contains two forms of small interstitial dermatan sulfate proteoglycans called DS-PGI (biglycan) and DS-PGII (decorin).[32,33] Analogous forms of these proteoglycans have been isolated from several other connective tissues.[34-40] The amino acid sequences of biglycan and decorin have been determined.[41-44] Native intact articular cartilage biglycan has a molecular weight of 100,000 and a core protein with a molecular weight of 37,280. Two dermatan sulfate chains (molecular weight, 30,000) are attached to serine residues at positions 5 and 11 at the NH_2-terminus of the protein core. Native intact decorin has a molecular weight of 67,000 and a core protein with a molecular weight of 36,383. A single dermatan sulfate chain is attached to the serine residue at position 4.

Analogous proteoglycans from different tissues such as skin, cartilage, and bone possess the same core protein with an identical amino acid sequence, but contain glycosaminoglycan chains that differ greatly in their iduronic acid content. Thus, skin and cartilage decorin carry dermatan sulfate chains with 85% and 40% iduronic acid,[33] respectively, whereas bone decorin carries chondroitin sulfate chains that contain only glucuronic acid and no iduronic acid residues. These differences in glycosaminoglycan chain structure must be regulated by tissue-specific mechanisms. Some of the biologic activities of these two proteoglycans are directly related to the iduronic acid content of their dermatan sulfate chains. However, the significance of the dramatic difference in glycosaminoglycan chain structure in different tissues has only recently been appreciated and is not understood.

Dermatan sulfate proteoglycans are multifunctional molecules that bind to collagens, fibronectin, growth factors, and a variety of other macromolecules. The noncovalent association of a dermatan sulfate proteoglycan with another macromolecule may be mediated by the binding of the core protein to the protein moiety of the second macromolecule, by the binding of the second macromolecule to the glycosaminoglycan chains of a dermatan sulfate proteoglycan, or by both. The binding of the dermatan sulfate proteoglycan affects the biochemical properties and biologic functions of the second macromolecule. The dermatan sulfate proteoglycans appear to regulate, augment, or inhibit the biologic functions of other macromolecules.

Localization of the Dermatan Sulfate Proteoglycans in Extracellular Matrix

The distribution of decorin and biglycan in developing fetal tissues has been examined.[45,46] To the best of our knowledge, there has been no immunohistochemical or electron microscopic study of the distribution and localization of decorin and biglycan in postnatal and mature articular cartilage and the changes in the localization and concentration of these molecules with aging. In fetal tissues, biglycan appears to be localized in the cell surface of a variety of cell types, whereas decorin is distributed throughout the extracellular matrix of tissues, both in the spaces between collagen fibrils and on the surfaces of collagen fibrils.

Poole and associates[45] described the immunohistochemical localization of decorin in developing bovine fetal epiphyseal cartilage. In bovine fetal epiphyseal cartilage, decorin was uniformly and widely distributed throughout the epiphyseal cartilage. Postnatally, at 10 months and 18 months, decorin was concentrated primarily at the articular surface; it was no longer uniformly distributed through the extracellular matrix of the epiphyseal cartilage, but was distributed in a splotchy fashion in the pericellular matrix of chondrocytes and in the interterritorial matrix.

Bianco and associates[46] compared the localization of biglycan and decorin in human fetal epiphyseal and articular cartilage, growth plate cartilage, and other tissues. Antibodies were prepared to synthetic peptides corresponding to the nonhomologous amino acid sequences in the NH_2-terminal regions of decorin and biglycan core proteins. Specifically, a rabbit antiserum LF-15 was raised against a synthetic peptide corresponding to amino acid residues 11 to 24 of biglycan, and a rabbit antiserum LF-30 was raised against a synthetic peptide corresponding to residues five to 17 of human decorin. Immunohistochemical studies of the cartilage of the bones of the hand of 14- to 17-week-old human fetuses were then examined. The articular surface of the developing epiphysis stained heavily for biglycan but not for decorin, whereas the epiphyseal cartilage below the surface stained heavily for decorin but only weakly for biglycan. In the growth plate, decorin and biglycan were present around cells and in the extracellular matrix of the zone of proliferating chondrocytes, but neither biglycan nor decorin was present in the extracellular matrix of the hypertrophic zone or in the spicules of calcified cartilage. Poole and associates[45] also noted that decorin disappeared from the extracellular matrix of the hypertrophic zone and calcified cartilage.

Electron microscopic studies have shown that dermatan sulfate proteoglycans are localized on the surfaces of collagen fibrils.[47-52] In tendon stained with cupromeronic blue, dermatan sulfate proteoglycans on the surface of collagen fibrils appear as densely stained elongated filaments disposed in two different orientations. Some of the dermatan sulfate proteoglycans are randomly oriented and appear to form a network on the surface of the collagen fibril. Other dermatan sulfate proteoglycans are transversely oriented, at right angles to the long axis of the fibril. The transversely oriented dermatan sulfate proteoglycan filaments are spaced at regular intervals at the d bands of the collagen fibril.[49]

In addition to these electron microscopic studies, which demonstrate an ultrastructural association of the dermatan sulfate proteoglycans with collagen fibrils, biochemical studies have shown that decorin binds to collagen fibrils.

For example, Brown and Vogel[53] examined the binding of decorin from bovine tendon to type I collagen fibrils. Native soluble collagen with intact telopeptides was prepared from bovine tendon by extraction with acetic acid. Decorin labeled with radioactive sulfur dioxide was prepared from the medium of cell cultures from bovine fetal tendon, grown in the presence of radioactive sulfur dioxide. The binding of native intact decorin, its core protein, and its free glycosaminoglycan chains to the type I collagen were compared. Decorin was mixed with type I collagen before fibrillogenesis was initiated. The mixtures were then incubated at 37 C to induce fibrillogenesis. After 24 hours, when fibrillogenesis was complete, the collagen fibrils were sedimented by centrifugation, and the amounts of unbound decorin in the supernatant and bound decorin associated with the sedimented collagen fibrils were determined. Similar studies were carried out using pepsin-solubilized collagen and preformed fibrils formed from native intact soluble collagen with intact telopeptides. In each case, the results were essentially the same.

Both intact decorin and its core protein bound to type I collagen fibrils. Free glycosaminoglycan chains did not bind to a significant degree. The binding of the decorin to type I collagen was maximal at an ionic strength of 0.05 to 0.15, and the proteoglycan was not dissociated by increasing the salt concentration to 2 M.

Scatchard plot analysis of one experiment using type I collagen with intact telopeptides yielded a linear plot and a K_a of $3.3 \times 10^7 M^{-1}$, and indicated 0.054 decorin binding sites per collagen monomer, suggesting that a collagen fibril consisting of 20 collagen monomers binds one molecule of decorin. Experiments using pepsin-solubilized type I collagen yielded similar plots and values for K_a, suggesting that collagen telopeptides are not involved in the binding of decorin to type I col-

Table 1 Collagen types in adult articular cartilage*

Molecules	Molecular Formula	% of Total Collagen	Distribution
Fibril-forming			
Type II	[α1(II)]₃	95	Throughout
Type XI/V	[α1(XI)α2(XI)α3(XI)]	3	Throughout
Short-helix			
Type VI	[α1(VI)α2(VI)α3(VI)]	0 to 1	May be concentrated pericellularly
Type IX	[α1(IX)α2(IX)α3(IX)]	1	Throughout
Type X	[α1(X)]₃	1	Zone of calcified cartilage only

*Based on analyses of bovine articular cartilage. (Reproduced with permission from Eyre DR, Wu J-J, Apone S: A growing family of collagens in articular cartilage: Identification of 5 genetically distinct types. *J Rheumatol* 1987;14(suppl 14):25–27.)

lagen. However, in other experiments, somewhat different results were obtained. When the decorin concentration was extended over a much lower range, Scatchard plots suggested the presence of two types of binding sites, one with a $K_a = 2.1 \times 10^7 M^{-1}$ and the other with a $K_a = 3 \times 10^7 M^{-1}$. Additional experiments indicated that decorin does not bind to type I collagen with intact telopeptides.

Dermatan Sulfate Proteoglycans Inhibit the Attachment of Cells to Fibronectin and Other Substrata

Studies from several laboratories indicate that dermatan sulfate proteoglycans inhibit the attachment of cells to fibronectin and/or the cell-binding domain of fibronectin.[54–58] Because dermatan sulfate proteoglycans bind to and cover specific regions on the surface of collagen fibrils, one must ask whether dermatan sulfate proteoglycans shield cell adhesion sites on the surfaces of collagen fibrils, inhibiting the adhesion of both eukaryotic cells and bacteria to the attachment sites on collagen fibrils. If this is the case, degradation of dermatan sulfate proteoglycans may be an important step in the biochemical mechanism involved in the bacterial adhesion that occurs in bacterial arthritis.

Cartilage Collagens

The different genetic types of collagen identified in articular cartilage are listed in Table 1.[59] Type II collagen is the most abundant and forms the basic framework of the extracellular matrix. However, a number of other molecular species of collagen have been identified in cartilage in recent years. Types IX and XI are especially notable in that they are also cartilage-specific proteins that are co-expressed with type II collagen. Growing evidence points to an intimate copolymerization and covalent interaction among collagen types II, IX, and XI in cartilage matrix.

Type II Collagen

The type II collagen molecule is a homotrimer of α1(II) chains, the product of the COL2A1 gene. Its molecular dimensions and polymeric

213

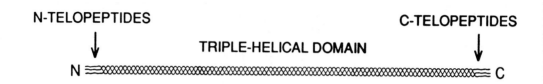

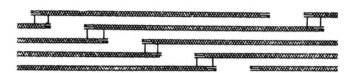

Fig. 4 *Structure of the type II collagen molecule (**top**) and its cross-linked polymer, the 67–nm periodic fibril (**bottom**). All class I collagens (types I, II, III, V, and XI) have these basic molecular and fibrillar forms.*

form, a 67–nm repeat banded fibril by electron microscopy, resemble closely those of the other major class I fibril-forming collagens, types I and III (Fig. 4).

The tensile strength of the collagen then depends on intermolecular cross-linking. The principal cross-linking residues in the mature fibril are hydroxylysyl pyridinoline residues.[60] These trivalent cross-links form by a further reaction of the divalent ketoamines that are the initial products of lysyl oxidase-mediated cross-linking in growing cartilage.

With development and maturation of cartilage tissue, the diameter of the type II fibrils increases from less than 20 nm in fetal tissue to a range of 50 to 100 nm or more in adult human articular cartilage.[50,61] The diameters remain thin, however, in the uppermost tangential zone of the tissue where the fibrils lie primarily parallel to the plane of the articular surface. The collagen fibrillar network provides a cohesive framework in which the large, aggregating proteoglycans (aggrecans) are entrapped and to which the small proteoglycans (decorin and biglycan) appear to bind specifically.[47-53]

It was shown recently that two forms of COL2A1 mRNA are apparently expressed by variable splicing of the primary transcript. One contains and the other lacks the cysteine-rich exon 2 coding domain.[62] These appear to be differentially expressed in different tissue during development. The functions of these splicing variants are not yet known.

There is a growing evidence that type IX collagen and possibly type XI collagen contribute critically to the organization and mechanical stability of the type II collagen fibrillar network.

N-PROPEPTIDE

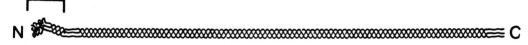

Fig. 5 *Structure of the type XI collagen molecule. Unlike type I and II collagen molecules, the N-propeptide domain is retained in the functioning molecule in the extracellular matrix.*

Type XI Collagen

Type XI collagen was originally discovered in a salt-precipitated fraction (1.2 M sodium chloride) of pepsin-solubilized cartilage collagen.[63] Three distinct α chains were resolved: α1(XI) (initially called 1α), α2(XI) (2α), and α3(XI) (3α) in a ratio of 1:1:1. The α3(XI) chain is indistinguishable in primary sequence from α1(II).[64] The α1(XI) chain shows close sequence homology to α1(V) but is, nevertheless, a distinct gene product; α2(XI) is also a distinct gene product. The three chains probably form primarily a heterotrimeric native molecule of composition [α1(XI)α2(XI)α3(XI)], at least in young cartilage, though a spectrum of chain combinations is possible.

The functioning molecule in the extracellular matrix retains its N-propeptide extensions judging by sodium dodecyl sulfate-polyacrylamide gel electrophoresis of neutral salt and denaturant extracts of cartilage.[65] As with the other class I collagens, the N-propeptide sequences of α1(XI) and α2(XI) include a short segment of triple helix (GlyXY) and an amino terminal noncollagenous domain (Fig. 5). Retention of the N-propeptide may prevent the growth of fibrils laterally.

Type XI collagen seems to be the equivalent protein, in cartilages based on type II collagen, to type V collagen in tissues based on type I collagen. The situation is more complicated, however. During the maturation of articular cartilage, the type XI collagen fraction contains an increasing concentration of the α1(V) chain, apparently at the expense of α1(XI).[64] By contrast, in bone the α1(XI) chain accumulates in the type V collagen fraction at the expense of α1(V) with increasing age from fetal to adult bone.[66] The significance of these apparent developmental switches in gene expression from α1(XI) to α1(V) and vice versa is unknown. The stoichiometry of α-chain yields implies the existence of hybrid heterotrimeric molecules in which α1(V) and α1(XI) can be substituted for each other.

In adult articular cartilage, therefore, type XI collagen may consist of more than one molecular species assembled from the various chain types in the collagen XI/V family of gene products.

Type XI collagen is clearly polymerized and cross-linked by the lysyl oxidase mechanism, but even in mature tissue the cross-links seem to remain as immature divalent ketoamines.[67]

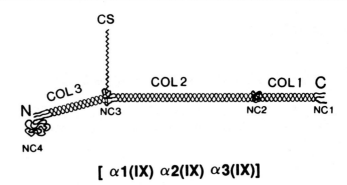

$$[\ \alpha1(IX)\ \ \alpha2(IX)\ \ \alpha3(IX)]$$

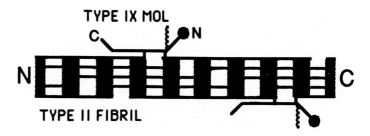

Fig. 6 *Domain structure of the type IX collagen molecule (**top**). Most molecules function in the extracellular matrix in covalent linkage to the surface of type II collagen fibrils (**bottom**).*

Type IX Collagen

Type IX collagen accounts for about 1% of the collagenous protein in adult mammalian articular cartilage but 10% or more in fetal cartilage, the amount decreasing with increasing cartilage maturity.[68] It is a proteoglycan and a collagen. The molecule has a single site of attachment for a chondroitin sulfate chain on the α2(IX) chain in the NC3 domain, shown by chemical analysis[69] and by predictions from the chick α2(IX) cDNA sequence.[70,71] All molecules of type IX collagen may not bear chondroitin sulfate chains, however. The molecule is a heterotrimer of three distinct gene products, α1(IX), α2(IX), α3(IX). It consists of three triple-helical domains, COL 1, COL 2, and COL 3 (Fig. 6). The α1(IX) chain is expressed in different forms in different tissues as a result of variable mRNA splicing.[72]

Cross-linking sites have been identified in the COL 2 domain to which the telopeptides of type II collagen can covalently attach.[73,74] One site is within a few amino acid residues of the N-terminus of COL 2. All three chains in this domain have at least one hydroxylysine residue to which the α1(II) N-telopeptide cross-linking sequence can attach.[75] In addition, an $\alpha1(II)$ N-telopeptide attachment site is located farther into the COL 2 triple helix but only in $\alpha3(IX)$. The stoichiometric yield of cross-linked peptides indicates that essentially every type IX collagen molecule in fetal or adult bovine articular cartilage can be covalently linked through at least one site to molecules of type II collagen. The chemistry of the cross-linking is similar to that between type II collagen molecules, with ketoamines formed initially that mature to hydroxypyridinium residues. Moreover, the aldehyde precursors originate in the type II collagen telopeptides, which interact with the above specific triple-helix sites in type IX collagen. Electron microscopy has shown that molecules of type IX collagen decorate the surface of type II collagen fibrils in chick cartilage.[76]

In summary, the findings imply that type IX collagen provides a covalent interface between the surface of the type II collagen fibril and the interfibrillar proteoglycan domain. It has also been proposed[66,77] that type IX collagen provides covalent links between type II collagen fibrils that could enhance the mechanical stability of the network and help prevent the entrapped large, aggregating proteoglycans from swelling it.

Recent work has shown that the matrix metalloproteinase, stromelysin, can cleave the type IX collagen molecule through its NC2 domain,[78,79] and can also cleave type II collagen molecules at sites just within their telopeptide cross-linking residues. This protease, which is expressed by chondrocytes and other connective tissue cells when stimulated by interleukin-1, has the potential, therefore, to strip type IX collagen molecules from the surface of type II collagen fibrils. Recent experiments also show that stromelysin treatment causes the collagen network of articular cartilage to swell.[79] Its potential role as a collagenolytic enzyme in the normal remodeling of cartilage and in cartilage degradation in disease clearly needs further study.

Type X Collagen

Collagen type X is another short-helix collagen molecule that consists of a single triple-helix domain with a globular C-terminal extension and shorter nonhelical sequences at the N-terminus.[80,81] It is restricted in expression to the hypertrophic zone of the growth plates of growing animals and the deep calcified layer of mature articular cartilages. The molecule is a homotrimer, $[\alpha1(X)]_3$. Its polymeric form is as yet undefined, but the $\alpha1(X)$ protein sequence is closely homologous to that of type VIII collagen,[82] which forms a distinctive hexagonal lattice in Descemet's membrane of the eye and in other endothelial basal laminae.

The content of type X collagen in the calcified zone of articular cartilage is about 1% of the total collagen. The main framework of the extracellular matrix consists of types II, IX, and XI collagens as in uncalcified cartilage.

Type VI Collagen

Collagen type VI, another short-helix collagen molecule, is widely distributed in small amounts in most types of connective tissue.[83] Small

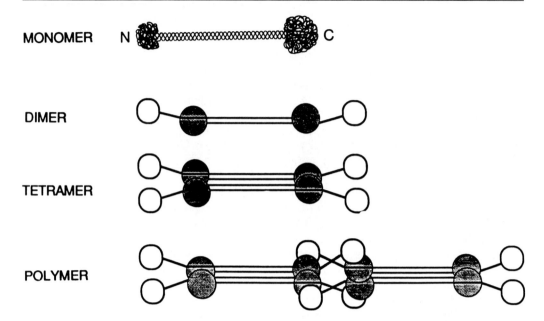

Fig. 7 *Structures of the type VI collagen molecule and its dimer, tetramer, and polymer.*

amounts of the protein can be extracted from articular cartilage. It forms a distinctive microfibril, aggregates of which can present a 100–nm periodicity (Fig. 7).

Type VI collagen molecules form disulfide-bonded tetramers, but do not appear to form the aldehydic cross-links that are characteristic of the other collagen types. The protein can largely be extracted from tissue by denaturing solvents.[84] Three distinct chains, α1(VI), α2(VI), and α3(VI), have been characterized at the protein and gene levels. There is evidence for variable splicing of the α2(VI) and α3(VI) mRNAs,[85] so tissue-specific forms of the molecule may exist. There are also several arginine-glycine-aspartic acid (RGD) sequences in each chain,[86] implying cell-binding properties. Enrichment, pericellularly around the chondrocytes, of articular cartilage has been reported.[87] Increased amounts of type VI collagen have been found in articular cartilage in an experimental model of osteoarthrosis.[88]

References

1. Yamada KM: Fibronectin domains and receptors, in Mosher DF (ed): *Fibronectin.* San Diego, Academic Press, 1989, pp 47–121.
2. Hook M, Switalski LM, Wadstrom T, et al: Interactions of pathogenic microorganisms with fibronectin, in Mosher DF (ed): *Fibronectin.* San Diego, Academic Press, 1989, pp 295–308.
3. Mayne R, Burgeson RE (eds): *Structure and Function of Collagen Types.* Orlando, Academic Press, 1987.

4. Smith RL, Schurman DJ: Biochemical mechanisms underlying cartilage destruction in infectious arthritis, in Ewing JW (ed): *Bristol-Myers/Zimmer Orthopaedic Symposium: Articular Cartilage and Knee Joint Function: Basic Science and Arthroscopy.* New York, Raven Press, 1990, pp 197–211.

5. Hascall VC: Proteoglycans: The chondroitin sulfate/keratan sulfate proteoglycan of cartilage, in *ISI Atlas of Science: Biochemistry. Volume I.* 1988, pp 189–198.

6. Hascall VC, Kimura JH: Proteoglycans: Isolation and characterization. *Methods Enzymol* 1982;82:769–800.

7. Rosenberg LC, Hellmann W, Kleinschmidt AK: Electron microscopic studies of proteoglycan aggregates from bovine articular cartilage. *J Biol Chem* 1975;250:1877–1883.

8. Buckwalter JA, Rosenberg LC: Electron microscopic studies of cartilage proteoglycans: Direct evidence for the variable length of the chondroitin sulfate-rich region of proteoglycan subunit core protein. *J Biol Chem* 1982;257:9830–9839.

9. Hardingham TE, Muir H: The specific interaction of hyaluronic acid with cartilage proteoglycans. *Biochim Biophys Acta* 1972;279:401–405.

10. Hascall VC, Heinegård D: Aggregation of cartilage proteoglycans: I. The role of hyaluronic acid. *J Biol Chem* 1974;249:4232–4241.

11. Hardingham TE, Muir H: Hyaluronic acid in cartilage and proteoglycan aggregation. *Biochem J* 1974;139:565–581.

12. Hardingham TE: The role of link-protein in the structure of cartilage proteoglycan aggregates. *Biochem J* 1979;177:237–247.

13. Tang L-H, Rosenberg LC, Reiner A, et al: Proteoglycans from bovine nasal cartilage: Properties of a soluble form of link protein. *J Biol Chem* 1979;254:10523–10531.

14. Choi HU, Tang L-H, Johnson TL, et al: Proteoglycans from bovine nasal and articular cartilages: Fractionation of the link proteins by wheat germ agglutinin affinity chromatography. *J Biol Chem* 1985;260:13370–13376.

15. Tang L-H, Rosenberg LC, Reihanian H, et al: Proteoglycans from bovine fetal epiphyseal cartilage: Sedimentation velocity and light scattering studies of the effect of link protein on proteglycan aggregate size and stability. *Connect Tissue Res* 1989;19:177–193.

16. Rosenberg LC, Tang L-H, Pal S, et al: Proteoglycans of bovine articular cartilage: Studies of the direct interaction of link protein with hyaluronate in the absence of proteoglycan monomer. *J Biol Chem* 1988;26:18071–18077.

17. Hardingham TE, Muir H, Kwan MK, et al: Viscoelastic properties of proteoglycan solutions with varying proportions present as aggregates. *J Orthop Res* 1987;5:36–46.

18. Mow VC, Mak AF, Lai WM, et al: Viscoelastic properties of proteoglycan subunits and aggregates in varying solution concentrations. *J Biomech* 1984;17:325–338.

19. Maroudas A: Physicochemical properties of articular cartilage, in Freeman MAR (ed): *Adult Articular cartilage*, ed 2. Kent, England, Pitman Medical Publishing, 1979, pp 215–290.

20. Doege K, Sasaki M, Horigan E, et al: Complete primary structure of the rat cartilage proteoglycan core protein deduced from cDNA clones. *J Biol Chem* 1987;262:17757–17767.

21. Halberg DF, Proulx G, Doege K, et al: A segment of the cartilage proteoglycan core protein has lectin-like activity. *J Biol Chem* 1988;263:9486–9490.

22. Heinegård D, Hascall VC: Aggregation of cartilage proteoglycans: III. Characteristics of the proteins isolated from trypsin digests of aggregates. *J Biol Chem* 1974;249:4250–4256.

23. Bonnet F, Dunham DG, Hardingham TE: Structure and interactions of cartilage proteoglycan binding region and link protein. *Biochem J* 1985;228:77–85.

24. Perkins SJ, Miller A, Hardingham TE, et al: Physical properties of the hyaluronate binding region of proteoglycan from pig laryngeal cartilage: Densitometric and small-angle neutron scattering studies of carbohydrates and carbohydrate-protein macromolecules. *J Mol Biol* 1981;150:69–95.

25. Neame PJ, Christner JE, Baker JR: The primary structure of link protein from rat chondrosarcoma proteoglycan aggregate. *J Biol Chem* 1986;261;3519–3535.

26. Déak F, Kiss I, Sparks KJ, et al: Complete amino acid sequence of chicken cartilage link protein deduced from cDNA clones. *Proc Natl Acad Sci USA* 1986;83:3766–3770.

27. Doege K, Hassell JR, Caterson B, et al: Link protein cDNA sequence reveals a tandemly repeated protein structure. *Proc Natl Acad Sci USA* 1986;83:3761–3765.

28. Rhodes C, Doege K, Sasaki M, et al: Alternative splicing generates two different mRNA species for rat link protein. *J Biol Chem* 1988;263:6063–6067.

29. Neame PJ, Périn J-P, Bonnet F, et al: An amino acid sequence common to both cartilage proteoglycan and link protein. *J Biol Chem* 1985;260:12402–12404.

30. Bonnet F, Périn J-P, Lorenzo F, et al: An unexpected sequence homology between link proteins of the proteoglycan complex and immunoglobulin-like proteins. *Biochim Biophys Acta* 1986;873:152–155.

31. Perkins SJ, Nealis AS, Dudhia J, et al: Immunoglobulin fold and tandem repeat structures in proteoglycan N-terminal domains and link protein. *J Mol Biol* 1989;206:737–753.

32. Rosenberg LC, Choi HU, Tang L-H, et al: Isolation of dermatan sulfate proteoglycans from mature bovine articular cartilages. *J Biol Chem* 1985;260:6304–6313.

33. Choi HU, Johnson TL, Pal S, et al: Characterization of the dermatan sulfate proteoglycans, DS-PGI and DS-PGII, from bovine articular cartilage and skin isolation by octyl-sepharose chromatography. *J Biol Chem* 1989;264:2876–2884.

34. Vogel KG, Fisher LW: Comparisons of antibody reactivity and enzyme sensitivity between small proteoglycans from bovine tendon, bone, and cartilage. *J Biol Chem* 1986;261:11334–11340.

35. Vogel KG, Evanko SP: Proteoglycans of fetal bovine tendon. *J Biol Chem* 1987;262:13607–13613.

36. Fisher LW, Hawkins GR, Tuross N, et al: Purification and partial characterization of small proteoglycans I and II, bone sialoproteins I and II, and osteonectin from the mineral compartment of developing human bone. *J Biol Chem* 1987;262:9702–9708.

37. Sampaio L de O, Bayliss MT, Hardingham TE, et al: Dermatan sulphate proteoglycan from human articular cartilage: Variation in its content with age and its structural comparison with a small chondroitin sulphate proteoglycan from pig laryngeal cartilage. *Biochem J* 1988;254:757–764.

38. Simionescu D, Iozzo RV, Kefalides NA: Bovine pericardial proteoglycan: Biochemical, immunochemical, and ultrastructural studies. *Matrix* 1989;9:301–310.

39. Scott PG, Nakano T, Dodd CM, et al: Proteoglycans of the articular disc of the bovine temporomandibular joint: II. Low molecular weight dermatan sulphate proteoglycan. *Matrix* 1989;9:284–292.

40. Fedarko NS, Termine JD, Young MF, et al: Temporal regulation of hyaluronan and proteoglycan metabolism by human bone cells in vitro. *J Biol Chem* 1990;265:12200–12209.

41. Fisher LW, Termine JD, Young MF: Deduced protein sequence of bone small proteoglycan I (biglycan) shows homology with proteoglycan II (decorin) and several nonconnective tissue proteins in a variety of species. *J Biol Chem* 1989;264:4571–4576.

42. Neame PJ, Choi HU, Rosenberg LC: The primary structure of the core protein of the small, leucine-rich proteoglycan (PGI) from bovine articular cartilage. *J Biol Chem* 1989;264:8653–8661.

43. Krusius T, Ruoslahti E: Primary structure of an extracellular matrix proteoglycan core protein deduced from cloned cDNA. *Proc Natl Acad Sci USA* 1986;83:7683–7687.

44. Day AA, McQuillan CI, Termine JD, et al: Molecular cloning and sequence analysis of the cDNA for small proteoglycan II of bovine bone. *Biochem J* 1987;248:801–805.

45. Poole AR, Webber C, Pidoux I, et al: Localization of a dermatan sulfate proteoglycan (DS-PGII) in cartilage and the presence of an immunologically related species in other tissues. *J Histochem Cytochem* 1986;34:619–625.

46. Bianco P, Fisher LW, Young MF, et al: Expression and localization of the small proteoglycans biglycan and decorin in developing human skeletal and nonskeletal tissues. *J Histochem Cytochem* 1990;38:1549–1563.

47. Scott JE: Collagen-proteoglycan interactions: Localization of proteoglycans in tendon by electron microscopy. *Biochem J* 1980;187:887–891.

48. Scott JE, Orford CR, Hughes EW: Proteoglycan-collagen arrangements in developing rat tail tendon: An electron microscopical and biochemical investigation. *Biochem J* 1981;195:573–581.

49. Scott JE, Orford CR: Dermatan sulphate-rich proteoglycan associates with rat tail-tendon collagen at the d band in the gap region. *Biochem J* 1981;197:213–216.

50. Scott JE: The periphery of the developing collagen fibril: Quantitative relationships with dermatan sulphate and other surface-associated species. *Biochem J* 1984;218:229–233.

51. Scott JE: Proteoglycan histochemistry: A valuable tool for connective tissue biochemists. *Coll Relat Res* 1985;5:541–575.

52. Scott JE, Hughes EW: Proteoglycan-collagen relationships in developing chick and bovine tendons: Influence of the physiological environment. *Connect Tissue Res* 1986;14:267–278.

53. Brown DC, Vogel KG: Characteristics of the in vitro interaction of a small proteoglycan (PG II) of bovine tendon with type I collagen. *Matrix* 1990;9:468–478.

54. Rosenberg LC, Choi HU, Poole AR, et al: Biological roles of dermatan sulphate proteoglycans, in *Functions of the Proteoglycans (Ciba Foundation Symposium 124)*. New York, John Wiley & Sons, 1986, pp 47–68.

55. Lewandowska K, Choi HU, Rosenberg LC, et al: Fibronectin-mediated adhesion of fibroblasts: Inhibition by dermatan sulfate proteoglycan and evidence for a cryptic glycosaminoglycan-binding domain. *J Cell Biol* 1987;105:1443–1454.

56. Mugnai G, Lewandowska K, Choi HU, et al: Ganglioside-dependent adhesion events of human neuroblastoma cells regulated by the RGDS-dependent fibronectin receptor and proteoglycans. *Exp Cell Res* 1988;175:229–247.

57. Schmidt G, Robenek H, Harrach B, et al: Interaction of small dermatan sulfate proteoglycan from fibroblasts with fibronectin. *J Cell Biol* 1987;104:1683–1691.

58. Lebaron R, Bidanset DJ, Rosenberg L, et al: Effects of small galactosaminoglycan-containing proteoglycans. *J Cell Biol*, in press.

59. Eyre DR, Wu J-J, Apone S: A growing family of collagens in articular cartilage: Identification of 5 genetically distinct types. *J Rheumatol* 1987;14(suppl 14):25–27.

60. Eyre DR, Oguchi H: The hydroxypyridinium crosslinks of skeletal collagens: Their measurement, properties and a proposed pathway of formation. *Biochem Biophys Res Commun* 1980;92:403–410.

61. Lane JM, Weiss C: Review of articular cartilage collagen research. *Arthritis Rheum* 1975;18:553–562.

62. Ryan MN, Sandell LJ: Differential expression of a cysteine-rich domain in the amino-terminal propeptide of type II (cartilage) procollagen by alternative splicing of mRNA. *J Biol Chem* 1990;265:10334–10339.

63. Burgeson RE, Hollister DW: Collagen heterogeneity in human cartilage: Identification of several new collagen chains. *Biochem Biophys Res Commun* 1979;87:1124–1131.

64. Eyre DR, Wu J-J: Type IX or $1\alpha2\alpha3\alpha$ collagen, in Mayne R, Burgeson RE (eds): *Structure and Function of Collagen Types*. Orlando, Academic Press, 1987, pp 261–281.

65. Morris NP, Bächinger HP: Type XI collagen is a heterotrimer with the composition (1α, 2α, 3α) retaining non-triple-helical domains. *J Biol Chem* 1987;262:11345–11350.

66. Niyibizi C, Eyre DR: Identification of the cartilage $\alpha1(XI)$ chain in type V collagen from bovine bone. *FEBS Lett* 1989;242:314–318.

67. Wu J-J, Eyre DR: Cartilage type IX collagen is cross-linked by hydroxypyridinium residues. *Biochem Biophys Res Commun* 1984;123:1033–1039.

68. Eyre DR, Wu J-J, Niyibizi C: The collagens of bone and cartilage: Molecular diversity and supramolecular assembly, in Cohn DV, Glorieux FH, Martin TJ (eds): *Calcium Reglation and Bone Metabolism: Basic and Clinical Aspects*. Amsterdam, Excerpta Medica, 1990, vol 10, pp 188–194.

69. Huber S, Winterhalter KH, Vaughan L: Isolation and sequence analysis of the glycosaminoglycan attachment site of type IX collagen. *J Biol Chem* 1988;263:752–756.

70. McCormick D, van der Rest M, Goodship J, et al: Structure of the glycosaminoglycan domain in the type IX collagen-proteoglycan. *Proc Natl Acad Sci USA* 1987;84:4044–4048.

71. van der Rest M, Mayne R, Ninomiya Y, et al: The structure of type IX collagen. *J Biol Chem* 1985;260:220–225.

72. Muragaki Y, Nishimura I, Henney A, et al: The $\alpha1$ (IX) collagen gene gives rise to two different transcripts in both mouse embryonic and human fetal RNA. *Proc Natl Acad Sci USA* 1990;87:2400–2404.

73. Eyre DR, Apon S, Wu J-J, et al: Collagen type IX: Evidence for covalent linkages to type II collagen in cartilage. *FEBS Lett* 1987;220:337–341.

74. van der Rest M, Mayne R: Type IX collagen proteoglycan from cartilage is covalently cross-linked to type II collagen. *J Biol Chem* 1988;263:1615–1618.

75. Wu J-J, Eyre DR: Covalent interactions of type IX collagen in cartilage. *Connect Tissue Res* 1989;20:241–246.

76. Vaughan L, Mendler M, Huber S, et al: D-periodic distribution of collagen type IX along cartilage fibrils. *J Cell Biol* 1988;106:991–997.

77. Müller-Glauser W, Humbel B, Glatt M, et al: On the role of type IX collagen in the extracellular matrix of cartilage: Type IX collagen is localized to intersections of collagen fibrils. *J Cell Biol* 1986;102:1931–1939.

78. Okada Y, Konomi H, Yada T, et al: Degradation of type IX collagen by matrix metalloproteinase 3 (stromelysin) from human rheumatoid synovial cells. *FEBS Lett* 1989;244:473–476.

79. Wu J-J, Lark MW, Chun LE, et al: Molecular sites of stromelysin cleavage in collagen types II, IX, X, and XI of cartilage. *J Biol Chem* 1991;266:5625–5628.

80. Schmid TM, Conrad HE: A unique low molecular weight collagen secreted by cultured chick embryo chondrocytes. *J Biol Chem* 1982;257:12444–12450.

81. Ninomiya Y, Gordon M, van der Rest M, et al: The developmentally regulated type X collagen gene contains a long open reading frame without introns. *J Biol Chem* 1986;261:5041–5050.

82. Yamaguchi N, Benya PD, van der Rest M, et al: The cloning and sequencing of α1(VIII) collagen cDNAs demonstrate that type VIII collagen is a short chain collagen and contains triple-helical and carboxyl-terminal nontriple-helical domains similar to those of type X collagen. *J Biol Chem* 1989;264:16022–16029.

83. Timpl R, Engle J: Type VI collagen, in Mayne R, Burgeson RE (eds): *Structure and Function of Collagen Types.* Orlando, Academic Press, 1987, pp 105–143.

84. Wu J-J, Eyre DR, Slayter HS: Type VI collagen of the intervertebral disc: Biochemical and electron-microscopic characterization of the native protein. *Biochem J* 1987;248:373–381.

85. Chu M-L, Zhang RZ, Pan TC, et al: Mosaic structure of globular domains in the human type VI collagen α3 chain: Similarity to von Willebrand factor, fibronectin, actin, salivary proteins, and aprotinin type protease inhibitors. *EMBO J* 1990;9:385–393.

86. Aumailley M. Mann K, von der Mark H, et al: Cell attachment properties of collagen type VI and Arg-Gly-Asp dependent binding to its α2(VI) and α3(VI) chains. *Exp Cell Res* 1989;181:463–474.

87. Poole CA, Ayad S, Schofield JR: Chondrons from articular cartilage: I. Immunolocalization of type VI collagen in the pericellular capsule of isolated canine tibial chondrons. *J Cell Sci* 1988;90:635–643.

88. McDevitt CA, Pahl JA, Ayad S, et al: Experimental osteoarthritic articular cartilage is enriched in guanidine soluble type VI collagen. *Biochem Biophys Res Commun* 1988;157:250–255.

Chapter 16

Bioartificial Neural Prostheses for Parkinson's Disease

Moses Goddard, MD

Recent studies of Parkinson's disease have demonstrated that transplantation of small populations of specific cell types into the brains of affected patients or experimental animals may have some value for ameliorating the symptoms of this movement disorder. Unfortunately, conventional human transplantation techniques require the use of allograft or autograft tissue, both of which are associated with significant difficulties. Among these are the limited availability of allograft donors, the need for immunosuppression of allograft recipients, and the complications related to retrieving appropriate autograft tissue from elderly patients. An alternative approach developed for cellular grafts uses encapsulation of the cells in semipermeable polymer membranes to isolate the graft tissue from the host immune system while allowing exchange of small-molecule nutrients and cellular products across the wall of the capsule.

The concept of transplanting dopamine-producing neural or paraneural tissue into specific dysfunctional areas of the central nervous system has received considerable attention recently as a potential therapy for Parkinson's disease, a movement disorder characterized by progressively severe tremor, muscular rigidity, and bradykinesia. Although the specific etiology of the disease in most cases remains obscure, the pathophysiology is known to be related to the loss of dopaminergic neurons in the midbrain structure known as the substantia nigra. These neurons normally project their axons to the corpus striatum in the forebrain where they are the only significant source of the neurotransmitter dopamine, which is used by the striatal cells. When a sufficient number of cells projecting from the substantia nigra to the striatum are lost as the disease progresses, the dopamine available is no longer adequate for normal neurologic function, and the patient demonstrates the symptoms of Parkinson's disease.

In most cases, patients can be treated for a number of years by resupplying the striatum with dopamine through oral administration of its precursor, levodopa, which is converted to dopamine by the presynaptic terminals of dopaminergic cells that remain within the striatum. Eventually, however, most patients become intolerant of the increasing doses of levodopa and the other drugs required, and are forced to balance progressively intermittent and incomplete therapeutic action against dystonias and other unpleasant side effects. Many patients are either totally disabled by the disease or experience long and often unpredictable "off periods" of immobility several times per day because drug therapy cannot be regulated well enough. This pharmacologic loss of effectiveness has been attributed to several factors, including fluctuating and unreliable delivery of the dopamine precursor to the target structure, progressive loss of the ability of the striatal cells to metabolize levodopa to dopamine, and inability of the striatal cells to respond to the levels of the neurotransmitter deliverable by systemic administration.

Direct Transplantation

Some investigators have hypothesized that transplantation of viable dopamine-producing cells directly into the striatum may resolve the imperfections of oral drug delivery. Experiments during the late 1970s using rodent and primate models of Parkinson's disease demonstrated that very small amounts of transplanted dopaminergic tissue were associated with improvement of neurotoxin-induced, experimental Parkinson's lesions.[1-3] On the basis of these early results, clinicians in a number of centers around the world proceeded with transplantation experiments for human idiopathic Parkinson's disease, and in some cases obtained promising results that generally consisted of partial but often temporary improvement of symptoms.[4-6] So although both the animal and the human data apparently proved that neural transplantation may, in principle, be used to relieve Parkinson's disease symptoms, the technique is far from ready for routine use, and a number of critical questions remain concerning how the transplants actually achieve their effect and how the performance of the transplants can be improved and made more reliable.

One of the important issues in transplantation therapy is that even in the best cases of grafts implanted with conventional transplantation techniques, it is possible at best to demonstrate only extremely small amounts of viable transplanted tissue in or near the striatum, although there may be clear symptomatic improvement associated with the procedure. In these cases it is difficult to maintain that the functional improvement is the result of dopamine produced by the graft, and it seems likely that the improvement in striatal activity may be the result of trophic factors that originate either from the graft or, possibly, from adjacent neural tissue injured during the transplantation procedure. Whether or not this is the case, most investigators believe that long-term graft viability is probably desirable, and a number of laboratories are currently evaluating methods to accomplish this.[7]

A second major issue concerns significant problems associated with most of the potential sources of transplant tissue. Tissue for both human and nonhuman primate experiments has so far been taken from autologous adrenal glands, allogeneic fetal midbrain, or allogeneic adult adrenal glands. The most commonly used tissue for the human experiments has been from autologous adrenal glands retrieved during the transplantation procedure. Unfortunately, this technique has been associated with high morbidity and mortality related to the adrenalectomy and poor graft viability when the tissue is obtained from typically elderly patients with Parkinson's disease. Adult and fetal allogeneic tissues have both proved effective experimentally; however, they are both subject to a chronic shortage of available donors and require the use of immunosuppressive drugs to maintain graft viability (although a few investigators believe that immunosuppression may not be necessary for transplantation of fetal tissue into the brain). Further, it appears unlikely that an ethical consensus will be reached that allows the use of fetal tissue for routine transplantation, at least in the United States.

Encapsulation

In response to these problems, our laboratory has developed several techniques for enclosing small populations of dopaminergic cells (as well as other cell types) within semipermeable polymer capsules. These capsules allow unrestricted passage of molecules with a molecular weight of less than 50,000. These include oxygen, water, dopamine, and nutrients. At the same time, the polymer membrane is able to prevent cells, antibodies, and other large molecules of the host immune system from reaching the cells within the capsule and also to prevent the escape of either cells or large-molecule antigens from the graft. Use of these capsules then allows implantation of "immunoprotected" and fully contained cellular grafts that are nourished by diffusion of oxygen and other substrates across the wall of the membrane from the adjacent host tissues, and whose cellular products, including dopamine, are allowed to diffuse out to the surrounding area. This technique is presently being used to provide long-term viability of functional xenografts in both rodent[8-10] and primate[11] models without the use of immunosuppressive therapy.

The principal encapsulation technique currently being developed for possible human application uses asymmetric, tubular membranes that are spun from the copolymer, poly (acrylonitrile vinylchloride), with internal diameters from 300 to 500 μ. The wall of the capsule consists of a continuous, condensed inner membrane that forms the selectively permeable barrier. This membrane is mechanically supported by an outer, radially oriented trabecular layer and either a continuous or a fenestrated outer skin (Fig. 1). The wall thickness of the capsules ranges from 50 to 150 μ, depending on mechanical and diffusion requirements.

The system can be configured to allow loading of the membranes with cells at several different stages in the fabrication and implantation process, including the period when the capsule is being formed (that

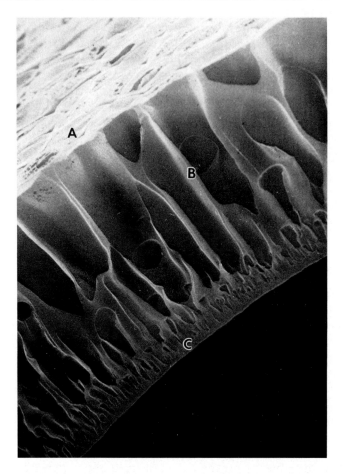

Fig. 1 *Scanning electron micrograph of a cross section of the capsule wall, without cells, showing the fenestrated outer skin (A), the radially oriented trabecular wall (B), and the continuous, selectively permeable inner skin (C) (× 100).*

is, precipitated around the cells) or when the capsule is completely formed but not yet sealed. Each alternative has its own advantages for experimental or therapeutic applications. Devices can also be fabricated that permit removing or replacing encapsulated cells implanted in a host without disturbing the active portion of the membrane.

Use of immunoisolated, polymer-encapsulated grafts permits far greater freedom in selecting the source of dopaminergic cells than can be allowed with unprotected transplants. Functional improvement has been demonstrated in experimental Parkinson's disease models using xenografts of fetal mouse midbrain, bovine adrenal chromaffin cells, and a cell line known as PC12 derived from a rat pheochromocytoma. However, there is no reason to believe that any culturable cell population could not be used as an encapsulated graft, provided that the

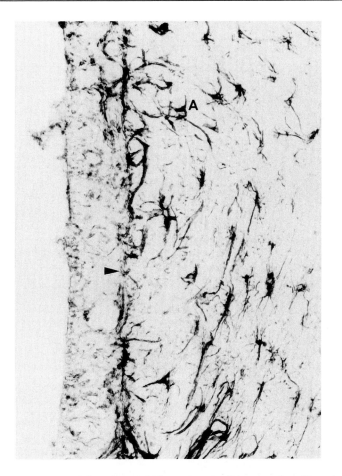

Fig. 2 *Frozen section of the polymer-glial reaction interface more than 12 weeks after implantation in the parietal cortex of a rat. The slide has been stained for reactive astrocytes (A) with antisera to glial fibrillary acidic protein and demonstrates a reactive layer extending approximately 50 μ from the capsule surface (× 320).*

cells produce appropriate neurotransmitter and/or trophic factors. Further, it appears possible that the membranes are able to provide sufficiently secure containment of the grafted cells to allow transplantation of potentially tumor-forming, genetically engineered cell lines that could offer improved production of dopamine or specific trophic factors.[12]

The polymer-encapsulated grafts can be surgically implanted by routine stereotaxic neurosurgical techniques that allow the devices to be placed within the target structures with an accuracy of ± 1 mm under magnetic resonance imaging or computed tomographic guidance. The length and number of capsules and the spacing between implant locations required in humans is currently unknown; however, experience

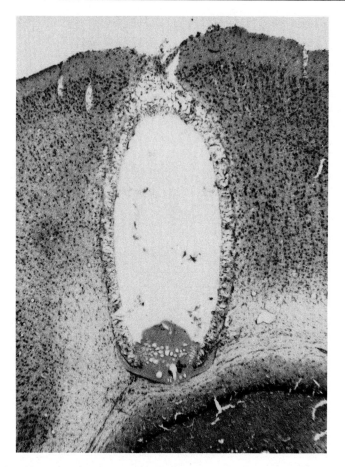

Fig. 3 *Frozen section of an empty, unsealed capsule one year after implantation in the parietal cortex of a rat and stained with glial fibrillary acidic protein demonstrates the absence of any apparent disturbance of the normal neuronal architecture adjacent to the implant (× 100).*

in primates has demonstrated that capsules 400 μ in diameter and 1 cm long can be placed at 3–mm intervals throughout the striatum without apparent adverse effects.

Inflammatory Reactions

Probably the most critical functional and therapeutic problem facing this technique is the need to minimize host inflammatory reactions to the capsule. Any incompatibility between the host tissue and the capsule material or contaminants on its surface can result in the formation of sufficient amounts of fibrosis to act as a diffusion barrier, limiting the availability of oxygen for the grafted cells and interfering with diffusion of the cellular products to the surrounding brain. Early studies using this encapsulation system for transplantation of experimental thymocyte and pancreatic islet grafts demonstrated that this is a potential problem for free-floating, intraperitoneal implants because central portions of the grafted cell mass became necrotic in association with increasing thickness of the fibroblastic reaction around the implant.[13,14]

Fortunately, capsules implanted in the brain have produced less severe inflammatory reactions than those implanted in peripheral sites. Longitudinal biocompatibility studies done two to 54 weeks after implantation in rodents have shown some evidence of a peripheral-type inflammatory response with fibroblasts and macrophages appearing adjacent to the polymer as long as 12 weeks after implantation. However, these cell types are much less common than they are in intraperitoneal implants, and the amount of collagen deposited on the surface of the material is minimal by transmission electron microscopy. There was no evidence of host tissue necrosis adjacent to the capsules even very early after implantation. Foreign body giant cells, which are the usual peripheral inflammatory cells associated with biomaterials, were not observed in association with the brain implants at any time. The inflammatory response, which is more characteristic of the central nervous system and which does occur with encapsulated transplants in the brain, consists of an increased density of microglia and reactive astrocytes that initially extend several hundred micrometers from the surface of the capsule. After 12 weeks, however, only a neuroglial cell layer two to four cells thick is present (Fig. 2). This extremely mild reaction produces no visible alteration in the architecture of the adjacent brain after one year of implantation (Fig. 3) and does not appear to result in any significant diffusion barrier, provided that the outside of the capsule is not contaminated. Further evidence of the relatively undisturbed nature of neural tissue near the capsule is provided by the observation of an apparently normal cortical neuropil within 30 to 40 μ of the polymer and normal synapses within 3 to 5 μ of the material.[15]

The emerging concept of bioartificial prostheses for neural transplantation, cell-seeded vascular grafts, the artificial pancreas, and a variety of organ replacements clearly places far greater demands on the biomaterials used in terms of soft-tissue reaction than do more conventional applications, such as large-diameter vascular grafts and cemented or screw-fixed orthopaedic prostheses. It appears that in immunoprotected central nervous system grafts, the inflammatory and fibrotic response to the material is attenuated, at least to some degree, by the specialized immune system of the brain, and that this seems to contribute to the success of the grafts in experimental models. The same degree of graft viability and function will probably be much more difficult to achieve in peripheral implantation sites, which may require some sort of immunomodulation, possibly in the form of local release of factors from the implant, for satisfactory soft-tissue integration.[14]

References

1. Perlow MJ, Freed WJ, Hoffer BJ, et al: Brain grafts reduce motor abnormalities produced by destruction of nigrostriatal dopamine system. *Science* 1979;204:643–647.

2. Björklund A, Stenevi U: Reconstruction of the nigrostriatal dopamine pathway by intracerebral nigral transplants. *Brain Res* 1979;177:555–560.

3. Morihisa JM, Nakamura RK, Freed WJ, et al: Adrenal medulla grafts survive and exhibit catecholamine-specific fluorescence in the primate brain. *Exp Neurol* 1984;84:643–653.

4. Madrazo I, Drucker-Colín R, Díaz V, et al: Open microsurgical autograft of adrenal medulla to the right caudate nucleus in two patients with intractable Parkinson's disease. *N Engl J Med* 1987;316:831–834.

5. Goetz CG, Olanow CW, Koller WC, et al: Multicenter study of autologous adrenal medullary transplantation to the corpus striatum in patients with advanced Parkinson's disease. *N Engl J Med* 1989;320:337–341.

6. Lewin R: Cloud over Parkinson's therapy. *Science* 1988;240:390–392.

7. Watts RL, Bakay RAE, Herring CJ, et al: Preliminary report on adrenal medullary grafting and cografting with sural nerve in the treatment of hemiparkinson monkeys. *Prog Brain Res* 1990;82:581–591.

8. Aebischer P, Winn SR, Galletti PM: Transplantation of neural tissue in polymer capsules. *Brain Res* 1988;448:364–368.

9. Aebischer P, Tresco P, Winn SR, et al: Long-term cross-species brain transplantation of a polymer encapsulated dopamine-secreting cell line. *Exp Neurol* 1991;111:269–275.

10. Aebischer P, Winn SR, Tresco P, et al: Transplantation of polymer encapsulated neurotransmitter secreting cells: Effect of the encapsulation technique. *J Biomech Eng*, in press.

11. Aebischer P, Goddard M, Timpson R, et al: Polymer encapsulated PC12 cells transplanted in MPTP lesioned primates. *Soc Neurosci Abstr* 1990;16:963.

12. Wolff JA, Fisher LJ, Xu L, et al: Grafting fibroblasts genetically modified to produce L-dopa in a rat model of Parkinson's disease. *Proc Natl Acad Sci USA* 1989;86:9011–9014.

13. Aebischer P, Russell PC, Christenson L, et al: A bioartificial parathyroid. *ASAIO Trans* 1986;32:134–137.

14. Christenson L, Aebischer P, McMillan P, et al: Tissue reaction to intraperitoneal polymer implants: Species difference and effects of corticoid and doxorubicin. *J Biomed Mater Res* 1989;23:705–718.

15. Winn SR, Aebischer P, Galletti PM: Brain tissue reaction to permselective polymer capsules. *J Biomed Mater Res* 1989;23:31–44.

Future Directions

This section has focused on the structure and composition of human and synthetic biomaterials, as well as the interactions at the interface. The effect that the collagen and proteoglycan of articular cartilage and the collagen, bone matrix, and high mineral concentration of bone has on bacterial adherence and growth needs to be determined. Proteoglycan aggregate is degraded by bacterial enzymes. Do the breakdown products serve as an improved substratum, which enhances colonization and bacterial growth?

The Race for the Surface

Initially, at the time of implantation of a sterile biomaterial, no bacterial or host cells are adherent. A race for the surface begins immediately to determine whether host or bacterial cells will colonize the device. The initial events are most important, because they dictate further interactions and need to be characterized in terms of adsorption of host macromolecules to the implant surface. These macromolecules and other serum constituents will modulate succeeding events in wound healing, inflammation, and adhesion of cells and bacteria. Host cellular adhesion mechanisms are incompletely understood. In order to design biomaterial implants that enhance host cell adhesion and possibly deter bacterial adhesion, more must be learned about eukaryotic cellular adhesion mechanisms. It may be discovered that bacteria and host cells have similar or identical adhesion mechanisms, or alternatively, each may have a unique binding process. The regulation of

this process by breakdown products from the biomaterial or host should be evaluated. What proteins are induced during adhesion? How are the synthesis and processing of adhesion proteins regulated? The existence of specific bonding sites on biomaterials for host cells and bacteria and the possibility of enhancing or blocking these domains should be determined.

Implant Design

Biomaterials, which are foreign bodies, accordingly cause a host immune response, which by interfering with optimal tissue ingrowth can contribute to infection. The role that biomaterials play in modulating inflammation and immune response must be better characterized, focusing on how composition and release of components into the local environment affects these processes. Components released from the implant, both initially and as wear debris, may be found to have specific effects on macrophages and neutrophils. What are the positive and negative interactions associated with a biodegradable implant versus a permanent one? Specific areas to analyze include the mechanism by which biomaterial composition and chemical and physical characteristics affect the process. What are the specific effects of local change in pH and ion products (type and valence) from metals in local and distant tissues (quantity, complexed forms, location in vivo)? The systemic effects need to be better understood.

Macroporosity and microtexture of the implant must be optimized. Implant shape

233

and elastic modulus should be adjusted to diminish stress concentration and micromotion at the interface. New biomaterials should be developed that preferentially direct cellular adherence as opposed to bacterial adherence. Standards must be designated and enforced concerning cleaning, sterilization, and handling of implants.

Surface Preconditioning

Can the implant surface be preconditioned before insertion to enhance eukaryotic cell adhesion? What impact do prosthetic coatings such as calcium phosphate or titanium nitrates have on immediate and long-term host cell function? Do compounds such as fluoride affect bacterial attachment and cellular adhesion? Could host cells be used to precoat biomaterials in vitro and thus decrease bacterial colonization? Are implant-modified or disease-modified biologic fluids significantly different from unperturbed fluids? Could they be used to precoat the device?

Timing of Infections

Biomaterial infections are not clearly defined with respect to timing. Implant infections may be caused by seeding at the time of implantation. Late infections can result from new activity of quiescent organisms, or late hematogenous contamination can occur. If both processes occur, knowledge about the relative incidence of each is valuable to improve prevention and treatment modalities. Are nonadherent organisms virulent in the presence of a biomaterial?

Allografts as Substrate

Better characterization of allografts with regard to their physical and mechanical properties postprocessing but before implantation is necessary. The effects of harvesting, handling, cleaning, and sterilization on the implant and the resulting interactions with microorganisms and host cells is imprecisely understood. Of equal importance is the understanding of the effects of processing on allograft composition, breakdown, and integration.

Collaboration With Dental Research

In many respects, experience with implants is similar in dental and orthopaedic settings. Comparisons should be made to create a broader knowledge base. Critical issues related to the staging of load application and the introduction of tension, compression, and shear forces along the interface need to be cross-correlated for osseous and fibro-osseous integrated implant conditions.

Similar collaborative research could open the doors for exciting alternative biomaterial uses in orthopaedics. Use of semipermeable polymer membranes may allow transfer of allograft, xenograft, or engineered cell lines to specific host sites requiring long-term release of growth factors or other chemical mediators without the use of immunosuppressive therapy.

Cell Culture and In Vivo Models

Finally, there is a critical need for the development of relevant cell culture and in vivo models. The problems associated with cell culture include the type of substrate used, the composition and physical characteristics of the particulates used, primary versus immortalized cell lines, cell type, the use of serum-free or serum-containing media, time-course and dose-response characteristics, and competition between bacterial and host cells in culture in the presence and absence of antibiotics. Different in vivo models should be designed to take into consideration differences between surgical implantation and hematogenous infections. Improved histologic methods are needed to allow more complete description of cell response to changes in material composition and design, over time, following implantation. It is hoped that better experimentation methods and further research will foster the design of improved biomaterial implants, with better host tissue integration and a sharply reduced risk of infection.

Section Four
Host Defenses

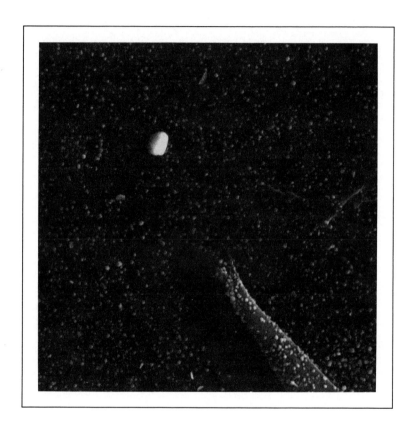

Introduction

Craig L. Levitz, BA
John L. Esterhai, Jr, MD

An understanding of the events that lead up to osteomyelitis and the host defenses that counter infection of the bone is particularly important in orthopaedic procedures, where the surgeon is often faced with severe, contaminated wounds. The difficulty in delivering antibiotics to the site of the infected bone further complicates treatment. In addition to the hypotension, disseminated intravascular coagulation, multiorgan failure, and shock that all physicians must be concerned with in association with any bacteremia, the orthopaedic surgeon must deal with the bone resorption, remodeling and resultant mechanical failure, the almost certain failure of bone grafts, and the need to remove essential "hardware" that are the result of bone infection.[1,2] Furthermore, the increasing use of biomaterials, in the form of prosthetic implants and biomedical polymers, and the need to develop biomaterials that will not contribute to the infectious process necessitates an understanding of the events that are triggered by surgical implantation of a foreign substance.

In the first chapter of this section, Petty reviews the mechanisms of immune defense and some of the ways these mechanisms are altered. The chapter begins with a discussion of the antibacterial proteins that are present in tissue fluid. It then describes the chemotaxis of phagocytic cells, phagocytosis, and bacterial killing, and highlights the role of lymphocytes, plasma cells, and antibodies in the immune response. The chapter concludes with some brief points concerning alteration of the immune response.

The implantation of biomaterials, regardless of the mechanism of implantation, initiates a response to the foreign material. Inflammatory and immune responses are generated. However, a modification of the host defense occurs to allow the acceptance of the biomaterial. The biocompatibility of biomaterials depends on the pathophysiologic conditions created by the implantation of the biomaterial and the extent to which these conditions alter the immune response. The initial events in the inflammatory response have been hypothesized to be especially important in controlling biocompatibility and tissue response.[3,4] The cell-cell and cell-tissue interactions at the biomaterial interface, including the adsorption of human blood proteins onto a material and the activation of specific cells involved in inflammatory and immune responses, have not been extensively studied or correlated with in vivo studies.[5,6]

The second chapter of this section, by Anderson and associates, deals with the biologic events in the biocompatibility of biomedical polymers. The authors suggest that the adsorption of proteins to the polymer surface elicits a cellular response that results in adhesion and cellular activation. Previous studies, as well as the results of recent work from our laboratory, are offered as evidence. Studies support the hypothesis that biomedical polymers and the proteins that adsorb to their surfaces alter the activation of macrophages and the synthesis of interleukin-l. The effect of these changes on the fibroblast is noted. In conclusion, the authors correlate with in vivo investigations the in vitro evidence of the role of the macrophage and the release of interleukin-1 in controlling the biocompatibility of biomedical polymers.

In the past, attention has been focused on infecting organisms and the antimicrobial drugs used to combat these organisms. Future advances may well depend on our ability to manipulate host defense mechanisms to combat the infectious etiology and to provide an environment that is less conducive to colonization and propagation of infection. Our ability to accomplish this requires an understanding of the factors involved in bone-cell communication and the role of these factors in bone's response to infection. While the specific triggering mechanisms for the host's response to bone infection, bone allograft implantation, fracture repair, and biomaterial implantation may differ, the mediators may be identical. Little is known about these factors, but cytokines, prostaglandins, and the lipopolysaccharide of the gram-negative bacterial cell wall (i.e., the endotoxin) are hypothesized to play a role in bone-cell communication and, possibly, in bone's response to infection.

It has been documented that prostaglandins stimulate bone resorption and bone formation. While the bone resorptive effects are part of the overall stimulation of bone remodeling, prostaglandins can stimulate independent bone formation.[7-9] Exogenously administered prostaglandin 2 stimulates chondrogenesis in mesenchymal chick limb bud cells. These mesenchymal cells release the different prostaglandins in significantly elevated amounts during the different stages of bone formation.[10,11]

Prostaglandins may play a role in the stimulation of dormant mesenchymal cells during fracture repair. There is a significant rise in local prostaglandin release following tibial fractures in rats.[12] Furthermore, fracture repair is retarded by nonsteroidal inflammatory drugs (NSAIDS), which inhibit prostaglandin synthesis.[13]

Nonunion, a frequent complication of osteomyelitis, may be caused by the generation of prostaglandin inhibitors or by interference with prostaglandin's normal interaction with bone cells. Elevated levels of prostaglandins demonstrated in experimentally induced osteomyelitis seems to favor the latter concept.[14] Osteoblasts have prostaglandin receptors and these cells are thought to be the primary producers of prostaglandins in bone. Prostaglandins exhibit both a direct inhibitory effect on osteoclasts and an indirect stimulation of osteoclasts by osteoblasts. Prostaglandin 2 has been shown to be complement dependent in its production.[15] The significant role of prostaglandins in the regulation of bone homeostasis and their specific interactions with osteoclasts suggest a role for prostaglandins in the immune response that needs to be examined. It is unknown whether bone allografts or biomaterials that are implanted during orthopaedic procedures have an effect on prostaglandin concentration.

While it is clear that bacterial endotoxin affects numerous target cells associated with the inflammatory and immune responses, including macrophages, neutrophils, and lymphocytes, the effect of lipopolysaccharide on bone cell function and communication and its mechanism of action is not clear.[16] It is known that bone macrophages and osteoblasts are activated by lipopolysaccharide.[17] It is suggested by the authors that lipopolysaccharide induces bone cell activation and that these activated cells secrete cytokines, which are the chemical mediators of lipopolysaccharide-induced interactions with the immune response in bone.

The most studied of the cytokines is interleukin-1. Tissue macrophages are known to produce interleukin-1. Interleukin-1 stimulates both lymphocytes and macrophages.[18] Because osteoclasts are related to macrophages, it seems likely that osteoclasts secrete and respond to interleukin-1 as part of the host's response to infection.

Interleukin-1 has been implicated in the destruction of cartilage and is a potent stimulator of osteoclastic bone resorption. It may mediate the bone destruction and fracture repair retardation that is associated with osteomyelitis. It has been suggested that prostaglandins may function as natural feedback inhibitors of interleukin-1. Evidence to the contrary includes the facts that piroxicam, a nonsteroidal anti-inflammatory drug, enhances the production of interleukin-1 inhibitors, and ibuprofen decreases gross tibial pathology in experimentally induced osteomyelitis.[19]

The third chapter, by Horowitz and associates, focuses on the effect of endotoxin on bone cell function, bone allograft incorporation, and fracture repair. This section examines the hypothesis put forward by the authors that molecules of bacterial origin activate host cells. Studies from their laboratory are presented that demonstrate the induction of cytokine-mediated events by lipopolysaccharide, specifically dealing with the cytokine, interleukin-1. The cellular source of interleukin-1 is also identified.

The discussion then moves on to consider the host response to bone allografts. The immune mechanisms that are responsible for acceptance or rejection of a bone allograft are highlighted. The authors explore the effect of lipopolysaccharide on cytokine secretion in the fracture callus. Their data suggest that the cytokines secreted by the fracture callus are the same as those secreted when normal bone encounters lipopolysaccharide and when immune cells respond to allogenic bone.

No discussion of bone's response to infection would be complete unless it addressed how the bone's response to infection is altered in the immunocompromised host. In the last chapter of this section, MacGregor addresses the host defense, the compromised host, and osteomyelitis. it is not known whether immunocompromised hosts have a direct impairment of the bone's ability to resist infection. The change in host response in the various immune-compromised states most probably differs depending on the site of alteration of the immune cascade. Studies of the incidence of osteomyelitis in different disease states provide evidence as to the specific cells that are important in bone's resistance to infection. These studies suggest that some cells that are normally part of the body's defense against infection are not important in bone. MacGregor identifies diseases and therapies that impair normal host defense mechanisms. He examines the function of host defenses in bone and concludes with a specific look at infection as an immune-compromising event in bone.

References

1. Morrison DC, Ryan JL: Endotoxins and disease mechanisms. *Annu Rev Med* 1987;38:417–432.
2. Morrison DC, Ulevitch RJ: The interaction of bacterial endotoxins or host mediation systems: A review. *Am J Pathol* 1978;93:526–617.
3. Anderson JM, Bonfield TL, Ziats NP: Protein adsorption and cellular adhesion and activation on biomedical polymers. *Int J Artif Organs* 1990;13:375–382.
4. Ziats NP, Pankowsky DA, Tierney BP, et al: Adsorption of Hageman factor (factor XII) and other human plasma proteins to biomedical polymers. *J Lab Clin Med* 1990, in press.
5. Andrade JD, Hlady V: Protein adsorption and materials biocompatibility: A tutorial review and suggested hypothesis. *Adv Polym Sci* 1986;79:1.
6. Horbett TA: Techniques for protein adsorption studies, in Williams DF (ed): *Techniques of Biocompatibility Testing.* Boca Raton, FL, CRC Press, 1986, vol II, pp 183–214.
7. Raisz LG, Martin TJ: Proteoglandins and bone, in Pech WA (ed): *Bone and Mineral Research.* New York, Elsevier Science Publishing Co., Inc., 1984, vol II, pp 286–310.
8. Nefussi JR, Baron B: PGE2 stimulates both resorption and formation of bone *in vitro*: Differential responses of the periosteum and the endosteum in fetal rat long bone cultures. *Anat Rec* 1985;211:9–16.
9. Li XJ, et al: Transient effects of subcutaneously administered prostaglandin E2 on cancellous and cortical bone in young adult dogs. *Bone* 1990;11:353.
10. Gay SW, Kosher RA: Prostaglandin synthesis during the course of limb cartilage differentiation *in vitro*. *J Embryol Exp Morp* 1984;89:367–382.
11. Wientroub S, Wahl LM, Feurstein N, et al: Changes in tissue concentration of prostaglandins during endochondral bone differentiation. *Bioch Biophys Res Comm* 1983;117:746–750.

12. Dekel S, et al: Release of prostaglandins from bone and muscle after tibial fracture. *J Bone Joint Surg* 1981;63B:185–189.

13. Allen HL, Wase A, Blar WT: Indomethacin and aspirin: Effect of nonsteroidal anti-inflammatory agents on the rate of fracture repair in the rat. *Acta Orthop Scand* 1980;51:595–600.

14. Rissing JP, Buxton TB: Effect of ibuprofen on gross pathology, bacterial count and levels of prostaglandin E_2 in experimental staphylococcal osteomyelitis. *J Infect Dis* 1986;154:627–630.

15. Raisz LG, Kream BE: Regulation of bone formation. *N Engl J Med* 1983;309:29–35.

16. Morrison DC, Ryan JL: Bacterial endotoxins and host immune responses. *Adv Immunol* 1979;28:293–450.

17. Horowitz MC, Einhorn TA, Philbrick W, et al: Functional and molecular changes in colony stimulation factor secretion by osteoblasts. *Connective Tissue Res* 1989;20:159–168.

18. Durum SK, Schmidt JA, Oppenheim JJ: Interleukin 1: An immunological perspective. *Annu Rev Immunol* 1985;3:263–287.

19. Herman JH, Sowder WG, Donaldson JB, et al: NSAID modulation of catabolin production reflects induction of interleukin-1 inhibitory activition. *Trans Orthop Res Soc* 1991;16:200.

Chapter 17

Resistance to Bacterial Infection

William Petty, MD

Immune function involves specific and nonspecific responses to encounters with a foreign configuration such as bacteria. Nonspecific responses, which are active almost immediately following bacterial exposure, include the activity of phagocytic cells and antibacterial proteins present in plasma and other tissue fluids (Fig. 1). The skin and mucous membrane barriers are also important components of nonspecific resistance to bacteria. Specific responses, which have a more delayed effect, are mediated by antibody (immunoglobulins) or sensitized lymphocytes.[1] It is obvious that the integrity of the skin and mucous membrane barriers is often lost during surgery or as a result of accidental trauma. It is less obvious, but no less true, that other components of immune defense may be impaired by many different factors. This chapter discusses the mechanisms of immune defense and some of the ways these mechanisms can be altered.

Antibacterial Proteins in Tissue Fluid

Antibacterial humoral substances include properdin, lysozyme, beta lysins, immunoconglutinins, C-reactive protein, transferrin, complement, and interferon. Since 1895, when Bordet[2] reported that serum was capable of lysis of bacteria, many reports have described bacterial-inhibiting proteins in normal tissue fluids.

The properdin system is a natural mechanism of normal serum that acts on many bacteria, viruses, protozoa, and fungi. The system includes complement, magnesium, and properdin, which is a beta globulin; all these components are essential for antibacterial action.[3,4]

Lysozyme is a heat stable enzyme, derived from leukocytes, that lyses gram-negative bacteria primarily, but has been reported to be cidal for micrococci as well.[5,6] Lysozyme levels are very low in tissue fluids from normal individuals, but they increase significantly during illness.[7,8] Lysozyme action is a true enzymatic process, in which the substance attacks the bacterial cell wall mucopeptides.[7,9] In addition

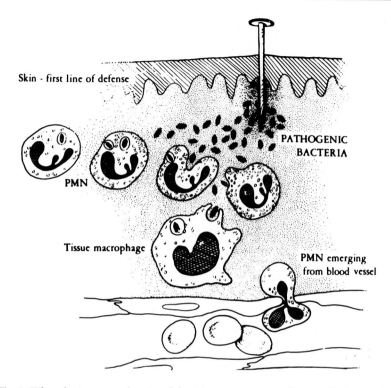

Fig. 1 *When the important barrier of the skin or mucous membrane is broken and bacteria enter the tissues, the activity of phagocytic cells is critical in eliminating bacteria from the tissues.*

to its direct cidal action, lysozyme enhances complement killing of gram-negative organisms.[10]

Beta lysins are heat-stable, low-molecular-weight, serum proteins that are cidal primarily for gram-positive bacteria.[11] Like lysozyme, they increase in amount during acute illness, but their lethal effect is mediated by causing a loss of functional integrity of the cell membrane.[12,13] Beta lysins are derived from platelets, and there is evidence that they may be important in resisting localized infections in vivo.[12–14]

Immunoconglutinins are antibodies produced in response to antigen complement combinations.[15] The antibodies produced are nonspecific in that they react with other antigens combined with complement.[15–19] Immunoconglutinins are not adsorbed by bacteria that have stimulated their production, a further indication of their nonspecificity.[15,17] There is evidence that immunoconglutinins significantly increase resistance to infection in vivo, and studies in humans indicate that immuno-conglutinin levels rise during bacterial illness and may be important in preventing many infections from reaching a clinical level.[17,19]

C-reactive protein determinations have been used for many years as a nonspecific indicator of infection. C-reactive protein has been demonstrated to enhance phagocytosis of many different bacteria and has a direct anti-bacterial activity in which it attacks cell wall polysaccharides. In vivo, the rise of C-reactive protein is closely correlated with an increase in resistance to bacterial infection.[20,21]

Transferrin is a protein contained in body fluids that combines with two atoms of iron per molecule. The normal serum level of transferrin is approximately 30 micromoles, which can combine with 60 micromoles of iron; thus, transferrin is only about one third saturated normally, so that it can easily deprive bacteria of the 0.3 to 4.0 micromoles of iron they require for normal metabolism. Growth of some bacteria has been directly correlated with the percentage saturation of transferrin, in vitro. In vivo, adding iron has caused a lowering of the LD_{50} for some bacteria in experimental animals.[22] Transferrin may be important in nonspecific resistance to bacteria by depriving bacteria of essential iron.

Though there is evidence that these nonspecific humoral substances may play an important role in bacterial resistance in vivo, most of the investigation of them has been in vitro. Their role in direct bacterial inhibition in vivo is yet to be verified. However, it is known that some of these humoral substances are important for chemotaxis, phagocytosis, and bacterial killing by leukocytes, which is the cornerstone of primary or nonspecific immune defense.[10,23-25]

One of the most important and thoroughly studied of the humoral antibacterial substances is complement (Fig. 2). Complement is not a single substance, but consists of eleven distinct serum proteins, which are designated by the symbols C1q, C1r, C1s, C2, C3, C4, C5, C6, C7, C8, and C9.[26-29] The various components of complement account for more than 10% of serum globulins. Most components are beta globulins with molecular weights between 100,000 and 200,000. Although these proteins do not contain lipid, most do contain carbohydrate.[30] The sites of synthesis of all the complement components is not known but it has been demonstrated that C3 and C6 are produced in the liver, C3 and C1q are produced by macrophages, and C1 is produced in the intestinal mucosa.[31-34]

Once initiated, the reactions of the complement sequence continue to completion.[26,27] Initiation of the complement sequence is classically considered to be caused by the interaction of cell surface antigens, antibody, and the three subunits of C1.[26,35] The complement sequence can also be initiated through the so-called alternate pathway by various types of damaged tissue.[30,36-38] This does not require activity of C1, C4, or C2. Either classical or alternate pathway complement activation leads to an active form of C567 and active fragments of C3 and C5, which are important for leukocyte chemotaxis, immune adherence, and phagocytosis.[23,24,26,29,39-42]

An important effect of the complement sequence is immune cytolysis. For cytolysis to occur, complement activity must continue through the C8 component, at which point a small amount of lysis occurs. Cell lysis is greatly enhanced by activity of C9.[26] Most studies

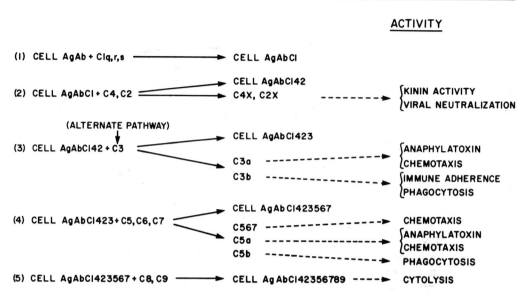

Fig. 2 *Complement reactions and activity of complement components resulting from complement activation.*

of cytolysis have been carried out with erythrocytes, but the same mechanisms are involved in bacterial lysis, which occurs primarily with gram-negative organisms.[10,43,44] Cellular lesions produced by complement activity have been demonstrated in *Escherichia coli* cells by electron microscope study.[44] There is evidence that complement may have a direct cidal effect on bacteria and does not require the presence of antibody.[33]

Complement is essential for, or enhances, chemotaxis, immune adherence, phagocytosis, and lysis of bacteria, all of which are important components of immune defense. Partial complement deficiencies of mild or moderate degree probably do not cause increased susceptibility to infection. Complete or nearly complete absence of complement proteins is rare but has been reported to be associated with frequent infections, especially with gram-negative organisms.[26,45]

Interferon is a low-molecular-weight (20,000 to 30,000) group of glycoproteins elaborated by a number of infected cells, including lymphocytes and other leukocytes, which protects cells from cytophilic parasites. It is antiviral to both DNA and RNA viruses by binding on the surface and inducing enzymes that inhibit translation of viral messenger RNA into viral protein. It is also protective against many tumor cells.

In addition to these antiviral and antitumor cell effects, interferon acts intracellularly to inhibit chlamydia, rickettsias, bacteria, fungi, and protozoa. Interferon activity is stimulated both by these cytophilic pathogens and by products produced by bacteria during growth.

Chemotaxis of Phagocytic Cells

It has been known for many years that monocytes or polymorphonuclear leukocytes accumulate in areas of inflammation, especially in tissue areas contaminated with bacteria. In 1888, Leber first observed that cells actively migrate toward such areas of inflammation.[46] It has been demonstrated both in vivo and in vitro that phagocytic cells migrate directionally in response to various substances.[7,36,37,47-52]

In vivo electron microscopic studies have revealed increased emigration of polymorphonuclear leukocytes from vessels in areas of inflammation.[53-56] By thrusting their pseudopods, the neutrophils actively migrate through vascular endothelium at the interendothelial junctions and possibly through the endothelial cytoplasm.[53] It is possible that this response is stimulated by factors similar to those that attract phagocytic cells.[37]

Several substances have been demonstrated to attract phagocytic leukocytes: (1) Lymphokines produced by lymphocytes; (2) factors from the phagocytic cells themselves; (3) factors generated by the sequential activation of complement; and (4) factors released by most bacteria during growth.[1,23,39,42,48,57-60] Either classical or alternate pathway complement activation leads to active forms of C3, C5, and C567.[26,36-39] Among the substances that stimulate the production of chemotactically active complement fragments are antigen-antibody complexes; gamma globulins; various damaged tissues, such as burned skin and damaged heart and liver; and lysosomes (granules) of phagocytic cells.[23,37,38]

The chemotactic factors from bacteria are not a portion of the bacterium itself, but a product elaborated during growth.[23,48] The factor is stable at 56 C and is probably of low molecular weight, on the order of 3600.

Chemotactic factors appear to interact with leukocytes by activating esterases on their surfaces, and two esterases are probably involved in bringing about the directional motility of the cells.[61-63] The cells migrate toward an increasing concentration gradient of the active chemotactic factors.[23,64]

The importance of chemotaxis in vivo is suggested by the findings that virulent brucellae, *Salmonella typhosa*, *Pseudomonas aeruginosa*, Serratia, and Tubercle bacillus all inhibit rather than stimulate chemotaxis.[65-67] In addition, chemotaxis has been shown to be depressed in patients who have rheumatoid arthritis and may correlate with the possible increased incidence of infection and probable increased mortality from infection in rheumatoid arthritis.[68]

Phagocytosis and Bacterial Killing

When a phagocytic cell reaches a foreign object, the object to be ingested is surrounded by pseudopods that gradually enclose it completely, until the particle occupies a vacuole that is limited by the invaginated cell membrane. This process appears to involve mechanisms much like those of motility.[69] Speed and amount of particle ingestion are inversely related to particle size, which is probably due to mechanical limitation imposed by the size of the phagocytic cell.[70] Leukocytes that have ingested particles exhibit an increased rate of phagocytosis.[71] Phagocytosis is an energy-requiring mechanism in which adenosine triphosphate is utilized. Glycolysis is the most important mechanism of energy production for polymorphonuclear leukocytes and most mononuclear leukocytes.[70,72]

Following phagocytosis, cytoplasmic granules are discharged from the cell cytoplasm into the vacuoles containing bacteria.[73-76] The granules may be considered lysosomes, because they consist of membrane-bound structures that contain a number of hydrolytic enzymes. The granules contain phagocytin (a bactericidal protein), lysozyme, cathepsin, acid phosphatase, alkaline phosphatase, nucleotidase, ribonuclease, deoxyribonuclease, and beta glucuronidase, all of which may have a detrimental effect on bacteria. The granule membrane fuses with the vacuole containing the bacteria and the granule contents are released into the vacuole. Vacuole membrane continuity is maintained so that the granule substances are not released into the leukocyte cytoplasm.[74,76] This process of degranulation usually occurs within 30 minutes of ingestion of bacteria and is directly related to the quantity of material engulfed.[74]

Several investigators have reported data to indicate that the cationic proteins in granules play an important part in bacterial death.[73,75-79] The increased respiratory and hexose monophosphate activity in phagocytizing cells results in hydrogen peroxide production, which has a direct cidal effect on many bacteria and has been shown to enhance bacterial killing by granule proteins and make bacteria more sensitive to lysis by lysozyme.[80-83] Lactoferrin is contained within granules and probably exerts a deleterious effect on bacteria by depriving them of essential iron.[77,84,85] Bacterial killing is often complete within five to ten minutes, and bacterial digestion is well along within 30 to 60 minutes of phagocytosis.[74,79]

Exoplasmosis is the process by which phagocytic cells rid themselves of indigestible particles remaining following bacterial digestion.[76] Phagocytosis and bacterial killing is not a suicidal process and, after phagocytosis, the leukocytes appear to remain healthy.[74,76] Following phagocytosis, there is a marked decrease in motility and increase in aggregation of leukocytes, which facilitate recruitment and retention of phagocytic cells in areas of microbial invasion.[86]

Lymphocytes and Plasma Cells

Lymphocytes function as effector cells or release biologically active mediators in cell-mediated immune responses. In addition, they act as regulator cells in the production of humoral antibody. Stimulated lymphocytes release migration inhibitory factor, which increases the number of phagocytic macrophages, and chemotactic factors, which also increases the number of phagocytes in areas of injury or contamination. Lymphotoxic or growth inhibitory factors, which are important in inhibiting growth of mammalian cells, may also be important in defense against bacteria. There are two primary types of lymphocytes, B-lymphocytes and T-lymphocytes. The B-lymphocytes are important in the production of antibody; T-lymphocytes are responsible for cell mediated immunity. The T-lymphocytes effect their action by direct cytotoxicity, by elaboration of cytotoxin, or by antibody-dependent cytotoxicity.[1] Plasma cells have an extensive endoplasmic reticulum in their cytoplasm, a finding characteristic of cells active in protein synthesis. They have been shown to store and release immunoglobulin and are probably the primary site of antibody synthesis.[1] These processes of lymphocytes and plasma cells are critical to host defense mechanisms in general and to resistance to infection specifically.[87-90]

Antibody

Immunoglobulins are proteins that function as specific antibodies and are responsible for the specific humoral aspects of immunity. Immunoglobulin molecules have many similar structural, biologic, and antigenic characteristics; but their antibody function is highly specific because of differences in primary amino acid sequence. In man, five different immunoglobulin classes are known. They are designated by the letters G, A, M, D, and E.[1]

Immunoglobulins of class G are present in larger amounts than any of the other immunoglobulins. They reach significant levels in both the intravascular and extravascular spaces and have a relatively long half-life of 23 days. This class of immunoglobulins is thought to be the most important in immunity to infection involving blood-borne dissemination, whether bacterial, viral, fungal, or protozoal.[1]

The second most abundant immunoglobulins are those of class A. These proteins are especially important in providing immune activity in secretory fluids from the skin and respiratory, genitourinary, and gastrointestinal tracts.[1]

The M immunoglobulins are restricted, by their large molecular size, almost entirely to the intravascular space. These immunoglobulins are very effective in the agglutination of particulate antigens, such as bacteria. Following antigenic exposure, this class of immunoglobulins is the first to reach significant levels and they appear to be most important in the first few days after exposure to antigen. Immunoglobulins D and E are involved in hypersensitivity and allergic reactions but their importance in resistance to infectious agents has not been established.[1]

Immunoglobulins have direct effects on invading bacteria. These effects include agglutination, precipitation, immobilization, and lysis. In addition, they enhance other aspects of immune function, including immune adherence, phagocytosis, and the actions of complement.

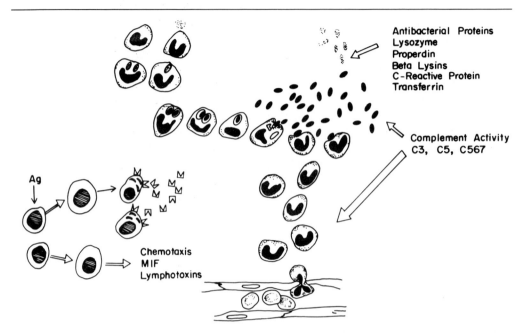

Fig. 3 *Components of antibacterial defense include antibacterial proteins, complement reactions, phagocytosis and bacterial killing by leukocytes, the activities of immunoglobulins, and the activities of lymphocytes (Ag = antigen; MIF = migration inhibitory factor).*

Alteration of Immune Response

It is accepted that size of inoculum, virulence of an infecting agent, and the defensive responses of a host are important in determining whether or not infection is established. Because of the marked beneficial effects of antimicrobial agents, physicians tend to focus their attention more on the infecting agent than on the responses of the host. However, Hirsch[80] has stated that host resistance, not exposure to the parasite, is the prime determinate of infectious disease. Many events may cause an alteration in the normal function of immune defense activities, including nutritional deficiencies or excesses, various disease states, and many forms of medical treatment.[42,68,80,91-102]

A physician treating infections or involved in surgery where infection is a potential complication should be aware of the normal mechanisms of immune defense against infection as well as the effects that nutritional deficiency states, disease states, and various treatment methods have on the function of the immune system (Fig. 3). This knowledge provides for a rational consideration of the importance of the host, as well as the invading organism, in the prevention and treatment of infection.

References

1. Bellanti JA: *Immunology II*, ed 2. Philadelphia, WB Saunders, 1978.

2. Bordet J: Les leucocytes et les propriétés actives du sérum chez les vaccinés. *Ann Inst Pasteur* 1895;9:462–506.

3. Hinz CF Jr, Wedgwood RJ, Pilemer L: The properdin system and immunity: XV. Some biologic effects of the administration of zymosan and other polysaccharides to rabbits, and the presence of antibodies to zymosan in human and rabbit serum. *J Lab Clin Med* 1969;57:185–198.

4. Wardlaw AC, Pillemer L: The properdin system and immunity: V. The bactericidal activity of the properdin system. *J Exp Med* 1956;103:553–575.

5. Noller EC, Hartsell SE: Bacteriolysis of Enterobacteriaceae: I. Lysis by four lytic systems utilizing lysosomes. *J Bacteriol* 1961;81:482–491.

6. Wardlaw AC: The complement-dependent bacteriolytic activity of normal human serum: I. The effect of pH and ionic strength and the role of lysozyme. *J Exp Med* 1962;115:1231–1249.

7. Inoue K, Tanigawa Y, Takubo M, et al: Quantitative studies on immune bacteriolysis: II. The role of lysozyme in immune bacteriolysis. *Biken J* 1959;2:1–20.

8. Tew JG, Hess WM, Donaldson DM: Lysozyme and beta-lysin release stimulated by antigen-antibody complexes and bacteria. *J Immunol* 1969;102:743–750.

9. Mandelstam J: Isolation of lysozyme-soluble mucopeptides from the cell wall of *Escherichia coli*. *Nature* 1961;189:855–856.

10. Muschel LH, Jackson JE: Activity of the antibody-complement system and lysozyme against rough gram negative organisms. *Proc Soc Exp Biol Med* 1963;113:881–884.

11. Johnson FB, Donaldson DM: Purification of staphylocidal beta-lysin from rabbit serum. *J Bacteriol* 1968;96:589–595.

12. Matheson A, Donaldson DM: Alterations in the morphology of *Bacillus subtilis* after exposure to beta-lysin and ultraviolet light. *J Bacteriol* 1968;95:1892–1902.

13. Myrvik QN, Leake ES: Studies on antibacterial factors in mammalian tissues and fluids: IV. Demonstration of two nondialyzable components in the serum bactericidin system for *Bacillus subtilis*. *J Immunol* 1960;84:247–250.

14. Jensen RS, Tew JG, Donaldson DM: Extracellular beta-lysin and muramidase in body fluids and inflammatory exudates. *Proc Soc Exp Biol Med* 1967;124:545–549.

15. Bienenstock J, Bloch KJ: Some characteristics of human immunoconglutinin. *J Immunol* 1966;96:637–645.

16. Ingram DG: The conglutination phenomenon: XIV. The resistance enhancing effect of conglutinin and immuno-conglutinin in experimental bacterial infections. *Immunology* 1959;2:334–345.

17. Ingram DG: The conglutination phenomenon: XIII. *In vivo* interactions of conglutinin and experimental bacterial infection. *Immunology* 1959;2:322–333.

18. Ingram DG: The production of immuno-conglutinin: III. Factors affecting the response to autostimulation in mice. *Can J Microbiol* 1962;8:335–344.

19. Ingram DG, Barker H, McLean DM, et al: The conglutination phenomenon: XII. Immuno-conglutinin in experimental infections of laboratory animals. *Immunology* 1959;2:268–282.

20. Kindmark CO: Stimulating effect of C-reactive protein on phagocytosis of various species of pathogenic bacteria. *Clin Exp Imunol* 1971;8:941–948.

21. Patterson LT, Harper JM, Higginbotham RD: Association of C-reactive protein and circulating leukocytes with resistance to *Staphylococcus aureus* infection in endotoxin-treated mice and rabbits. *J Bacteriol* 1968;95:1375–1379.

22. Weinberg ED: Role of iron in host-parasite interactions. *J Infect Dis* 1971;124:401–410.

23. Boyden SV, North RJ, Faulkner SM: Complement and the activity of phagocytes, in Wolstenholme GEW, Knight J (eds): *Complement* (Ciba Foundation Symposium). Boston, Little Brown, 1965, pp 190–213.

24. Nelson DS: Immune adherence, in Wolstenholme GEW, Knight J (eds): *Complement* (Ciba Foundation Symposium). Boston, Little Brown, 1965, pp 222–237.

25. Nishioka K, Linscott WD: Components of guinea pig complement: I. Separation of a serum fraction essential for immune hemolysis and immune adherence. *J Exp Med* 1963;118:767–793.

26. Cooper NR, Polley MJ, Müller-Eberhard HJ: Biology of complement, in Samter M (ed): *Immunological Diseases*, ed 2. Boston, Little Brown, 1971, vol 1, pp 289–331.

27. Kabat EA, Mayer MM: *Experimental Immunochemistry*, ed 2. Springfield, Charles C Thomas, 1961.

28. Lachmann PJ, Hobart MJ, Aston WP: Complement technology, in Weir DM (ed): *Handbook of Experimental Immunology*, ed 2. Oxford, Blackwell Scientific Publications, 1972, vol 1, pp 5.1–5.17.

29. Nelson RA Jr, Jensen J, Gigli I, et al: Methods for the separation, purification, and measurement of nine components of hemolytic complement in guinea-pig serum. *Immunochemistry* 1966;3:111–135.

30. Hurley JV: Acute inflammation: The effect of concurrent leucocytic emigration and increased permeability on particle retention by the vascular wall. *Br J Exp Pathol* 1964;45:627–633.

31. Alper CA, Johnson AM, Birtch AG, et al: Human C3: Evidence for the liver as the primary site of synthesis. *Science* 1969;163:286–288.

32. Colten HR, Gordon JM, Rapp HJ, et al: Synthesis of the first component of guinea pig complement by columnar epithelial cells of the small intestine. *J Immunol* 1968;100:788–792.

33. Rother KO, Rother U, Philipps ME, et al: Further studies on sites on production of C' components, abstract. *J Immunol* 1968;101:814.

34. Stecher VJ, Morse JH, Thorbecke GJ: Sites of production of primate serum proteins associated with complement system. *Proc Soc Exp Biol Med* 1967;124:433–438.

35. Mayer MM: Mechanism of haemolysis by complement, in Wolstenholme GEW, Knight J (eds): *Complement* (Ciba Foundation Symposium). Boston, Little Brown, 1965, pp 4–32.

36. Hurley JV, Spector WG: Endogenous factors responsible for leucocytic emigration *in vivo*. *J Pathol Bacteriol* 1961;82:403–420.

37. Hurley JV: Substances promoting leukocyte emigration. *Ann NY Acad Sci* 1964;116:918–935.

38. Ryan GB, Hurley JV: The chemotaxis of polymorphonuclear leukocytes towards damaged tissues. *Br J Exp Pathol* 1966;47:530–536.

39. Becker EL: The relationship of the chemotactic behavior of the complement-derived factors, C3a, C5a, and C567, and a bacterial chemotactic factor to their ability to activate the proesterase 1 of rabbit polymorphonuclear leukocytes. *J Exp Med* 1972;135:376–387.

40. Morelli R, Rosenberg LT: The role of complement in the phagocytosis of *Candida albicans* by mouse peripheral blood leukocytes. *J Immunol* 1971;107:476–480.

41. Ruddy S, Austen KF: C_3 inactivator of man: I. Hemolytic measurement by the inactivation of cell-bound C_3. *J Immunol* 1969;102:533–543.

42. Shin HS, Snyderman R, Friedman E, et al: Chemotactic and anaphylatoxic fragment cleaned from the fifth component of guinea pig complement. *Science* 1968;162:361–363.

43. Humphrey JH, Dourmashkin RR: Electron microscope studies of immune cell lysis, in Wolstenholme GEW, Knight J (eds): *Complement* (Ciba Foundation Symposium). Boston, Little Brown, 1965, pp 175–186.

44. Medhurst FA, Glynn AA, Dourmashkin RR: Lesions in *Escherichia coli* cell walls caused by the action of mouse complement. *Immunology* 1971;120:441–450.

45. Alper CA, Propp RP, Johnston RB Jr, et al: Genetic aspects of human C'3, abstract. *J Immunol* 1968;101:816–817.

46. Leber T: Ueber die Entstehung der Entzündung und die Wirkung der entzündungserrengentden Schädlichkeiten. *Fortschr Med* 1888;6:460–464.

47. Boyden S: The chemotactic effect of mixtures of antibody and antigen on polymorphonuclear leucocytes. *J Exp Med* 1962;115:453–466.

48. Keller HU, Sorkin E: Studies on chemotaxis: V. On the chemotactic effect of bacteria. *Int Arch Allergy* 1967;31:505–517.

49. Keller HU, Sorkin E: Studies on chemotaxis: I. On the chemotactic and complement-fixing activity of gamma-globulins. *Immunology* 1965;9:241–247.

50. Keller HU, Sorkin E: Studies on chemotaxis: IV. The influence of serum factors on granulocyte locomotion. *Immunology* 1966;10:409–416.

51. Thomas L: Possible role of leucocyte granules in the Schwartzman and Arthus reactions. *Proc Soc Exp Biol Med* 1964;115:235–240.

52. Wilkinson PC, Borel JF, Stecher-Levin VJ, et al: Macrophage and neutrophil specific chemotactic factors in serum. *Nature* 1969;222:244–247.

53. Florey HW, Grant LH: Leucocyte migration from small blood vessels stimulated with ultraviolet light: An electron-microscope study. *J Pathol Bacteriol* 1961;82:13–17.

54. Machesi VT, Florey HW: Electron micrographic observations on the emigration of leucocytes. *Q J Exp Physiol* 1960;45:343–348.

55. Spector WG, Willoughby DA: The inflammatory response. *Bacteriol Rev* 1963;27:117–154.

56. Williamson JR, Grisham JW: Electron microscopy of leukocytic margination and emigration in acute inflammation in dog pancreas. *Am J Pathol* 1961;39:239–256.

57. Harris H: Mobilization of defensive cells in inflammatory tissue. *Bacteriol Rev* 1960;24:3–15.

58. Hill JH, Ward PA: C_3 leukotactic factors produced by a tissue protease. *J Exp Med* 1969;130:505–518.

59. Ward PA: A plasmin-split fragment of C_3 as a new chemotactic factor. *J Exp Med* 1967;126:189–206.

60. Ward PA, Lepow IH, Newman LJ: Bacterial factors chemotactic for polymorphonuclear leukocytes. *Am J Pathol* 1968;52:725–736.

61. Lepow IH, Naff GB, Pensky J: Mechanisms of activation of C'I and inhibition of CI esterase, in Wolstenholme GEW, Knight J (eds): *Complement* (Ciba Foundation Symposium). Boston, Little Brown, 1967, pp 74–90.

62. Ward PA, Becker EL: Mechanisms of the inhibition of chemotaxis by phosphonate esters. *J Exp Med* 1967;125:1001–1020.

63. Ward P, Becker EL: The deactivation of rabbit neutrophils by chemotactic factor and the nature of the activatable esterase. *J Exp Med* 1968;1217;693–709.

64. Nelson RD, Quie PG, Simmons RL: Chemotaxis under agarose: A new and simple method for measuring chemotaxis and spontaneous migration of human polymorphonuclear leukocytes and monocytes. *J Immunol* 1975;115:1650–1656.

65. Elberg SS, Schneider P: Directed leucocyte migration in response to infection and other stimuli. *J Infect Dis* 1953;93:36–42.

66. Martin SP, Chaudhuri SN: Effect of bacteria and their products on migration of leukocytes. *Proc Soc Exp Biol Med* 1952;81:286–288.

67. Martin SP, Pierce CH, Middlebrook G, et al: The effect of tubercle bacilli on the polymorphonuclear leucocytes of normal animals. *J Exp Med* 1950;91:381–392.

68. Mowat AG, Baum J: Chemotaxis of polymorphonuclear leukocytes from patients with rheumatoid arthritis. *J Clin Invest* 1971;50:2541–2549.

69. Brewer DB: Electron microscopy of phagocytosis of staphylococci. *J Pathol Bacteriol* 1963;86:299–303.

70. North RJ: The uptake of particulate antigens. *J Reticuloendothel Soc* 1968;5:203–229.

71. Cohn ZA, Morse SI: Functional and metabolic properties of polymorphonuclear leucocytes: I. Observations on the requirements and consequences of particle ingestion. *J Exp Med* 1960;111:667–687.

72. Karnovsky ML: Metabolic basis of phagocytic activity. *Physiol Rev* 1962;42:143–168.

73. Cohn ZA, Hirsch JG: The isolation and properties of the specific cytoplasmic granules of rabbit polymorphonuclear leucocytes. *J Exp Med* 1960;112:983–1004.

74. Hirsch JG, Cohn ZA: Degranulation of polymorphonuclear leucocytes following phagocytosis of microorganisms. *J Exp Med* 1960;112:1105–1014.

75. Zeya HI, Spitznagel JK: Cationic proteins of polymorphonuclear leukocyte lysosomes: I. Resolution of antibacterial and enzymatic activities. *J Bacteriol* 1966;91:750–754.

76. Zucker-Franklin D, Hirsch JG: Electron microscope studies on the degranulation of rabbit peritoneal leukocytes during phagocytosis. *J Exp Med* 1964;120:569–576.

77. Gladstone GP, Walton E: Effect of iron on the bactericidal proteins from rabbit polymorphonuclear leukocytes. *Nature* 1970;227:849–851.

78. Hirsch JG: Antimicrobial factors in tissues and phagocytic cells. *Bacteriol Rev* 1960;24:133–140.

79. Hirsch JG: Phagocytin: A bactericidal substance from polymorphonuclear leucocytes. *J Exp Med* 1956;103:589–611.

80. Hirsch JG: The phagocytic defence system. *Symp Soc Gen Microbiol* 1972;22:59–74.

81. McRipley RJ, Sbarra AJ: Role of the phagocyte in host-parasite interactions: XI. Relationship between stimulated oxidative metabolism and hydrogen peroxide formation, and intracellular killing. *J Bacteriol* 1967;94:1417–1424.

82. McRipley RJ, Sbarra AJ: Role of the phagocyte in host-parasite interactions: XII. Hydrogen peroxide-myeloperoxidase bactericidal system in the phagocyte. *J Bacteriol* 1967;94:1425–1430.

83. Miller TE: Killing and lysis of gram-negative bacteria through the synergistic effect of hydrogen peroxide, ascorbic acid, and lysosome. *J Bacteriol* 1969;98:949–955.

84. Baggiolini M, De Duve C, Masson PL, et al: Association of lactoferrin with specific granules in rabbit heterophil leukocytes. *J Exp Med* 1970;131:559–570.

85. Gladstone GP, Walton E: The effect of iron and haematin on the killing of staphylococci by rabbit polymorphs. *Br J Exp Pathol* 1971;152:452–464.

86. Bryant RE, DesPrez RM, VanWay MH, et al: Studies on human leukocyte motility: I. Effects of alterations in pH, electrolyte concentration, and phagocytosis on leukocyte migration, adhesiveness, and aggregation. *J Exp Med* 1966;124:483–499.

87. David JR: Lymphocytic factors in cellular hypersensitivity, in Good RA, Fisher DW (eds): *Immunobiology: Current Knowledge of Basic Concepts in Immunology and Their Clinical Applications.* Stamford, Sinauer Associates, 1971, pp 146–156.

88. Gowans JL: Immunobiology of the small lymphocyte, in Good RA, Fisher DW (eds): *Immunobiology: Current Knowledge of Basic Concepts in Immunology and Their Clinical Applications.* Stamford, Sinauer Associates, 1971, pp 18–27.

89. Mackaness GB: Cell-mediated immunity to infection, in Good RA, Fisher DW (eds): *Immunobiology: Current Knowledge of Basic Concepts in Immunology and Their Clinical Applications.* Stamford, Connecticut, Sinauer Associates, 1971, pp 45–54.

90. Panush RS, Anthony CR: Effects of acetylsalicylic acid on normal human peripheral blood lymphocytes: Inhibition of mitogen- and antigen-stimulated incorporation of tritiated thymidine. *Clin Exp Immunol* 1976;23:114–125.

91. Beisel WR: Magnitude of the host nutritional responses to infection. *Am J Clin Nutr* 1977;30:1236–1247.

92. DaMert GJ, Sohnle PG: Effect of chloramphenicol on in vitro function of lymphocytes. *J Infect Dis* 1979;139:220–224.

93. Elek SD, Conen PE: The virulence of *Staphylococcus pyogenes* for man: A study of the problems of wound infection. *Br J Exp Pathol* 1957;38:573–586.

94. Faulk WP, Vitale JJ: Immunology, in Schneider HA, Anderson CE, Coursin DBB (eds): *Nutritional Support of Medical Practice.* Hagerstown, Maryland, Harper & Row, 1977, pp 341–346.

95. McHugh MI, Wilkinson R, Elliott RW, et al: Immunosuppression with polyunsaturated fatty acids in renal transplantation. *Transplantation* 1977;24:263–267.

96. Park SK, Brody JI, Wallace HA, et al: Immunosuppressive effect of surgery. *Lancet* 1971;1:53–55.

97. Pickering LK, Ericsson CD, Kohl S: Effect of chemotherapeutic agents on metabolic and bactericidal activity of polymorphonuclear leukocytes. *Cancer* 1978;42:1741–1746.

98. Preud'homme J-L: Immunoproliferative disorders, in Bach J-F (ed): *Immunology.* New York, John Wiley & Sons, 1978, pp 754–780.

99. Rogers AE, Herndon BJ, Newberne PM: Induction by dimethylhydrazine of intestinal carcinoma in normal rats and rats fed low levels of vitamin A. *Cancer Res* 1973;33:1003–1009.

100. Sellmeyer E, Bhettay E, Truswell AS, et al: Lymphocyte transformation in malnourished children. *Arch Dis Child* 1972;47:429–435.

101. Velez H, Restropo A, Vitale JJ, et al: Folic acid deficiency secondary to iron deficiency in man: Remission with iron therapy and a diet low in folic acid. *Am J Clin Nutr* 1966;19:27–36.

102. Vitale JJ: The impact of infection on vitamin metabolism: An unexplored area. *Am J Clin Nutr* 1977;30:1473–1477.

Chapter 18

The Biocompatibility of Biomedical Polymers

James M. Anderson, MD, PhD
Kazuhiro Yamaguchi, MD
Tracey Bonfield, PhD
Nicholas P. Ziats, PhD

Introduction

Biomaterials require injection, insertion, or surgical implantation, each of which injures the tissues or organs involved. The surgical procedure initiates a response to injury by the body and activates mechanisms to maintain homeostasis. The extent of these reactions is a measure of the host response to the biomaterial and may ultimately determine its biocompatibility and bioacceptability. The initial events in the inflammatory response may be especially important in controlling biocompatibility and tissue response, including human blood protein adsorption to biomaterials and subsequent cellular adhesion and activation.[1,2] Although protein adsorption has been well described for single proteins or combinations of proteins, it has not been extensively studied in human blood.[3,4] Our view is that there is concurrent adsorption of many proteins to a surface. These changes may involve the displacement of proteins such as fibrinogen, high-molecular-weight kininogen, and Hageman factor.[5,6] Alternatively, proteins such as Hageman factor and factor VIII/vWF may concurrently adsorb to and desorb from surfaces at various rates, resulting in different surface concentrations of proteins. The adsorbed protein layer is probably composed of coagulation proteins of the intrinsic and extrinsic pathways, complement proteins, fibrinolytic proteins and other proteins found in high concentrations in blood.

After protein adsorption, cells interact with the protein-coated polymer surfaces.[7-10] These interactions characterize the inflammatory response, the intensity and duration of which determine the fate of the polymer implant.[8] The predominant cell type present in the inflammatory response varies with time after implantation. Generally, neutrophils predominate in the first several days after injury and then are replaced by monocytes. Neutrophils are short-lived, disappearing after 24 to 48 hours; neutrophil emigration is of short duration and chemotactic factors for neutrophil migration are activated early in the inflammatory response. Monocytes show different characteristics. After emigration from the vasculature, they differentiate into macrophages,

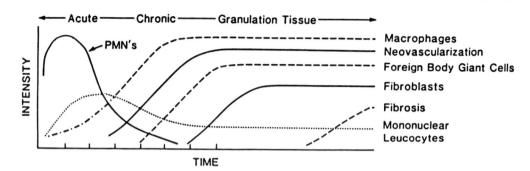

Fig. 1 *Cellular events during the acute and chronic phases of inflammation and wound healing. The intensity and duration (days) of the cellular response may be determined by the size and nature of the implanted material and host factors.*

and these cells are very long-lived (up to several months). Monocyte emigration may continue for days to weeks depending on the injury and implanted biomaterial, and chemotactic factors for monocytes are activated over long periods.

Figure 1 shows the general sequence of events after biomaterial implantation. Alterations in the magnitude or duration of these responses may compromise the functional capacity or permanent bioacceptance of the implant. The tissue response to implants depends, in part, on the extent of injury or the defect created by the implantation procedure. The size, shape, and chemical and physical properties of the biomaterial also may be responsible for variations in the intensity and duration of the inflammatory or wound healing process. Recent laboratory studies have focused on the humoral and cellular interactions that govern protein adsorption and cellular adhesion to the polymer and activation.[1,2,7-20]

Protein Adsorption Studies

When blood comes into contact with a polymer surface, one of the initial events is the adsorption of blood proteins onto the surface.[3-6] After protein adsorption, interactions between the protein-coated polymer surface and cells can lead to the adhesion and activation of cells on the polymer surface.[7-10] In blood, these interactions characterize the thrombotic response. In tissue, the interactions characterize the inflammatory response. In both cases, the intensity and duration of these interactions determine the fate of the biomedical polymer.

Materials used in orthopaedic procedures, such as metals and alloys, may produce thrombosis and/or embolism, probably because of instant protein adsorption followed by platelet and leukocyte adherence. Williams and associates[21,22] showed that albumin and fibrinogen adsorb differently on metals and that copper, gold, and silver adsorb and desorb proteins to a greater extent than iron. Other studies have shown adsorption of albumin to stainless-steel[23] and aluminum surfaces.[24] The recent studies by Sharma and Sunny[24] suggest that albumin adsorption is greater onto oxide layers than onto bare aluminum. In addition, they showed that in the presence of anti-Hageman factor (factor XII), fibrinogen and albumin adsorption to these surfaces increased. These observations support the role of coagulation factors as important proteins in adsorption phenomena.

Veerman and associates[25] showed that proteins such as albumin and fibrinogen are deposited on the surfaces of bone substitutes such as hydroxyapatite, β-whitlockite, titanium, and aluminum implanted intramuscularly into guinea pigs. They suggested that adsorbed proteins interact with cells such as macrophages and plasma cells. Sukenik and associates[26] have shown that the plasma protein fibronectin adsorbs to titanium and may be implicated in cellular and bacterial adhesion.

As stated previously, our view is that there is concurrent adsorption of many proteins to a polymer surface, followed by temporal changes in the type and concentration of proteins at the blood-surface interface. These proteins play a role in determining the thrombotic response as well as in cellular adhesion and activation. We have used this hypothesized series of events to probe various polymers for protein adsorption and cellular adhesion and activation. We consider these initial events to be important factors in protein-polymer, cell-polymer, cell-protein-polymer, and cell-cell interactions.

One of our goals was to determine the adsorption of human blood plasma proteins to various biomedical polymers, including experimental, reference, candidate, and clinically used materials. Our technique of identifying adsorbed proteins at the blood-surface interface[1,2,27,28] allows us to identify almost any protein found in human blood against which an antibody has been made. This provides a powerful means of identifying proteins important to the biocompatibility of materials. The adsorbed protein (antigen) is first identified by a specific interaction with the primary antibody, that is, rabbit or goat anti-human IgG, and then by the detecting antibody, either anti-rabbit or anti-goat IgG labeled with ^{125}I, in a radioimmunoassay. Blocking steps before incubation with the primary antibody and the detecting antibody are necessary. We currently use a solution of nonfat dry milk (15% weight/volume) in phosphate-buffered saline containing 3 mmol of ethylenediaminetetraacetic acid (EDTA) to block nonspecific binding of IgGs to the polymers or other proteins. These studies have been described in detail.[1,2,27,28]

Blood protein adsorption was determined in human blood from healthy individuals. Briefly, we obtained human citrated (0.01 M) platelet-poor plasma from four fasting healthy donors. The prepared plasma was pooled and frozen until use. Glass coverslips, 13 mm in diameter, were cleaned by rinsing twice in 70% alcohol for 15 minutes each time, followed by three rinses in distilled water. The polymers used in addition to glass were a polyurethane (Biomer) and polydimethylsiloxane. Disks (2 cm² and 15 mm in diameter) of polymer or glass were inserted into the bottom of 24–well polystyrene containers and a silicon rubber sleeve (16 mm in diameter) was placed over the material to prevent floating. The samples were rinsed once with phosphate-buffered saline and then incubated for 60 minutes with 1 ml of either 100% or 1% (diluted with phosphate-buffered saline) plasma at 37 C. Materials were also incubated with a purified solution of human fibrinogen (3 mg/ml), gamma globulin (10 mg/ml), or fibronectin (10 mg/ml).

After the plasma or protein was removed and the materials rinsed three times with phosphate-buffered saline, we added 2 ml of a milk solution (15% nonfat dry milk in phosphate-buffered saline with 2 mmol of EDTA sodium). The samples were refrigerated at 4 C overnight, and then rinsed three times with phosphate-buffered saline. Primary antibodies were obtained from rabbit anti-human IgG fractions. Stock solutions (10 mg/ml) were diluted 1:500 in phosphate-buffered saline containing 1% chicken egg albumin (ovalbumin) and 1 ml was added to each material for 60 minutes of incubation at 37 C. The samples were again rinsed with phosphate-buffered saline three times and the milk solution added before overnight refrigeration at 4 C. The samples were rinsed (three times) with phosphate-buffered saline and 1 ml of goat anti-rabbit IgG labeled with ^{125}I (7 µCi/ml, 250,000 cpm) was added to each material for 60 minutes of incubation at 37 C. After incubation, the samples were rinsed three times with phosphate-buffered saline and the silicon rubber sleeve removed; the materials were then placed into a clean test tube and counted in a gamma counter.

The data were expressed as counts per minute of ^{125}I binding of the second antibody to the primary antibody of the protein of interest, fibrinogen, IgG, or fibronectin. Alphafetoprotein and phosphate-buffered saline (1% ovalbumin) were used as the controls. Alphafetoprotein represented the background control for the primary antibodies and phosphate-buffered saline represented the control for background binding of ^{125}I to the materials.

For scanning electron microscopic analysis, we used a modification of a previously described method for immunogold labeling in which nonspecific protein-binding sites were blocked with 15% nonfat dry milk in phosphate-buffered saline with 2 mmol of EDTA sodium.[29] Unlabeled protein A (0.2 mg/ml) from *Staphylococcus aureus*, Cowan strain was added to this mixture to block Fc portions of adsorbed plasma immunoglobulins and the samples were incubated for one hour at 37 C. The samples were rinsed in phosphate-buffered saline and then incubated with primary antibodies (1:500) for one hour at 37 C. The samples were then rinsed in phosphate-buffered saline and fixed in 2.5% glutaraldehyde overnight at 4 C.

The samples were again rinsed in phosphate-buffered saline and then neutralized with 50 mmol of glycine for 20 minutes. Protein A-gold complex (10–nm gold beads) was diluted 1:75 with phosphate-buffered saline and incubated with samples for one hour at 37 C, after which the samples were rinsed with phosphate-buffered saline and then distilled water. We detected the gold beads by scanning microscopy, using

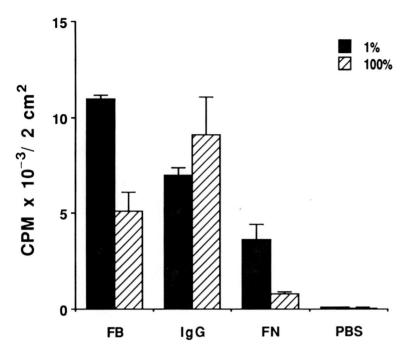

Fig. 2 *Adsorption of the proteins fibrinogen (FB), gamma globulin (IgG), and fibronectin (FN) from whole human plasma (100%) or diluted plasma (1%) onto glass after 60 minutes. PBS, phosphate-buffered saline.*

a method developed for light microscopy that employs silver enhancement (silver binds to any metal). The samples then underwent routine scanning electron microscopy at a working distance of approximately 22 mm and a 25–kV accelerating voltage.

Significant adsorption of fibrinogen, IgG, and fibronectin from both whole and diluted human plasma occurred on glass, a model hydrophilic (wettable) surface (Fig. 2). Our findings differed from those of Brash and associates,[27] who were unable to detect fibrinogen on glass surfaces after two to 180 minutes. They suggested that fibrinogen is rapidly adsorbed and then desorbed by the action of the proteolytic protein, plasmin. We also have observed that fibrinogen adsorbs in a relatively short time (less than one minute), but we have been able to detect immunologically reactive proteins even after one hour in static systems (Fig. 2), in recirculating systems,[1,2,27] and from retrieved human specimens[28] that have been implanted and exposed to blood for months. The differences between adsorption from whole plasma and diluted plasma may be explained by the competitive protein interactions described elsewhere.[5,6,30]

The other two polymers studied—a polyurethane used in a number of devices that come into contact with blood (catheters, heart-assist

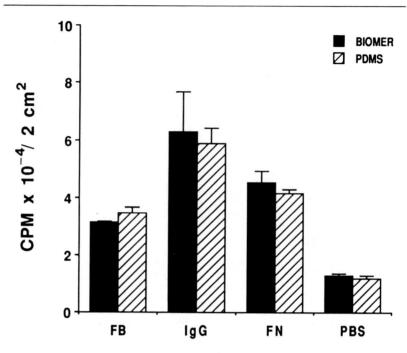

Fig. 3 *Adsorption of the purified proteins fibrinogen (FB), gamma globulin (IgG), and fibronectin (FN) onto polyurethane (Biomer) or polydimethylsiloxane (PDMS) after 60 minutes. PBS, phosphate-buffered saline.*

devices, and pumps) and polydimethylsiloxane, a silica-free material used as a reference material—both showed significant adsorption of purified proteins (Fig. 3). We used pure proteins to determine whether specific proteins could be identified on the material surfaces. We found more IgG (63,000 ± 14,000 cpm) than fibronectin (45,000 ± 4,000 cpm) or fibrinogen (31,000 ± 400 cpm) on the polyurethane (Fig. 3). The results were similar for polydimethylsiloxane, that is, we found more IgG than fibronectin and more fibronectin than fibrinogen.

These polymer-protein interactions were also evaluated by immunogold-labeling techniques.[27] The protein adsorption patterns for fibronectin (Fig. 4) and IgG (Fig. 5) on the same surfaces were suggestive of monolayer formation. Networks of fibronectin have been observed on some surfaces,[29] but we were not able to detect them, suggesting incomplete or altered protein adsorption.

The adsorption of proteins appears to elicit a cellular response. Kuwahara and associates[31] suggested that plasma proteins activate neutrophils, causing them to secrete superoxide anion, and Trezzini and associates[32] showed that fibrinogen can affect monocyte adherence as well as oxidative metabolism. Morley and Feuerstein[33] showed that platelets enhanced the spreading of polymorphonuclear cells to fibrinogen and albumin-coated disks.

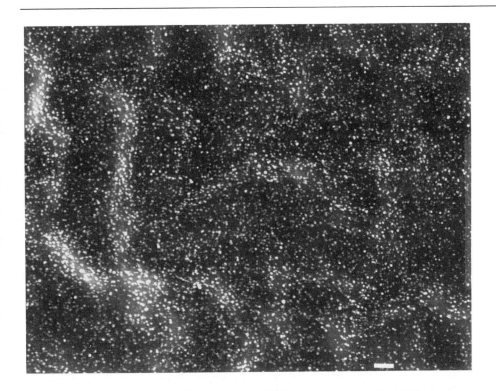

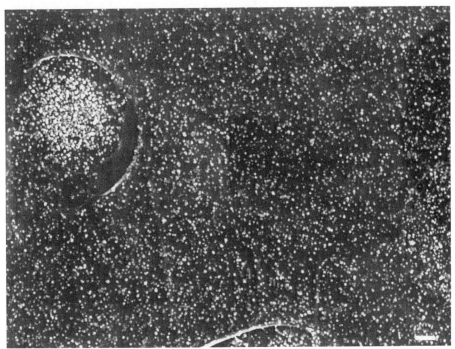

Fig. 4 *Scanning electron micrographs of purified fibronectin detected by immunogold labeling. Note that the beads are evenly distributed (bars = 1μ; × 4,000).* **Top,** *Adsorption onto polyurethane for 60 minutes.* **Bottom,** *Adsorption onto polydimethylsiloxane for 60 minutes.*

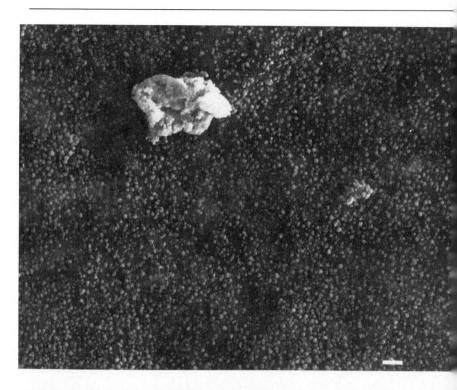

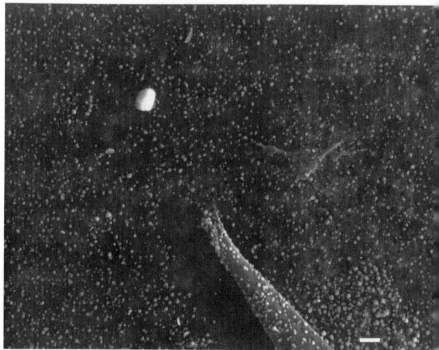

Fig. 5 *Scanning electron micrographs of purified IgG detected by immunogold labeling. Note that the beads are evenly distributed (bars = 1μ; × 4,000).* **Top**, *Adsorption onto polyurethane for 60 minutes.* **Bottom**, *Adsorption onto polydimethylsiloxane for 60 minutes.*

Thus, the adsorption of blood proteins to a biomedical polymer initiates cellular adhesion and activation. Those proteins that are deposited from blood onto the surface of a material can modulate the thrombotic-antithrombotic response. In tissue, proteins can modulate cellular adhesion and activation and thus the myriad of inflammatory mediators produced by the cells. These, in turn, ultimately influence the biocompatibility of that material.

Monocyte Adhesion and Activation on Biomedical Polymers

Cellular interactions occurring at tissue-implant interfaces have been a focus of attention because of the possible contribution of these interactions to determining the biocompatibility of implanted biomedical materials.[9,34] The complexity of these cellular interactions is amplified by the initial phenomenon of protein adsorption because of the intricate network of protein-polymer, protein-cell, and protein-polymer-cell responses.[3,35]

Macrophages

We studied the macrophage, which is common at the tissue-implant interface during foreign-body responses to implanted biomedical polymers,[8] because it produces many products with the potential to alter the inflammatory and wound-healing response to a prosthetic device. Recent attention has focused on growth factors, cytokines, and inhibitors produced by the macrophage and their roles at implant sites.[7,9] These growth factors have implications for polymer-associated wound healing, inflammatory, and immunologic responses.[36,37] Interleukin-1, a major product of activated macrophages, participates significantly in inflammatory responses. Interleukin-1 is multifunctional and mediates many of its effects by interaction with other cells, altering their functional capacity (Fig. 6). Cells that can be altered by interleukin-1 responsiveness include the fibroblast, which modulates proliferation, collagen and collagenase production, and the expression of endothelial cell intracellular adhesion molecules and interleukin-6.[38] It has been shown that interleukin-1 levels increase in patients who have undergone hemodialysis with polymeric regenerated cellulosic membranes, suggesting polymer alteration of macrophage activation.[39] Interleukin-1 has also been implicated in inflammatory diseases, including arthritis, suggesting its significance in modulating chondrocytes, osteoclasts, and osteoblasts during immunologic and inflammatory reactions.[40]

The modulatory capacity of biomedical polymers has been associated with macrophage activation and secretion of biologically active interleukin-1.[10,17] We cultured monocytes in vitro on the surfaces of various biomedical polymers: polyester (Dacron), polyethylene, polyurethane (Biomer), expanded polytetrafluoroethylene, and polystyrene. The monocytes were stimulated with lipopolysaccharide to

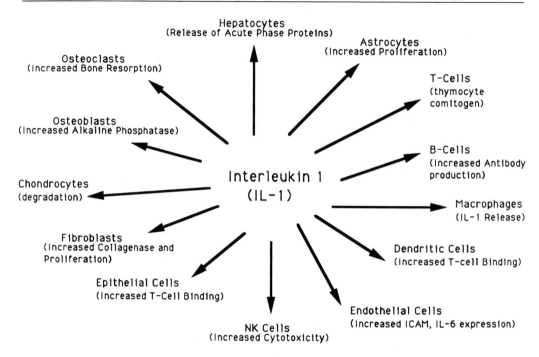

Fig. 6 *Cells responsive to interleukin-1 and their response.*

mimic the foreign-body reaction observed in vivo at the tissue-implant interfaces, as well as to aid in the activation of macrophages. The in vitro tissue culture system (5% fetal bovine serum with 10 μg/ml of lipopolysaccharide for 24 hours) maximized cell viability and culture supernatant activity.[17]

The biologic assay for functional interleukin-1 used mouse thymocytes. The assay involved the incorporation of tritiated-thymidine into mouse thymocytes as a result of interleukin-1 in the culture supernatant. The activity was compared to purified and crude interleukin-1 standards and was measured in units per milliliter.[10,17] The observations made from these functional data (Table 1) depended on the controls used for comparison. We used two controls, biomedical polymers without protein preadsorption and polystyrene. Interleukin-1 activity for these controls was comparable: 15 ± 10 units/ml and 13 ± 6 units/ml, respectively. When these same two polymers underwent preadsorption with fibrinogen or fibronectin, the activity was significantly enhanced to 710 ± 299 units/ml for polyurethane and 71 ± 16 units/ml for polyurethane, a 50–fold increase and a five-fold increase, respectively. Polyurethane and polyethylene that underwent preadsorption with fibronectin had 20 times and 30 times the functional activity of the polymer controls that did not undergo protein preadsorption. There appeared to be two effects: the protein pread-

Table 1 Interleukin-1 activity

Polymer	Protein Adsorbed*			
	None	**IgG**	**Fibrinogen**	**Fibronectin**
Polyurethane	15 ± 10	23 ± 1	203 ± 167	710 ± 299
Polydimethylsiloxane	20 ± 0.1	63 ± 8	386 ± 126	$1,847 \pm 1,301$
Expanded polytetrafluoroethylene	2 ± 1	6 ± 7	238 ± 32	$1,067 \pm 888$
Polyethylene	13 ± 6	17 ± 0.3	334 ± 64	72 ± 16
Polyester	16 ± 6	27 ± 12	562 ± 201	80 ± 27
Polystyrene	20 ± 5	74 ± 21	88 ± 23	$1,043 \pm 131$

*Mean units per milliliter $\pm$ SEM for No. = 3.

sorbed to the surface of the polymers enhanced macrophage activation and expression of functional interleukin-1 activity, and there was a polymer-dependent difference in the degree of enhancement.

Comparisons with the polystyrene control showed a protein-dependent suppression of interleukin-1 functional activity. Polyester and polyethylene had one-tenth the functional activity of polystyrene after preadsorption (72 ± 16 and 80 ± 27 units/ml, respectively, compared with $1,043 \pm 131$ units/ml). This suppression phenomenon was, however, both polymer- and protein-dependent. It was not observed in the absence of protein preadsorption, except in expanded polytetrafluoroethylene. These data suggest that suppression of interleukin-1 functional activity depended on polymer protein preadsorption, implying complex protein-polymer, protein-cell and protein-polymer-cell interactions.

Fibroblasts

We also tested monocyte culture supernatants for growth factors that may promote the growth of another cell type, implying the presence of paracrine growth-promoting potential.[20,41] We selected the fibroblast because of its significance in inflammation and wound healing at implant sites, as well as its responsiveness to interleukin-1. The culture supernatants were tested for fibroblast growth-promoting potential by means of two fibroblast assay systems. These different assay systems with the same fibroblast cell line were developed to measure "competence-like" and "progression-like" macrophage-derived fibroblast growth factors. Both competence and progression factors are required for the fibroblast to enter the cell cycle and proceed to DNA synthesis and eventual cellular proliferation. Competence factor activity implies the presence of growth factors that interact with the fibroblast in G_0 or G_1 of the cell cycle phase.[42] These include platelet-derived growth factor, fibroblast growth factors, and interleukin-6. Progression factor activity implies the presence of growth factors that act at or on the fibroblasts in the G_2 phase of the cell cycle. These include epidermal growth factor, insulin-like growth factor, and interleukin-1. The data obtained from the fibroblast competence and progression assays are summarized in Table 2.

These data can be simplified by categorizing the information into

Table 2 Competence and progression factor activity

Preadsorbed Protein	Polymer*		
	Polyurethane	Polydimethylsiloxane	Polystyrene
None	0/0	0/+	0/+
IgG	0/0	0/+	+/0
Fibronectin	0/0	0/+	+/0
Fibrinogen	0/0	0/+	+/+

*Values indicate interleukin-1 activity with $0 = <10$ units/ml and $+ = >10$ units/ml.

four groups on the basis of polymer and protein adsorption that altered the expression of competence and progression factor activity. These four possible conditions are no detectable interleukin-1 competence or progression factor activity (group 1), detectable competence factor activity without progression factor activity (group 2), progression factor activity without competence factor activity (group 3), and detectable activity of both competence and progression factors (group 4).

Polyurethane consistently fell into group 1 regardless of protein preadsorption, polydimethylsiloxane fell into group 3 before preadsorption and after preadsorption with fibronectin, fibrinogen, or albumin. Polystyrene also stimulated the monocytes to express variable competence and progression growth factor activity under conditions of protein adsorption.

It is not known whether monocyte-polymer interactions evoke the synthesis of any other growth factors or if there is preferential production of a specific growth factor. These studies, however, do support the hypothesis that biomedical polymers themselves, as well as the protein that adsorbs to their surfaces, can significantly alter the activation of macrophages and the synthesis of interleukin-1. These studies also support the hypothesis that alterations in macrophage activation may have the potential of altering other cell types, such as the fibroblast, that participate in wound healing, inflammatory, and foreign-body responses at the tissue implant site. These interactions, then, would have the potential of determining the biocompatibility of the implanted biomedical polymer.

In Vitro and In Vivo Correlations

To investigate further the role of the macrophage and the release of interleukin-1 in controlling biocompatibility in wound healing responses to biomedical polymers, we performed in vivo experiments directed at determining the extent of fibrous capsule formation surrounding subcutaneous implants of several polymers. Previous studies had suggested that differential interleukin-1 production and fibroblast-stimulating potential would result in variable in vivo fibrous capsule development.

Interleukin-1 is an important mediator of the inflammatory process, regulating fibroblast growth and proliferation and protein synthesis. By stimulating fibroblast activity, interleukin-1 induces the synthesis of the fibroblast product collagen.[43] However, because it has also been shown to stimulate collagenase production by cultured fibroblasts in human synovial cells, interleukin-1 must be a sensitive regulatory molecule capable of controlling the duration and extent of fibroblast activity. We anticipated that polymers producing low macrophage activation, low interleukin-1 production, and low fibroblast-stimulating potential would produce thin fibrous capsules in vivo and that, conversely, polymers producing high macrophage activation, high interleukin-1 production, and high fibroblast-stimulating potential would produce thick fibrous capsules in vivo. To test this hypothesis, we evaluated fibrous capsule formation around various subcutaneously implanted biomedical polymers.

Female Sprague-Dawley rats were anesthetized with diethyl ether, shaved, and scrubbed, and the polymer samples were implanted by tunneling immediately beneath the panniculus carnosus. The animals were killed after two, four, and eight weeks, and the entire implant site with adjacent tissue was removed and placed in buffered formaldehyde for histologic study with hematoxylin-eosin and Masson's trichrome staining of tissue sections prepared by standard paraffin-embedding and tissue-sectioning methods. This permitted the evaluation of changes in cellular and matrix composition and the organization of the fibrous capsule with time. Only sections taken from the midpoint of the implant site were studied. The thickness of the developing fibrous capsule on each side of the implant was determined.

Quantitative measurement of fibrous capsules surrounding the polymers showed polyethylene to have the thickest fibrous capsules at all times (0.178, 0.575, and 0.188 mm at two, four, and eight weeks, respectively), polydimethylsiloxane was intermediate (0.060, 0.165, and 0.107 mm), and polyurethane had the thinnest fibrous capsule (0.073, 0.086, and 0.079 mm). These results correlated with the in vitro studies of interleukin-1 production from macrophages and fibroblast-stimulating potential from supernatants of monocytes cultured on the polymers. Polyurethane generated a thin subcutaneous fibrous capsule with decreased amounts of collagen. Remarkably, the thickness of the fibrous capsule did not change significantly during the eight-week implantation period. The fibrous capsules for polyethylene and polydimethylsiloxane were thicker at all three times. The increase at four weeks was followed by condensation of the fibrous capsule at eight weeks.

Acknowledgment

This work was supported in part by grants HL-27277, HL-25239, and HL-33829 from the National Institute of Health.

References

1. Anderson JM, Bonfield TL, Ziats NP: Protein adsorption and cellular adhesion and activation on biomedical polymers. *Int J Artif Organs* 1990;13:375–382.
2. Ziats NP, Pankowsky DA, Tierney BP, et al: Adsorption of Hageman factor (factor XII) and other human plasma proteins to biomedical polymers. *J Lab Clin Med*, 1990;116:687–697.

3. Andrade JD, Hlady V: Protein adsorption and materials biocompatibility: A tutorial review and suggested hypothesis. *Adv Polym Sci* 1986;79:1–63.

4. Horbett TA: Techniques for protein adsorption studies, in Williams DF (ed): *Techniques of Biocompatibility Testing*. Boca Raton, CRC Press, 1986, vol 2, pp 183–214.

5. Vroman L: The life of an artificial device in contact with blood: Initial events and their effect on its final state. *Bull NY Acad Med* 1988;64:352–357.

6. Brash JL, Scott CF, ten Hove P, et al: Mechanism of transient adsorption of fibrinogen from plasma to solid surfaces: Role of the contact and fibrinolytic systems. *Blood* 1988;71:932–939.

7. Anderson JM, Miller KM: Biomaterial biocompatibility and the macrophage. *Biomaterials* 1984;5:5–10.

8. Anderson JM: Inflammatory response to implants. *ASAIO Trans* 1988;34:101–107.

9. Ziats NP, Miller KM, Anderson JM: *In vitro* and *in vivo* interactions of cells with biomaterials. *Biomaterials* 1988;9:5–13.

10. Bonfield TL, Colton E, Anderson JM: Plasma protein adsorbed biomedical polymers: Activation of human monocytes and induction of interleukin 1. *J Biomed Mater Res* 1989;23:535–548.

11. Marchant RE, Miller KM, Anderson JM: In vivo biocompatibility studies: V. In vivo leukocyte interactions with Biomer. *J Biomed Mater Res* 1984;18:1169–1190.

12. Spilizewski KL, Marchant RE, Anderson JM, et al: In vivo leucocyte interactions with the NHLBI-DTB primary reference materials: Polyethylene and silica-free polydimethylsiloxane. *Biomaterials* 1987;8:12–17.

13. Kottke-Marchant K, Anderson JM, Rabinovitch A, et al: The effect of heparin vs. citrate on the interaction of platelets with vascular graft materials. *Thromb Haemost* 1985;54:842–848.

14. Kottke-Marchant K, Anderson JM, Rabinovitch A: The platelet reactivity of vascular graft prostheses: An *in vitro* model to test the effect of preclotting. *Biomaterials* 1986;7:441–448.

15. Kottke-Marchant K, Anderson JM, Miller KM, et al: Vascular graft-associated complement activation and leukocyte adhesion in an artificial circulation. *J Biomed Mater Res* 1987;21:379–397.

16. Kottke-Marchant K, Anderson JM, Umemura Y, et al: Effect of albumin coating on the *in vitro* blood compatibility of Dacron arterial prostheses. *Biomaterials* 1989;10:147–155.

17. Miller KM, Anderson JM: Human monocyte/macrophage activation and interleukin 1 generation by biomedical polymers. *J Biomed Mater Res* 1988;22:713–731.

18. Miller KM, Huskey RA, Bigby LF, et al: Characterization of biomedical polymer-adherent macrophages: Interleukin 1 generation and scanning electron microscopy studies. *Biomaterials* 1989;10:187–196.

19. Miller KM, Rose-Caprara V, Anderson JM: Generation of IL-1–like activity in response to biomedical polymer implants: A comparison of in vitro and in vivo models. *J Biomed Mater Res* 1989;23:1007–1026.

20. Miller KM, Anderson JM: In vitro stimulation of fibroblast activity by factors generated from human monocytes activated by biomedical polymers. *J Biomed Mater Res* 1989;23:911–930.

21. Williams DF, Askill IN, Smith R: Protein absorption and desorption phenomena on clean metal surfaces. *J Biomed Mater Res* 1985;19:313–320.

22. Williams RL, Williams DF: Albumin adsorption on metal surfaces. *Biomaterials* 1988;9:206–212.

23. van Enckevort HJ, Dass DV, Langdon AG: The adsorption of bovine serum albumin at the stainless-steel/aqueous solution interface. *J Collagen Interf Sci* 1984;98:138–143.

24. Sharma CP, Sunny MC: Albumin adsorption onto aluminium oxide and polyurethane surfaces. *Biomaterials* 1990;11:255–257.

25. Veerman ECI, Suppers RJF, Klein CPAT, et al: SDS-PAGE analysis of the protein layers adsorbing *in vivo* and *in vitro* to bone substituting materials. *Biomaterials* 1987;8:442–448.

26. Sukenik CN, Balachander N, Culp LA, et al: Modulation of cell adhesion by modification of titanium surfaces with covalently attached self-assembled monolayers. *J Biomed Mater Res* 1990;24:1307–1323.

27. Brash JL, Uniyal S, Chan BMC, et al: Fibrinogen-glass interactions: A synopsis of recent research, in Gebelein CG (ed): *Polymeric Materials and Artificial Organs* (ACS Symposium Series 256). Washington, DC, American Chemical Society, 1984, pp 45–61.

28. Park K, Simmons SR, Albrecht RM: Surface characterization of biomaterials by immunogold staining: Quantitative analysis. *Scanning Microsc* 1987;1:339–350.

29. Pankowsky DA, Ziats NP, Topham NS, et al: Morphologic characteristics of adsorbed human plasma proteins on vascular grafts and biomaterials. *J Vasc Surg* 1990;11:599–606.

30. Ziats NP, Topham NS, Pankowsky DA, et al: Analysis of protein adsorption on retrieved human vascular grafts using immunogold labelling with silver enhancement. *Cells Mater*, 1991;1:73–82.

31. Kuwahara T, Markert M, Wauters JP: Proteins adsorbed on hemodialysis membranes modulate neutrophil activation. *Artif Organs* 1989;13:427–431.

32. Trezzini C, Jungi TW, Maly FE, et al: Low-affinity interaction of fibrinogen carboxy-gamma terminus with human monocytes induces an oxidative burst and modulates effector functions. *Biochem Biophys Res Commun* 1989;165:7–13.

33. Morley DJ, Feuerstein IA: Adhesion of polymorphonuclear leukocytes to protein-coated and platelet adherent surfaces. *Thromb Haemost* 1989;62:1023–1028.

34. Lydon MJ, Minett TW, Tighe BJ: Cellular interactions with synthetic polymer surfaces in culture. *Biomaterials* 1985;6:396–402.

35. Baier RE, Dutton RC: Initial events in interactions of blood with a foreign surface. *J Biomed Mater Res* 1969;3:191–206.

36. ten Dijke P, Iwata KK: Growth factors for wound healing. *Bio/Technology* 1989;7:793–798.

37. Wahl SM, Wong H, McCartney-Francis N: Role of growth factors in inflammation and repair. *J Cell Biochem* 1989;40:193–199.

38. Durum SK, Oppenheim JJ, Neta R: Immunophysiologic role of interleukin 1, in Oppenheim JJ, Shevach EM (eds): *Immunophysiology: The Role of Cells and Cytokines in Immunity and Inflammation*. New York, Oxford University Press, 1990, pp 210–225.

39. Lonnemann G, Bingel M, Koch KM, et al: Plasma interleukin-1 activity in humans undergoing hemodialysis with regenerated cellulosic membranes. *Lymphokine Res* 1987;6:63–70.

40. Snyderman R, Pike MC: Structure and function of monocytes and macrophages, in McCarty DJ (ed): *Arthritis and Allied Conditions: A Textbook of Rheumatology*, ed 11. Philadelphia, Lea & Febiger, 1989, pp 306–335.

41. Bonfield TL, Colton E, Anderson JM: Fibroblast stimulation by monocytes cultured on protein adsorbed biomedical polymers: I. Biomer and polydimethylsiloxane. *J Biomed Mater Res*, 1991;25:165–175.

42. Nemeth GG, Bolander NE, Martin GR: Growth factors and their role in wound and fracture healing, in Barbul A, Pines E, Caldwell M, et al (eds): *Growth Factors and Other Aspects of Wound Healing: Biological and Clinical Implications.* New York, Alan R Liss, 1988, pp 1–17.

43. Singh JP, Adams LD, Bonin PD: Mode of fibroblast growth enhancement by human interleukin-1. *J Cell Biol* 1988;106:813–819.

Chapter 19

Effect of Endotoxin (Lipopolysaccharide) on Bone Cell Function, Bone Allograft Incorporation, and Fracture Repair

Mark C. Horowitz, PhD
Robert L. Jilka, PhD
Thomas A. Einhorn, MD

Introduction

Postoperative infection can be a serious and, in some cases, life-threatening complication. This is particularly true for orthopaedic procedures, in which the severity of the wound, the use of prosthetic implants, and the difficulty in delivering antibiotics to the site of infection in sequestered necrotic bone can interfere with treatment. Infection of the bone, most notably bacterial sepsis, is associated with a series of events leading to bone loss and mechanical failure. The deleterious effects of infection, which are most pronounced when associated with bone grafting, almost always result in failure of the graft.

Invading organisms, bacteria in particular, produce enzymes, exotoxins, and, especially, endotoxins, which initiate a cascade of host-mediated events. At the organism level, infection with gram-negative bacteria can lead to pathophysiology characterized by hypotension, intravascular coagulation, multisystem organ failure, and shock.[1,2] At the cellular level, these events include induction of opsonic antibody, enzymatic degradation, activation of the fibrinolytic pathway, loss of vasculature, and eventual cell death leading to bone necrosis. It is our hypothesis that, in addition to this pathway, another set of events occurs that leads to cell activation rather than cell death. We assume that these two sets of events occur either sequentially or in tandem and may be part of the same cascade. Moreover, they may have aspects that are similar to those events induced by antigen-specific activation of immune cells, especially those associated with allograft reactivity. Many of the cell types, particularly the soluble mediators, are identical. While the specific triggering mechanism for each of these events may differ, it appears that a commonality may exist between the host's response to bone infection, bone allograft implantation, and fracture repair (Fig. 1).

During infection, the series of events that are induced may be initiated by bacterial endotoxin (lipopolysaccharide). It is well recognized that lipopolysaccharide exerts potent effects on a variety of target cells associated with both nonspecific inflammatory and specific immune

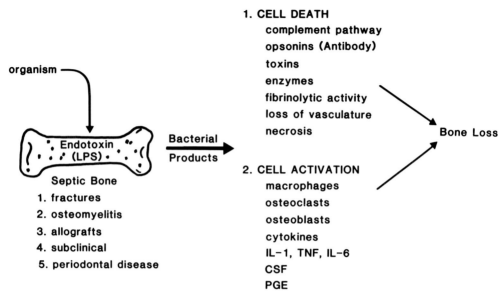

organism

1. CELL DEATH
complement pathway
opsonins (Antibody)
toxins
enzymes
fibrinolytic activity
loss of vasculature
necrosis

Endotoxin
(LPS)

Bacterial
Products

Bone Loss

Septic Bone
1. fractures
2. osteomyelitis
3. allografts
4. subclinical
5. periodontal disease

2. CELL ACTIVATION
macrophages
osteoclasts
osteoblasts
cytokines
IL-1, TNF, IL-6
CSF
PGE

Fig. 1 *Effect of endotoxin (lipopolysaccharide) on bone.*

responses, including macrophages, neutrophils, and B lymphocytes.[3] A similar response should be observed during bone infections. In addition to the cells normally associated with inflammatory foci, bone macrophages and osteoblasts are activated by lipopolysaccharides, as evidenced by cell proliferation, cytokine secretion, and increased bone resorption.[4,5] Moreover, because of the close physical association of bone to bone marrow, exposure of bone to infection results in a similar exposure to the bone marrow.

Because cells of both the hematopoietic and stromal cell lineage respond to bacterial endotoxin, exposure of bone cells to lipopolysaccharides from invading organisms results in the activation of cells from many different systems.[6] As part of this activation, cells secrete a genetically predetermined (and therefore specific) set of cytokines. These cytokines function initially in a paracrine fashion to amplify the activation, and they function secondarily to initiate associated cell activation. Certain of these biological response modifiers may also act in an autocrine manner to regulate the response. Some cytokines are involved in the induction of osteoclastic bone resorption; others are involved in bone cell maturation, which results in increased numbers of osteoclasts and possibly macrophages. A clear example of this is the response of bone cells to lipopolysaccharides and their subsequent interactions. We will present evidence that lipopolysaccharide induces bone cell activation and that these activated cells secrete cytokines that are involved in bone remodeling. A relationship will be established between the cells and cytokines that mediate the host's response to infected bone allografts, the activation of bone cells, and the regulation of fracture repair.

Activation of Bone Cells by Lipopolysaccharide

The purpose of reconstructive orthopaedic procedures is to restore a specific part of the musculoskeletal system to normal functioning. This may involve a wide range of approaches, including both non-biological biomaterials (metals, ceramics, and plastics) and biological biomaterials (cadaver derived frozen bone, lyophilized osteochondral allografts, and autologous bone as graft material). In all of these cases, with a possible caveat relating to the inflammatory response to the autograft, it is the host's response to the material that is critical to the successful outcome of the procedure. Therefore, modification of the host's response, either positively or negatively, is an important consideration. Infection can be a serious negative factor.

To examine our hypothesis that molecules of bacterial origin activate host cells, we will confine our discussion to a consideration of lipopolysaccharide. This is done for a number of reasons, not the least of which is the fact that gram-negative organisms represent the causative agent responsible for a significant percentage of orthopaedic infections, and lipopolysaccharide is produced by most gram-negative organisms. In addition, cells of various phenotypes, lineages, and states of maturation are sensitive to lipopolysaccharides.

Lipopolysaccharide is pyrogeneic and induces a vigorous inflammatory response.[7,8] Lipopolysaccharide is also a potent activator of immune cells that stimulates B but not T lymphocyte proliferation. This proliferation is followed by polyclonal immunoglobulin secretion.[9,10] Lipopolysaccharide directly activates macrophages to secrete interleukin-1, granulocyte-macrophage colony stimulating factor, tumor necrosis factor, and interleukin-6.[11-16] These cytokines all have bone cell stimulating activity. Lipopolysaccharide activates target cells through an 80 kD cell surface binding protein that may represent a lipopolysaccharide receptor.[17,18] This binding protein can be identified on all responsive cells.[18,19] Because lipopolysaccharide is such an effective stimulus to immune cells, can this molecule also stimulate normal bone cells to secrete cytokines? If it can, are these cytokines bone active and are they similar to those secreted by either bone cells or immune cells activated during conditions not associated with sepsis? If the answers to these questions are "yes," then it may be hypothesized that there is a biologically conserved response throughout bone to bacterial endotoxin.

To address this question we prepared isolated bone cells by sequential collagenase digestion from the calvaria of normal newborn mice.[20-22] Bone cells were seeded at either high (2×10^5/cm^2) or low (0.4×10^5/cm^2) density and cultured to confluence (Table 1). High-density cells reached confluence overnight, but five to seven days were

Table 1 Cellular composition of bone cell populations seeded at high or low density

Cells	High Density	Low Density
Osteoblast precursors or osteoblasts	80–90%	>90%
Mononuclear phagocytes	5–10%	<1%
Osteoclasts	0.1–0.2%	Undetectable
	Only following induction with PTH	No effect with PTH
	Resorb bone	No bone resorption
Other	Unknown	Unknown

required for the low-density cells to reach confluence. The monolayers were washed and cultured in the presence or absence of lipopolysaccharide (10 μg/ml) for 48 hours, at which time the conditioned media was collected and tested for the presence of cytokines. Although both populations consisted primarily of osteoblast and osteoblast precursors (more than 90%), they differed considerably in mononuclear cell content. The high-density population contained 5% to 10% mononuclear phagocytes, and osteoclasts could be detected in the presence of exogenously added parathyroid hormone. In contrast, no macrophages or osteoclasts were observed in the low-density population, even when parathyroid hormone was added.[23] These data suggest that a low seeding density does not support the growth of macrophage precursors, macrophages, or osteoclasts.

To illustrate our hypothesis of how lipopolysaccharide induces cytokine-mediated events, we will confine our discussion to the data concerning interleukin-1. Where appropriate, other relevant cytokines will be mentioned. Interleukin-1 has been selected for a number of reasons. Interleukin-1 is a potent stimulator of osteoclastic bone resorption; osteoblasts have high affinity surface membrane receptors for interleukin-1; interleukin-1 can modulate both immune and hematopoietic cell function.[24-27] Interleukin-1 activity was determined in a two-stage bioassay. LBRM cells, a T cell lymphoma line, secrete interleukin-2 only in the presence of interleukin-1 and phytohemagglutinin, which functions as a co-mitogen. Therefore, a titration of test conditioned media was added to LBRM cells and cultured in the presence or absence of phytohemagglutinin for 24 hours. At that point, 50 μl of conditioned media was transferred to a second set of tissue culture wells to which the interleukin-2 dependent T cell line CTLL (2 × 10⁴) was added.[28] The interleukin-2 activity was measured after 48 hours by ^{3}H-thymidine incorporation by the CTLL cells.

Conditioned media from low- and high-density calvarial cells cultured in the absence of lipopolysaccharide showed no detectable interleukin-1 activity, which suggests that the cells do not constitutively secrete interleukin-1. Conditioned media from cells cultured at low density in the presence of lipopolysaccharides also showed no detectable interleukin-1 activity. However, conditioned media from high-density cells cultured in the presence of lipopoysaccharides contained significant levels of interleukin-1 activity (Fig. 2).

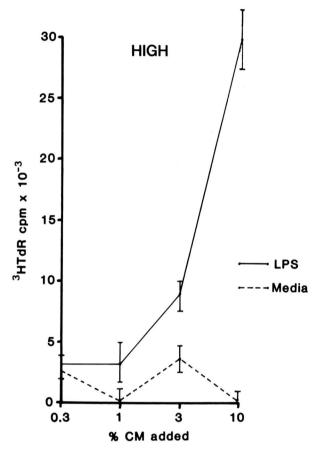

Fig. 2 *IL-1 secretion by high density seeded calvarial cells. Neonatal mouse calvarial cells (from sequential collagenase digestion, population 3–5) were seeded at high density and cultured in the presence (solid line) or absence (broken line) of 10 μg/ml of lipopolysaccharide for 48 hours. The conditioned media was collected and tested for interleukin-1 activity (³HTdR = tritiated thymidine density ratio).*

To demonstrate that this activity was caused by interleukin-1, polyclonal goat antimouse interleukin-1α or anti-interleukin-1β antibody was added to the LBRM half of the assay culture. The anti-interleukin-1 antibodies were provided by Dr. Thomas Kupper, Washington University, St. Louis. Conditioned media from cells cultured with lipopolysaccharides served as a positive control. Data in Figure 3 show that antibody to interleukin-1α blocked all the interleukin-1 activity. Neither antibody to interleukin-1β nor normal goat serum (negative control) had any inhibitory activity. These data strongly suggest that the activity observed is caused by interleukin-1α.

Inhibitors of interleukin-1 and interleukin-1 receptors have been identified, cloned, and expressed.[29–32] The presence of an inhibitor in

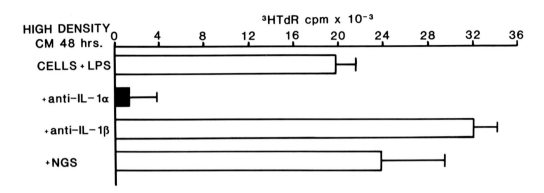

Fig. 3 *Interleukin-1a secretion by high density calvarial cells. Antibodies and normal goat serum were used at equivalent dilutions (³HTdR = tritiated thymidine density ratio).*

the conditioned media from the low-density cells may have precluded our ability to detect interleukin-1 activity. To test this possibility, predetermined stimulating doses of interleukin-1 were cultured with conditioned media from either low-density cells or MC3T3-E1 cells (Fig. 4). MC3T3 is a cloned murine osteoblast cell line that is very similar to primary low-density seeded cells.[33] To ensure that the concentration of conditioned media was sufficient, preliminary experiments were conducted, which showed that the concentrations of conditioned media used had detectable interleukin-1 activity if they were derived from high-density seeded cells. No diminution of the interleukin-1 activity was observed, which suggested the absence of an interleukin-1 inhibitor.

In summary, the data presented thus far indicate that the high-density population of calvarial cells, and not the low-density population, contain the cell or cells responsible for interleukin-1 secretion. The activity detected was, in fact, caused by interleukin-1, and the failure of the low-density conditioned media to stimulate could not be attributed to the presence of an interleukin-1 inhibitor. Interleukin-1 is secreted by the high-density cells only following activation and not constitutively.

The next step in the development of the hypothesis was to identify the cellular source of interleukin-1 in the high-density population. This was particularly important because conflicting reports have been published on the ability of different bone cell populations to secrete interleukin-1. We have addressed this issue by examining a large number of osteoblasts from different sources, including cell lines, osteosarcomas, and primary cells of mouse, rat, and human origin. In all cases, conditioned media from lipopolysaccharide-activated cells failed to show detectable levels of interleukin-1, with the exception of high-

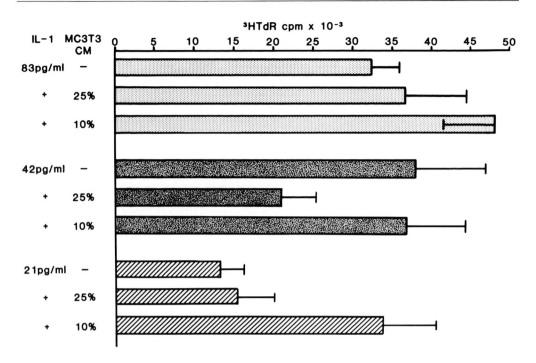

Fig. 4 *Absence of an interleukin-1 inhibitor from bone cell conditioned media. Recombinant human interleukin-1α was used. MC3T3 conditioned media was prepared by culturing confluent cell monolayers for 48 hours and collecting the media (³HTdR = tritiated thymidine density ratio).*

density seeded primary cells. The interleukin-1 assay can detect levels of interleukin-1 between 1 and 10 pg/ml. We have also examined some of these cells by Northern blot analysis and could not detect interleukin-1 mRNA in any of the samples, even following activation with lipopolysaccharides. Taken together, our data suggest that osteoblasts and osteoblast precursors are not a source of interleukin-1.

It is now recognized that within the population of bone cells there exists a subpopulation of bone macrophages.[23,34] Because macrophages in other tissue are a known source of interleukin-1, it was possible that the macrophages in bone were also a source of interleukin-1. To test this possibility, high-density cells were treated with the monoclonal antibody B23.1, which is specific for postmonoblastic mononuclear phagocytes.[35] The cells were washed and complement was added to kill the antibody-bearing population of cells.[36] The remaining cells were washed and cultured in the presence or absence of lipopolysaccharides for 48 hours and the conditioned media tested for interleukin-1 activity. Conditioned media from cells treated with complement only and lipopolysaccharide (positive control) contained interleukin-1 activity. However, conditioned media from cells treated with B23.1 plus com-

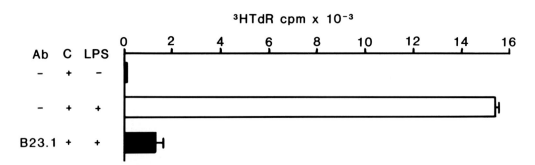

Fig. 5 *B23.1-bearing bone cells (macrophages) secrete interleukin-1. High density seeded cells were washed and incubated with B23.1 for 30 minutes at 37 C. The monolayers were washed and cultured in rabbit serum (diluted 1:10) as a source of complement. Monolayers cultured in complement alone served as a control (³HTdR = tritiated thymidine density ratio).*

plement and lipopolysaccharides contained no detectable interleukin-1 activity (Fig. 5). B23.1 is not cytotoxic for murine osteoblasts (M.C. Horowitz and R.L. Jilka, unpublished data). These data, in conjunction with the inability of osteoblasts to secrete interleukin-1, strongly suggest that bone macrophages, and not osteoblasts, are a major source of interleukin-1 in bone.

Recent evidence has shown that osteoclasts are members of the macrophage lineage.[37-40] Therefore, it is important to keep in mind that osteoclasts may also be a source of interleukin-1 in bone. However, no direct data are available to support or deny this supposition.

Having determined that osteoblasts are not a source of interleukin-1, we next asked whether or not they are capable of secreting other biologically active cytokines in response to lipopolysaccharides. To partially address this question, low-density primary mouse bone cells were cultured with lipopolysaccharides (as described previously) and the conditioned media tested for the presence of granulocyte-macrophage colony stimulating factor and macrophage colony stimulating factor. Colony stimulating factor activity was determined by measuring ³H-thymidine incorporation by factor-dependent cell lines, as previously described.[41,42] Primary cells secreted both granulocyte-macrophage colony stimulating factor (Fig. 6, *left*) and macrophage colony stimulating factor (Fig. 6, *right*) following exposure to lipopolysaccharides, but did not secrete either of these cytokines constitutively. These data indicate that osteoblasts, cultured under the same conditions in which they failed to show interleukin-1 activity, are fully capable of secreting other biologically active products. This suggests that, in a manner similar to T lymphocytes, osteoblasts can be distinguished from other bone cells on the basis of the cytokines they secrete.[43,44]

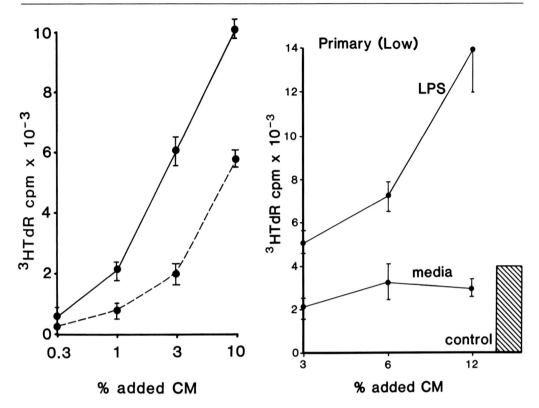

Fig. 6 *Primary osteoblasts secrete granulocyte macrophage-colony stimulating factor and macrophage-colony stimulating factor. **Left,** Granulocyte macrophage-colony stimulating factor activity was determined by culturing varying concentrations of conditioned media with 10⁴ HT-2 cells (T cell clone) for 48 hours (solid line represents conditioned media from 48-hour cultures and the broken line represents conditioned media from 96-hour cultures, control was less than 113 ± 15 SEM); **Right,** Macrophage-colony stimulating factor activity was determined by culturing varying concentrations of conditioned media with 10⁵ C3H/HeJ bone marrow cells for 72 hours. C3H/HeJ was selected because it fails to respond directly to lipopolysaccharide (³HTdR = tritiated thymidine density ratio). (Reproduced with permission from Horowitz MC, Coleman DL, Flood PM, et al: Parathyroid hormone and lipopolysaccharide induce murine osteoblast-like cells to secrete a cytokine indistinguishable from granulocyte-macrophage colony-stimulating factor. J Clin Invest 1989;83:149–157.)*

The Host Response to Bone Allograft

Bone allografts are used frequently to repair a variety of bone defects, including those resulting from trauma or tumor resection. Large numbers of procedures are performed using allogeneic bone chips or powder to repair smaller cystic defects, including those associated with periodontal defects. Large allografts are harvested from cadavers, treated with cryoprotectants and stored frozen. Alternatively, these grafts may be preserved by lyophilization. Bone chips or powder are most often prepared from lyophilized bone under sterile conditions. Grafted bone presents three distinct, but related, problems for the recipient. First, the graft presents a unique biomaterial, which has the ability to bind bacteria and provide a focus for bacterial growth. Second, the graft is a foreign body and by definition induces a foreign-body response. This response is characterized by a cellular infiltrate at the graft site, composed initially of neutrophils and macrophages, followed by T and B lymphocytes.[45,46] The inflammatory response is antigen nonspecific. Third, depending on the specific graft, the host mounts an immune response, comprised of an initial antigen specific response followed by a series of antigen nonspecific responses.

The fates of bone allografts, specifically large segmental grafts, fall into four basic categories. First, the allograft may be fully incorporated into the host skeleton and function in a physiologically normal fashion. The graft provides a physical scaffolding, is slowly resorbed by the host bone cells and is replaced with new bone. This new bone formation may be stimulated by proteins sequestered in the graft that are either released over time or are released following some active process such as bone resorption. This outcome occurs between 50% and 90% of the time, depending on the model evaluated and parameters equated with success. The fact that so many allografts are incorporated in the absence of immunosuppressive therapy is of particular significance. In the second of the four categories, the bone allograft appears inert, little inflammatory response is observed following implantation and no significant cellular response is noted. For the most part, these grafts fail to incorporate, although a small percentage (less than 20%) do survive to serve some biomechanical function. In the third category, the graft is rejected as manifested by unopposed resorption and eventual dissolution of the implant in what appears to be an immunologically mediated response. This response is characterized by an inflammatory exudate at the graft site, followed by the appearance of serum antibodies to graft antigens and possibly the appearance of cytotoxic effector T lymphocytes.[47-50] In the fourth category of allografts, postoperative drainage occurs, if not overt infection, usually caused by gram-negative or gram-positive bacteria. Almost without exception this leads to graft failure. We would suggest that, despite antibiotic intervention, this failure, which occurs early, is rarely reversible.

What is meant by the rejection of a bone allograft? The mechanism of bone allograft rejection has unique aspects, which differentiate it from soft tissue rejection. Both the specialized matrix and the mineral present in bone must be removed. This suggests that specialized machinery must be in place to perform these functions. The cell primarily responsible for this function is the osteoclast. Like other members of the macrophage lineage, osteoclasts, once activated, will attach to the bone surface and secrete enzymes, which remove the matrix, and protons, which acidify and dissolve the mineral phase.[51] Therefore, the presence of the allograft must stimulate the osteoclast and its precursors to actively resorb bone.

Activation of osteoclasts by allogeneic bone may be explained in the

Outline 1   Potential graft antigens

1. Bone (mineral) reservoir for proteins
2. Matrix
   a. collagenous
   b. noncollagenous
3. Ligamentous attachment sites
4. Cells
   a. bone marrow
   b. bone (osteoblasts, osteoclasts, macrophages)
   c. stromal cells

following manner. Protein antigens are carried by the graft, even after long periods of storage at -70 C. Graft antigens may be inadvertently protected by the cryopreservation process itself, as well as by the retention of ligamentous structures used for attachment at the time of engraftment. A bone allograft is a composite tissue and is very complex from the biomaterial standpoint. Part of this complexity arises from the potential sources and numbers of antigens associated with the graft (Outline 1).

Although these tissues and their component proteins have the potential to present thousands of antigens, the most likely set of antigens are those encoded by the major histocompatibility complex.

The major histocompatibility complex encoded antigens most commonly associated with allograft reactivity are Class I (transplantation antigens, K and D region products in the mouse; HLA-A, B, and C in humans) and Class II (Ia antigens, Aα:Aβ; Eα:Eβ in the mouse; HLA-D in humans).[52] Class I antigens are composed of 44 kD transmembrane glycoproteins with a noncovalently associated 12 kD protein, β_2-microglobulin.[53] The Class I transplantation antigens are highly polymorphic, are found on virtually all nucleated cells, and function as targets for cytotoxic (CD8[+]) T lymphocytes.[54] Class II antigens, which are also highly polymorphic, are generally found as cell-surface antigens composed of two transmembrane glycoproteins of 27–29 kD (light or β chain) and 33–35 kD (heavy or α chain), both encoded by the major histocompatibility complex. Class II antigens are found primarily on B lymphocytes and on populations of activated T lymphocytes. High densities of class II antigens are also found on antigen-presenting cells such as dendritic cells and cells of the macrophage/myeloid lineage.[55,56] Class II antigens are key elements in the control of T cell response to antigen, functioning as part of the antigen complex recognized by the T cell receptor of regulatory CD4[+] T lymphocytes (Fig. 7).[57,58]

It cannot be ruled out, however, that antigens other than major histocompatibility complex encoded proteins are contributing to this response. Antibodies to nonmajor histocompatibility complex encoded antigens can be detected in the circulation following grafting.[59,60] However, we believe that the recognition of major histocompatibility complex encoded antigens by the host's immune system (which results in the activation of T and B lymphocytes and macrophages) is the trigger

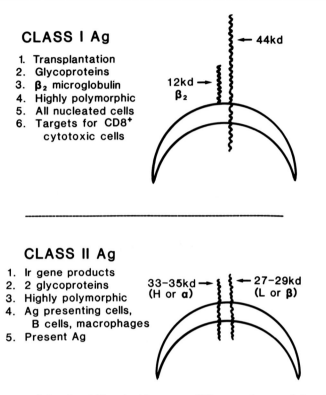

CLASS I Ag

1. Transplantation
2. Glycoproteins
3. β_2 microglobulin
4. Highly polymorphic
5. All nucleated cells
6. Targets for CD8[+] cytotoxic cells

44kd

12kd → β_2

CLASS II Ag

1. Ir gene products
2. 2 glycoproteins
3. Highly polymorphic
4. Ag presenting cells, B cells, macrophages
5. Present Ag

33–35kd → (H or α)

27–29kd (L or β)

Fig. 7 *Structure of class I and II major histocompatibility complex encoded antigens (Ag = antigen).*

that initiates the cascade of events that ultimately leads to incorporation or failure of the graft. Immune cell activation results in the elicitation of a variety of cytokines. These cytokines were first identified as being involved in amplification of T cell responses (IL-1), cytotoxic activity (tumor necrosis factor α) and stimulation of hematopoietic activity (granulocyte-macrophage colony stimulating factor, macrophage colony stimulating factor, and interleukin-6). As demonstrated in the previous section, these same factors are closely associated with bone cell functions, such as osteoclastogenesis (granulocyte-macrophage colony stimulating factor, macrophage colony stimulating factor, and interleukin-6), osteoblast activation, and the induction of bone resorption (interleukin-1 and tumor necrosis factor). Therefore, immune cells activated by alloantigen secrete cytokines that are similar if not identical to those secreted by lipopolysaccharide-activated bone cells. Moreover, the cytokines themselves are active on the cells that secrete them.

Bone resorption must occur before new bone formation can begin. This is true both for normal bone remodeling and during most bone

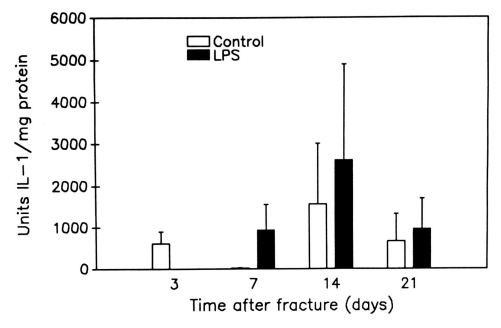

Fig. 8 *Interleukin-1 secretion by cultured fracture callus. Fracture callus derived interleukin-1 was determined by the LBRM assay.*

allograft responses. Therefore, if resorption must occur, then the critical event is not the resorption itself, but, rather, the regulation of that resorption. Too much resorption results in excessive bone loss and fracture. Too little resorption leads to an incompletely incorporated or inert graft, which will ultimately fail.

Cytokine Secretion by Fracture Callus

We have presented data suggesting that during bone infection caused by gram-negative bacteria the lipopolysaccharides present in the cell wall of the microorganism activate normal bone cells to secrete a genetically predetermined set of cytokines (e.g. osteoblasts secrete granulocyte-macrophage colony stimulating factor but not interleukin-1). These cytokines are similar to those secreted by immune cells activated by allografted bone. It is, therefore, possible that these and other cytokines play a central role in the regulation of bone remodeling under a variety of conditions. We have explored this possibility by studying the effect of lipopolysaccharides on the production of cytokines secreted by fracture callus. Fracture callus represents an excellent model of wound healing in hard tissue.

Closed fractures of rat femora were produced using the method of

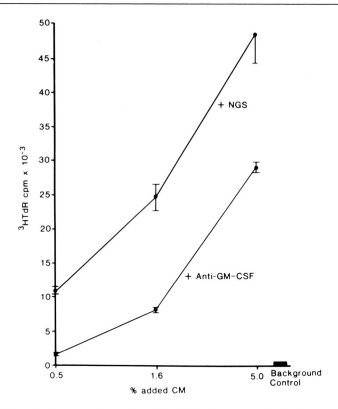

Fig. 9 *Granulocyte macrophage-colony stimulating factor secretion by fracture callus. Granulocyte macrophage-colony stimulating factor activity was determined by HT-2 cell proliferation. Neutralizing goat anti-mouse granulocyte macrophage-colony stimulating factor antibody (1:1000 diluton) was used to verify the presence of granulocyte macrophage-colony stimulating factor Normal goat serum at the same dilution as the antiserum was used as a control (³HTdR = tritiated thymidine density ratio).*

Bonnarens and Einhorn.[61] These fractures are ideal for these studies because of the low level of associated soft-tissue damage. Calluses, removed from the fracture site at various times postfracture, were cultured in the presence or absence of 10 μg/ml of lipopolysaccharide for 48 hours. The conditioned media were collected and tested for cytokine activity. Data in Figure 8 show the appearance of interleukin-1 activity in control fracture callus conditioned media, peaking at 14 days postfracture. This activity can be augmented by the addition of lipopolysaccharides. These results suggest that the trauma of breaking a bone is itself capable of inducing cytokine secretion by cells in the callus. Moreover, these cells can respond to lipopolysaccharides as evidenced by increased interleukin-1 secretion.

Data in Figure 9 indicate that the fracture callus conditioned media induces the proliferation of HT-2 cells. HT-2 cells are a factor-depen-

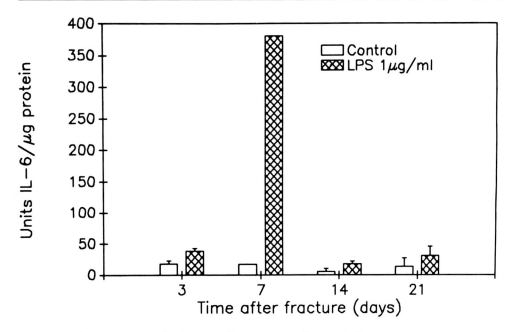

Fig. 10 *Interleukin-6 secretion by fracture callus. Fracture callus interleukin-6 activity was determined by culturing conditioned media with the interleukin-6 dependent cell line B9 (B cell hybridoma) for 72 hours. (Reprinted by permission of VCH Publishers, Inc., 220 East 23rd St., New York, N.Y., 10010 from: Aarden, DeGroot, Schaap, et al. Production of hybridoma growth factor by human monocytes. Eur J Immunol. 1987;17:1411–1416.)*

dent cell line that proliferate in response to granulocyte-macrophage colony stimulating factor.[41] This proliferation is partially blocked by the addition of neutralizing antibody to granulocyte-macrophage colony stimulating factor, thus demonstrating the presence of granulocyte-macrophage colony stimulating factors in the conditioned media. The anti-granulocyte-macrophage colony stimulating factor was provided by Dr. Jolanda Schures, DNAX Research Institute.

In addition to interleukin-1 and granulocyte-macrophage colony stimulating factor, fracture callus conditioned media was assayed for the presence of interleukin-6. Interleukin-6 activity was measured by the incorporation of ^{3}H-thymidine into the factor-dependent cell B cell hybridoma known as B9.[62] Data in Figure 10 show constitutive secretion of interleukin-6 by cells in the fracture callus. A peak of interleukin-6 activity can be detected in the conditioned media at seven days postfracture, but only in the presence of lipopolysaccharides. Therefore, it appears that lipopolysaccharides can regulate cytokine secretion from fracture calluses, although this is highly dependent on the individual cytokine.

These data suggest that the physical trauma of fracturing a bone is a sufficient signal to cells present in fracture callus to induce them to secrete certain cytokines. The amount of cytokines secreted is increased if lipopolysaccharide is present. Therefore, the presence of lipopolysaccharides, which under normal circumstances is provided by infecting microorganisms, could adversely affect the ability of fractures to heal and, subsequently, to bear mechanical load.

It is obvious that infection has a deleterious effect on any orthopaedic intervention. However, understanding the mechanism of infection can provide not only better methods for eradicating the source of infection, but also, as in the case of lipopolysaccharides, can provide us with tools to study bone's response to infection and to understand bone cell interactions in a more general sense.[63] Our data suggest that the cytokines secreted by cells present in fracture callus are identical to those secreted when normal bone cells encounter lipopolysaccharides and when immune cells respond to allogeneic bone. This suggests that a variety of induction signals can activate bone cells to secrete a specific set of cytokines. Because the cytokines remain the same as the induction signals vary, these factors may represent, as they do in other systems, for example, the immune system, a common language for bone cell communication. The end result could be regulation of bone remodeling.

References

1. Morrison DC, Ryan JL: Endotoxins and disease mechanisms. *Annu Rev Med* 1987;38:417–432.
2. Morrison DC, Ulevitch RJ: The effects of bacterial endotoxins on host mediation systems: A review. *Am J Pathol* 1978;93:527–617.
3. Morrison DC, Ryan JL: Bacterial endotoxins and host immune responses. *Adv Immunol* 1979;28:293–450.
4. Horowitz MC, Einhorn TA, Philbrick W, et al: Functional and molecular changes in colony stimulating factor secretion by osteoblasts. *Connect Tissue Res* 1989;20:159–168.
5. Hausmann E, Weinfeld N, Miller WA: Effects of lipopolysaccharides on bone resorption in tissue culture. *Calcif Tissue Res* 1972;9:272–282.
6. Rennick D, Yang G, Gemmell L, et al: Control of hemopoiesis by a bone marrow stromal cell clone: Lipopolysaccharide- and interleukin-1-inducible production of colony-stimulating factors. *Blood* 1987;69:682–691.
7. Dinarello CA, Renfer L, Wolff SM: Human leukocytic pyrogen: Purification and development of a radioimmunoassay. *Proc Natl Acad Sci, USA* 1977;74:4624–4627.
8. Murphy PA, Simon PL, Willoughby WF: Endogenous pyrogens made by rabbit peritoneal exudate cells are identical with lymphocyte-activating factors made by rabbit alveolar macrophages. *J Immunol* 1980;124:2498–2501
9. Klein J: *Immunology: The Science of Self-Nonself Discrimination.* New York, Wiley, 1982, pp 376.
10. Moller G, Andersson J, Sjöberg O: Lipopolysaccharides can convert heterologous red cells into thymus-independent antigens. *Cell Immunol* 1972;4:416–424.
11. Thorens B, Mermod J-J, Vassalli P: Phagocytosis and inflammatory stimuli induce GM-CSF mRNA in macrophages through posttranscriptional regulation. *Cell* 1987;48:671–679.
12. Krakauer T, Oppenheim JJ: Interleukin 1 production by a human acute monocytic leukemia cell line. *Cell Immunol* 1983;80:223–229.

13. Duff GW, Atkins E: The detection of endotoxin by in vitro production of endogenous pyrogen: Comparison with limulus amebocyte lysate gelation. *J Immunol Methods* 1982;52:323–331.

14. Helfgott DC, May LT, Sthoeger Z, et al: Bacterial lipopolysaccharide (endotoxin) enhances expression and secretion of β2 interferon by human fibroblasts. *J Exp Med* 1987;166:1300–1309.

15. Horii Y, Muraguchi A, Suematsu S, et al: Regulation of BSF-2/IL-6 production by human mononuclear cells: Macrophage-dependent synthesis of BSF-2/IL-6 by T cells. *J Immunol* 1988;141:1529–1535.

16. Cerami A, Beutler B: The role of cachectin/TNF in endotoxic shock and cachexia. *Immunol Today* 1988;9:28–31.

17. Lei M-G, Morrison DC: Specific endotoxic lipopolysaccharide-binding proteins on murine splenocytes: I. Detection of lipopolysaccharide-binding sites on splenocytes and splenocyte subpopulations. *J Immunol* 1988;141:996–1005.

18. Roeder DJ, Lei M-G, Morrison DC: Endotoxic-lipopolysaccharide-specific binding proteins on lymphoid cells of various animal species: Association with endotoxin susceptibility. *Infect Immun* 1989;57:1054–1058.

19. Lei M-G, Morrison DC: Specific endotoxic lipopolysaccharide-binding proteins on murine splenocytes: II. Membrane localization and binding characteristics. *J Immunol* 1988;141:1006–1011.

20. Jilka RL: Parathyroid hormone-stimulated development of osteoclasts in cultures of cells from neonatal murine calvaria. *Bone* 1986;7:29–40.

21. Jilka RL, Cohn DV: Role of phosphodiesterase in the parathormone-stimulated adenosine 3', 5'-monophosphate response in bone cell populations enriched in osteoclasts and osteoblasts. *Endocrinology* 1981;109:743–747.

22. Centrella M, McCarthy TL, Canalis E: Transforming growth factor β is a bifunctional regulator of replication and collagen synthesis in osteoblast-enriched cell cutures from fetal rat bone. *J Biol Chem* 1987;262:2869–2874.

23. Jilka RL: Effects of PTH and lipopolysaccharide on osteoclast and mononuclear phagocyte development in cultured calvarial cells of normal and osteopetrotic (mi/mi) mice, abstract. *J Bone Miner Res* 1987;2:259.

24. Gowen M, Wood DD, Ihrie EJ, et al: An interleukin 1 like factor stimulates bone resorption in vitro. *Nature* 1983;306:378–380.

25. Rodan SB, Wesolowski G, Chin J, et al: IL-1 binds to high affinity receptors on human osteosarcoma cells and potentiates prostaglandin E2 stimulation of cAMP production. *J Immunol* 1990;145:1231–1237.

26. Durum SK, Schmidt JA, Oppenheim JJ: Interleukin 1: An immunological perspective. *Annu Rev Immunol* 1985;3:263–287.

27. Stanley ER, Bartocci A, Patinkin D, et al: Regulation of very primitive, multipotent, hemopoietic cells by hemopoietin-1. *Cell* 1986;45:667–674.

28. Zlotnik A, Daine B, Smith CA: Activation of an interleukin-1–responsive T-cell lymphoma by fixed P388D1 macrophages and an antibody against the Ag:MHC T-cell receptor. *Cell Immunol* 1985;94:447–453.

29. Dower SK, Call SM, Gillis S, et al: Similarity between the interleukin 1 receptors on a murine T-lymphoma cell line and on a murine fibroblast cell line. *Proc Natl Acad Sci USA* 1986;83:1060–1064.

30. Dower SK, Kronheim SR, March CJ, et al: Detection and characterization of high affinity plasma membrane receptors for human interleukin 1. *J Exp Med* 1985;162:501–515.

31. Prieur AM, Kaufmann MT, Griscelli C, et al: Specific interleukin-1 inhibitor in serum and urine of children with systemic juvenile chronic arthritis. *Lancet* 1987;2:1240–1242.

32. Arend WP, Welgus HG, Thompson RC, et al: Biological properties of recombinant human monocyte-derived interleukin-1 receptor antagonist. *J Clin Invest* 1990;85:1694–1697.

33. Sudo H, Kodama H-A, Amagai Y, et al: In vitro differentiation and calcification in a new clonal osteogenic cell line derived from newborn mouse calvaria. *J Cell Biol* 1983;96:191–198.

34. Horowitz M, Philbrick W, Jilka R: IL-1 release from cultured calvarial cells is due to macrophages, abstract. *J Bone Miner Res* 1989;4:S256.

35. LeBlanc PA, Biron CA: Mononuclear phagocyte maturation: A cytotoxic monoclonal antibody reactive with postmonoblast stages. *Cell Immunol* 1984;83:242–254.

36. Habu S, Yamauchi K, Gershon RK, et al: A non-T:non-B cell bears I-A, I-E, I-J, and Tla (Qa-1) determinants. *Immunogenetics* 1981;13:215–225.

37. Wiktor-Jedrzejczak WW, Ahmed A, Szczylik C, et al: Hematological characterization of congenital osteopetrosis in op/op mouse: Possible mechanism for abnormal macrophage differentiation. *J Exp Med* 1982;156:1516–1527.

38. Wiktor-Jedrzejczak W, Bartocci A, Ferrante AW Jr, et al: Total absence of colony-stimulating factor 1 in the macrophage-deficient osteopetrotic (op/op) mouse. *Proc Natl Acad Sci USA* 1990;87:4828–4832.

39. Felix R, Cecchini MG, Fleisch H: Macrophage colony stimulating factor restores in vivo bone resorption in the op/op osteopetrotic mouse. *Endocrinology* 1990;127:2592–2594.

40. Yoshida H, Hayashi SI, Kunisada T, et al: The murine mutation osteopetrosis is in the coding region of the macrophage colony stimulating factor gene. *Nature* 1990;345:442–444.

41. Horowitz MC, Coleman DL, Flood PM, et al: Parathyroid hormone and lipopolysaccharide induce murine osteoblast-like cells to secrete a cytokine indistinguishable from granulocyte-macrophage colony-stimulating factor. *J Clin Invest* 1989;83:149–157.

42. Morgan C, Pollard JW, Stanley ER: Isolation and characterization of a cloned growth factor dependent macrophage cell line, BAC1.2F5. *J Cell Physiol* 1987;130:420–427.

43. Mosmann TR, Cherwinski H, Bond MW, et al: Two types of murine helper T cell clone: I. Definition according to profiles of lymphokine activities and secreted poteins. *J Immunol* 1986;136:2348–2357.

44. Killar L, MacDonald G, West J, et al: Cloned, Ia-restricted T cells that do not produce interleukin 4(IL4)/B cell stimulatory factor 1(BSF1) fail to help antigen-specific B cells. *J Immunol* 1987;138:1674–1679.

45. Bonfiglio M, Jeter WS: Immunological responses to bone. *Clin Orthop* 1972;87:19–27.

46. Bonfiglio M: Repair of bone-transplant fractures. *J Bone Joint Surg* 1958;40A:446–456.

47. Burwell RG, Gowland G: Studies in the transplantation of bone: II. The changes occurring in the lymphoid tissue after homografts and autografts of fresh cancellous bone. *J Bone Joint Surg* 1961;43B:820–843.

48. Elves MW: Humoral immune response to allografts of bone. *Int Arch Allerg* 1984;47:708.

49. Burchardt H: The biology of bone graft repair. *Clin Orthop* 1983;174:28–42.

50. Innis PC, Randolph JP, Paskert JF, et al: Vascularized bone allografts: In vitro assessment of the cell-mediated and humoral response. *Trans Orthop Res Soc* 1987;12:116.

51. Baron R, Neff L, Louvard D, et al: Cell-mediated extracellular acidification and bone resorption: Evidence for a low pH in resorbing lacunae and localization of a 100–kD lysosomal membrane protein at the osteoclast ruffled border. *J Cell Biol* 1985;101:2210–2222.

52. Kaufmann JF, Auffray C, Korman AJ, et al: The class II molecules of the human and murine major histocompatibility complex. *Cell* 1984;36:1–13.

53. Strominger JL, Engelhard VH, Fuks A, et al: Biochemical analysis of products of the MHC, in Dorf ME (ed): *The Role of the Major Histocompatibility Complex in Immunobiology*. New York, Garland STPM Press, 1981, pp 115–172.

54. Hood L, Steinmetz M, Malissen B: Genes of the major histocompatibility complex of the mouse. *Annu Rev Immunol* 1983;1:529–568.

55. Steinman RM, Gutchinov B, Witmer MD, et al: Dendritic cells are the principal stimulators of the primary mixed leukocyte reaction in mice. *J Exp Med* 1983;157:613–627.

56. Shackelford DA, Kaufman JF, Korman AJ, et al: HLA-DR antigens: Structure, separation of subpopulations, gene cloning and function. *Immunol Rev* 1982;66:133–187.

57. Abbas AK: A reassessment of the mechanisms of antigen-specific T-cell-dependent B-cell activation. *Immunol Today* 1988;9:89–94.

58. Stevens TL, Bossie A, Sanders VM, et al: Regulation of antibody isotype secretion by subsets of antigen-specific helper T cells. *Nature* 1988;334:255–258.

59. Poole AR, Reiner A, Choi H, et al: Immunological studies of proteoglycan subunits from bovine nasal cartilage. *Trans Orthop Res Soc* 1979;4:56.

60. Yablon IG, Brandt KD, DelLellis RA: The antigeneic determinants of articular cartilage: Their role in the homograft rejection. *Trans Orthop Res Soc* 1977;2:91.

61. Bonnarens F, Einhorn TA: Production of a standard closed fracture in laboratory animal bone. *J Orthop Res* 1984;2:97–101.

62. Aarden LA, DeGroot ER, Schaap OL, et al: Production of hybridoma growth factor by human monocytes. *Eur J Immunol* 1987;17:1411–1416.

63. Vogel SN, Rosenstreich DL: LPS unresponsive mice as a model for analyzing lymphokine induced macrophage differentiation in vitro. *Lymphokines* 1981;3:149.

Chapter 20

Host Defenses, the Compromised Host, and Osteomyelitis

Rob Roy MacGregor, MD

Introduction

Infection develops in bone only when host defense mechanisms fail or are overwhelmed, allowing entry of organisms into the bone's normally sterile environment, where they proliferate in such a way that tissue is damaged and a self-sustaining infection becomes established. It is not known whether disorders that compromise the body's immune defenses directly impair the bone's ability to resist infection, nor is it certain that the incidence of osteomyelitis is higher in diseases of immunocompromise than in any other debilitating disease. However, whether there is specific immunocompromise or merely the "compromise" of normal barriers to infection in debilitated patients, it is clear that many diseases, conditions, and medical treatments predispose patients to the development of osteomyelitis. This chapter focuses on three areas: diseases and therapies that impair normal defenses, the function of host defenses in bone, and infection itself as a "compromising" event in bone.

Diseases and Therapies That Impair Normal Host Defenses

Nonimmune (Nonspecific) Defense Mechanisms

Colonization Resistance The organisms that normally colonize the body's nonsterile areas (skin, mucous membranes, and gastrointestinal and respiratory tracts) have adapted to gaining sustenance from the environment without causing disease. However, when they are suppressed by antibiotic treatment or by the influences of chronic disease on their environment, their ecologic niche is taken over by less efficient but more invasive organisms. The result is increased risk of tissue infection and extension into the bloodstream; the latter jeopardizes the bone.[1]

Natural Barriers The skin and mucous membranes are the body's first line of defense against the array of microbes with which we are in constant contact. These barriers are breached in many ways. For example, many devices and procedures devised to treat illness allow bacteria to bypass natural barriers and to spread to bone either by direct extension or by the hematogenous route. Common examples include surgical procedures, vascular and drainage catheters, nasogastric and endotracheal tubes, and appliances that abrade normal squamous epithelium. From an orthopaedic perspective, trauma is the major event that overwhelms natural barriers to infection, often directly inoculating environmental organisms into injured tissue, an inviting and hospitable environment for infection. Decubitus ulcers and vascular insufficiency often have the same effect.[1]

Neuromuscular Integrity   Intact neuromuscular function is critical to maintenance of the natural barriers to infection; stroke, overly aggressive sedation, paralysis, trauma, and neuromuscular diseases such as diabetes and leprosy often lead to bacterial entry through aspiration of upper airway contents into the lung or by damage to the skin. Both result in inoculation of bone, either directly or via bloodstream dissemination.[1]

Immune Defense Mechanisms

Specific immune defense has several components, each of which can be compromised by various disorders and therapies, with differing effects on resistance of bone to infection.

Acute Inflammation   Consisting of neutrophils, chemical mediators, and the vascular system that delivers them, acute inflammation is the body's major immune defense against bacteria and some fungi such as *Aspergillus* and *Candida* species. Congenital defects in neutrophil metabolism such as chronic granulomatous disease of childhood[2] and leukocyte adhesion deficiency syndrome[3] often lead to osteomyelitis, indicating the importance of normal neutrophil function in defense of bone. Although these syndromes have taught us a great deal about neutrophil physiology, they are uncommon clinical phenomena. Acquired neutrophil dysfunction occurs with much greater frequency. Probably chief among these defects is neutropenia, which can result from bone marrow neoplasms or be a direct result of cytotoxic therapy for tumors and autoimmune diseases, an undesired toxic or immune-regulated effect of other drug therapy (such as anti-inflammatory agents, antibiotics, and antihypertensives), and a complication of malnutrition and radiation therapy.[4] Also clinically common are disorders and treatments that interfere with neutrophil delivery to sites of infection. Trauma, radiation damage, and vascular diseases such as arteriosclerosis, vasculitis, and diabetes all prevent neutrophils from reaching sites of bacterial invasion. For example, many orthopaedic surgeons have had the frustrating experience of trying to deal with osteomyelitis secondary to overzealous radiation to the chest, jaw, or other sites characterized by marginal blood supply and subcutaneous bone. The marked improvement in outcome in the treatment of chronic osteomyelitis obtained from the direct application of local muscle flaps to the site is further evidence of the importance of an adequate vascular supply.[5] Finally, delivery is also commonly impeded by medical treatments, most notably by the powerful anti-inflammatory effects of glucocorticoid therapy.

Cell-Mediated Immunity   This system, which includes T lymphocytes, macrophages, natural killer cells, and lymphokines, is the body's primary defense against fungi, mycobacteria, herpesviruses, other intracellular organisms, and *Pneumocystis carinii*. Cell-mediated immunity can be impaired by congenital disorders, cytotoxic therapy, T-cell tumors, and immunosuppressive drugs such as prednisone and cyclosporine. However, disorders of cell-mediated immunity generally are not characterized by an increased incidence of osteomyelitis, and the role of cell-mediated immunity in bone immune defense is unclear. The most striking disorder of cell-mediated immunity today is the acquired immune deficiency syndrome (AIDS). Although a number of case reports have been published of osteomyelitis secondary to unusual pathogens in patients with AIDS,[6,7] the frequency is surprisingly low given the profound degree of immunosuppression in AIDS. This provides further practical evidence that cell-mediated immunity is not a major component of the bone's immune defense.

Humoral Defense   B lymphocytes, plasma cells, immunoglobulins, the complement system, and a host of other plasma proteins (such as lysozyme, transferrin, C-reactive protein, and properdin) work synergistically to defend against bacteria and some viruses. Some may work by blocking bacterial adhesions, preventing their attachment to endothelial surfaces. Humoral immunity can be compromised by congenital and acquired defects in B-cell and complement development,[8–10] by tumors of B-cell lines such as lymphoma, leukemia, multiple myeloma, and Waldenstrom's macroglobulinemia, by splenectomy, and to some degree by cytotoxic and steroid therapy. In addition, diseases leading to increased loss of immunoglobulins (nephrotic syndrome, protein-losing enteropathies) or depletion of complement factors can increase the risk of bacterial infections.

The Reticuloendothelial System   Composed of fixed tissue macrophages and opsonic antibodies, this system serves as the body's major defense for clearing the bloodstream of bacteria and fungi. It is impaired by disorders leading to shunting of blood around the liver, by splenectomy (which removes a major component of the reticuloendothelial system), sickle cell disease and other hemoglobinopathies (which causes a functional "autosplenectomy" through repeated splenic infarcts), chronic debilitating conditions, and perhaps by hyperalimentation (reticuloendothelial system "blockade"). Regardless of the pathophysiologic mechanism involved, any disease or treatment that causes the reticuloendothelial system to lose its ability to protect sterile body sites from hematogenously spread bacterial and fungal infection significantly increases the patient's risk for osteomyelitis.

Summary of Common Immunocompromised States

The most common host defense defects that predispose to the development of osteomyelitis include the following:

Diabetes It could be argued on the basis of the incidence of diabetic foot infection that diabetes is the most common predisposing cause of osteomyelitis in the United States today.[11,12] Although a number of defects in immune function have been reported in diabetes, none has been demonstrated consistently in the absence of ketoacidosis or marked serum hyperosmolarity. It seems probable that the major mechanisms for diabetic osteomyelitis are peripheral neuropathy and vascular insufficiency of the lower extremity, which account for roughly three quarters and one quarter of cases, respectively.[11] When secondary to neuropathy, diabetic osteomyelitis is basically a decubitus ulcer of the foot with direct extension into bone, and it responds well to debridement and appropriate antibiotics (as long as the pressure is removed from the bone). In contrast, osteomyelitis secondary to vascular insufficiency is rarely controlled without vascular reconstruction or amputation.[12]

Immunosuppression Immunosuppressive therapy, particularly that using prednisone in doses exceeding 30 mg/day, is another common predisposing cause of osteomyelitis. Supraphysiologic doses of steroids impede neutrophil delivery to sites of infection, reduce the integrity of the skin as a barrier, and are significantly associated with an increased risk of bacteremia. The fact that 6.5 million new prescriptions were written for prednisone alone in the United States in 1989 indicates the magnitude of the problem.[13]

Neutropenia Profound neutropenia is most commonly caused by cytotoxic drug treatments for neoplasia and inflammatory disorders, and is associated with a risk of bacteremia inversely proportional to the absolute neutrophil count: above 1,000 cells/μl, infection is not increased, but risk doubles at counts between 500 and 1,000 cells/μl and becomes extremely high when there are less than 500 cells/μl for prolonged periods.[4] Despite this risk, it is noteworthy that a recent review of 673 pediatric patients with leukemia only documented nine cases of osteomyelitis, a rate of 1.3%.[14]

Sickle Cell Anemia This condition is frequently complicated by osteomyelitis, which can be a complication of bone infarcts induced by sickle crises or present a difficult problem in differential diagnoses.[15,16] In children, these episodes are usually secondary to infection with gram-negative bacteria, particularly *Salmonella* species, in contrast to the usual gram-positive coccal osteomyelitis that occurs in children without this disease.

Locally Compromising Conditions Trauma, conditions such as coma, paralysis, and neuropathy, and the use of medical devices that provide passage across natural antibacterial barriers are major causes of inoculation of bone (often compromised further by injury) with bacteria. Events such as these (particularly trauma) may constitute the greatest threat of osteomyelitis.

Function of Host Defenses in Bone

The function of host defenses in bone itself is a neglected subject. The fact that osteomyelitis is a common complication of chronic granulomatous disease of childhood and of immunoglobulin disorders and yet is extremely rare in AIDS suggests that neutrophils and antibodies are important for bone defense, but that T cells are not particularly important. In addition, the fact that osteomyelitis is an unusual complication of bacterial endocarditis, despite sustained bacteremia, indicates that bone is ordinarily quite capable of protecting itself from organisms brought to it through the bloodstream. How is this accomplished? The resident cell types are not known to be antibacterial; although constant osteoclastic activity goes on, it is not clear whether or not these cells perform a resident macrophage function. Nor is it known whether or not bone matrix contains antibody or complement, and, if so, whether or not they are functional in this milieu. We do not know what effects collagen, chondroitin sulfate, other unique proteoglycans, and the mineral concentrations of bone have on bacterial growth and on host defense components that migrate through and reside in bone. Clearly, the bone's blood supply is critical for providing access to sites of bone damage for neutrophils, macrophages, and soluble mediators of inflammation. In fact, the marrow is richly supplied with macrophages, and may contribute significantly to the reticuloendothelial system and its cleansing of circulating blood. However, such phagocytosis, if not followed by effective intracellular killing of the organism, may actually predispose the bone to infection. Finally, primary protection of bone from hematogenous inoculation with bacteria may simply be a result of normal endothelial cell integrity, covering up underlying adhesin receptors on collagen and fibronectin,[17] maintaining a negative surface charge, and perhaps producing soluble adhesin receptors.

Infection as an Immunocompromising Event in Bone

Infection itself acts to interfere with immune function in bone. Soluble factors released by tissue damaged by bacteria, and bacterial products themselves, cause neutrophils to adhere to the endothelium, impeding flow and promoting clot formation. Mediators of inflammation cause increased endothelial permeability and increased extravascular volume in the rigid structure of the bone. These events impede blood flow to the infected bone, leading to infarction, further compromising the delivery of antibacterial cells and humoral defense factors. The infarcted bone actually serves as a foreign body nidus, providing sanctuary from host defense mechanisms for the developing infection.

Inflammation in bone has been better studied in injury secondary to fracture, where it increases vascular volume secondary to vasodilitation and new vessel formation[18] and subsequently leads to infiltration by neutrophils and monocytes that autolyze ground substance.[19] Thus, although bone seems able to protect itself from circulating bacteria under ordinary conditions, once the bone sustains injury from infection, trauma, or other cause of vascular compromise, the ensuing inflammatory events may well promote bacterial adhesion and work against host defense efforts to combat the infection. If so, treating such infections at an early stage with anti-inflammatory agents may be warranted.[20]

References

1. Tramont EC: General or nonspecific host defense mechanisms, in Mandell GL, Douglas RG Jr, Bennett JE (eds): *Principles and Practice of Infectious Diseases*, ed 3. New York, Churchill Livingstone, 1990, pp 33–40.
2. Tauber AL, Borregaard N, Simons ER, et al: Chronic granulomatous disease: A syndrome of phagocyte oxidase deficiencies. *Medicine* 1983;62:286–309.
3. Anderson DC, Springer TA: Leukocyte adhesion deficiency: An inherited defect in the Mac-1, LFA-1, and p150,95 glycoproteins. *Annu Rev Med* 1987;38:175–194.
4. Bodey GP, Buckley M, Sathe YS, et al: Quantitative relationships between circulating leukocytes and infection in patients with acute leukemia. *Ann Intern Med* 1966;64:328–340.
5. Fitzgerald RH Jr, Ruttle PE, Arnold PG, et al: Local muscle flaps in the treatment of chronic osteomyelitis. *J Bone Joint Surg* 1985;67A:175–185.
6. Goh BT, Jawad ASM, Chapman D, et al: Osteomyelitis presenting as a swollen elbow in a patient with the acquired immune deficiency syndrome. *Ann Rheum Dis* 1988;47:695–696.
7. Blumenthal DR, Zucker JR, Hawkins CC: *Mycobacterium avium* complex-induced septic arthritis and osteomyelitis in a patient with the acquired immunodeficiency syndrome. *Arthritis Rheum* 1990:33-757–758.
8. Reinherz EL, Cooper MD, Schlossman SF, et al: Abnormalities of T cell maturation and regulation in human beings with immunodefidciency disorders. *J Clin Invest* 1981;68:699–705.
9. Gottsegen DN: Pneumococcal osteomyelitis associated with IgG2 subclass deficiency. *Pediatr Infect Dis J* 1987;6:281–284.
10. Ross SC, Densen P: Complement deficiency states and infection: Epidemiology, pathogenesis and consequences of neisserial and other infections in an immune deficiency. *Medicine* 1984;63:243–273.
11. LoGerfo FW, Coffman JD: Current concepts: Vascular and microvascular disease of the foot in diabetes. Implications for foot care. *N Engl J Med* 1984;31:1615–1619.
12. Bamberger DM, Daus GP, Gerding DN: Osteomyelitis in the feet of diabetic patients: Long-term results, prognostic factors, and the role of antimicrobial and surgical therapy. *Am J Med* 1987;83:653–660.
13. Simonsen LLP: What are pharmacists dispensing most often? *Pharm Times* 1990;56:56–64.

14. Murphy RG, Greenberg ML: Osteomyelitis in pediatric patients with leukemia. *Cancer* 1988;62:2628–2630.

15. Engh CA, Hughes JL, Abrams RC, et al: Osteomyelitis in the patient with sickle-cell disease. *J Bone Joint Surg* 1971;53A:1–15.

16. Syrogiannopoulos GA, McCracken GH Jr,, Nelson JD: Osteoarticular infections in children with sickle cell disease. *Pediatrics* 1986;78:1090–1096.

17. Buxton TB, Horner J, Hinton A, et al: In vivo glycocalyx expression by *Staphylococcus aureus* phage type 52/52A/80 in *S. aureus* osteomyelitis. *J Infect Dis* 1987;156:942–946.

18. Wray JB, Lynch CJ: The vascular response to fracture of the tibia in the rat. *J Bone Joint Surg* 1959;41A:1143–1148.

19. Rhinelander FW, Baragry RA: Microangiography in bone healing. I. Undisplaced closed fractures. *J Bone Joint Surg* 1962;44A:1273–1298.

20. Rissing JP, Buxton TB: Effect of ibuprofen on gross pathology, bacterial count, and levels of prostaglandin E_2 in experimental staphylococcal osteomyelitis. *J Infect Dis* 1986;154:627–630.

Future Directions

The function of host defenses in bone is an important topic, and it needs to be examined in greater detail in the future. Patients with subacute bacterial endocarditis with sustained bacteremias have a surprisingly low incidence of osteomyelitis. Why is this so? There must be some mechanism by which bone normally resists infection. Future studies should examine how bone normally protects itself from organisms brought to it by the bloodstream. Much remains to be learned regarding the cells that are important in bone's resistance to infection. Further in vitro studies to better identify the involved cells are recommended.

Role of the Macrophage

It is now known that osteoclasts are members of the macrophage/monocyte cell lineage. Macrophages, through their phagocytic actions and the products they secrete, are normally integral parts of the host's response to inflammation and infection. Studies should be undertaken to determine if osteoclasts respond as protective cells and exhibit macrophage-like function.

Recently, a subpopulation of macrophages has been identified in bone. It has been hypothesized that these macrophages may be unable to complete digestion of bacteria and other organisms, and that this predisposes bone to infection. Future research should seek to clarify the role of bone macrophages in osteomyelitis and to determine if bone macrophages protect or predispose bone to infection.

The role of the unique components of the bone matrix is another area that merits exploration. The effects that collagen, chondroitin sulfate, other unique proteoglycans, and the high mineral concentration of bone have on bacterial growth and the interaction of these components with the host defense mechanisms needs to be determined. The identification of antibody or complement in bone's matrix would help explain bone's response to foreign organisms.

Cytokines

We are beginning to understand cell-cell communication in bone. The preceding chapters offer strong evidence for the role of interleukin-1 and lipopolysaccharide as mediators in the host's response to infection. Further attempts to define other factors that are released by bone cells or that interact with bone to mediate the immune response to infection are warranted. The role of interleukin-1 in the immune response needs to be clarified. Specific studies should include an examination of osteoclasts to determine whether or not they release interleukin-1. The role of interleukin-1 inhibitors and their efficacy in reducing the bony destruction associated with osteomyelitis should also be examined. The documentation of other diseases or physiologic states that are associated with elevated levels of cytokines may also prove helpful.

Prostaglandins

There is virtually no information regarding the role of prostaglandins in bone infection and the host's response to the infection. Previous studies have suggested a prominent role of prostaglandins as local mediators of bone remodeling and bone formation. Studies helpful in determining a role of prostaglandins in osteomyelitis would include determination of local prostaglandin levels at the site of infection. The effect of exogenously administered prostaglandins and clarification of the effect of nonsteroidal anti-inflammatory drugs on osteomyelitis and associated bone destruction and nonunion must be determined.

Growth Factors

We must continue to examine events at the interface between biomaterials and cells and tissues if we expect to develop the optimal implantation material. In the monocyte/macrophage interaction growth factors are secreted. Further studies should examine if there is preferential production of a specific growth factor. The alteration in the immune response induced by biomaterials has been shown to affect fibroblasts. It is not known if this alteration affects any other cell types that participate in wound healing, inflammation, or the foreign-body response.

Inflammatory events are induced by surgical implantation. If these inflammatory events can be shown to promote bacterial adhesion and impede host defenses, it would suggest a possible role for anti-inflammatory agents in limiting early infection. A hypothesis of interest cites the zone of foreign-body reaction at the implant/tissue interface to be particularly prone to the development of infection. If this proves to be true, what mechanism limits the proliferation of inflammatory cells in the foreign-body reaction in order to allow acceptance? In addition, the chronic activity of the cells at the biomaterial-tissue interface has to be examined. The identification of the importance of membrane charge, bacterial adhesion molecules, flow dynamics, and other physical factors on biomaterial and allograft acceptance may provide the basis for future therapeutic manipulations of the bone's defense against infection.

Allografts

With regard to the immune response to allografts, there clearly must be some alteration in the immune response that allows acceptance of the allograft. The preceding chapters have focused on the ability of cytokines to activate bone cells. Examination of the properties of allografts that increase or decrease cytokine levels would be useful. Attempts should be made to identify other induction signals that affect the relative activation of bone cells.

Immunocompromised Host

Research involving the immunosuppressed population should occupy much of our time in the next decade and beyond. It must be determined if immunocompromised patients are at increased risk for developing osteomyelitis. If this is so, studies should be directed at examining the mechanism—impairment of the immune mechanism versus local factors. Preferential organisms and sites of infection in immunocompromised patients should be noted.

It appears that osteomyelitis is very uncommon in AIDS patients with chronic sustained bacteremias and *Mycobacterium avium* complex. Why is this so? The incidence of osteomyelitis in AIDS patients in comparison with normal controls and other immune compromised states needs to be clarified.

Effect of Aging on Musculoskeletal Infection

We conclude with suggestions for research on a topic, aging, that has not been mentioned in our previous discussion. The immune system appears to age with the rest of our body. The following questions need to be answered. Does aging itself contribute to increased risk of osteomyelitis when patients are controlled for diseases that are associated with increased age? Do the cells involved in bone's defense against infection age at an accelerated rate? Is a mediator or a component of bone's matrix involved in bone's resistance to infection produced in decreased amounts in the elderly?

Section Five
Therapeutics

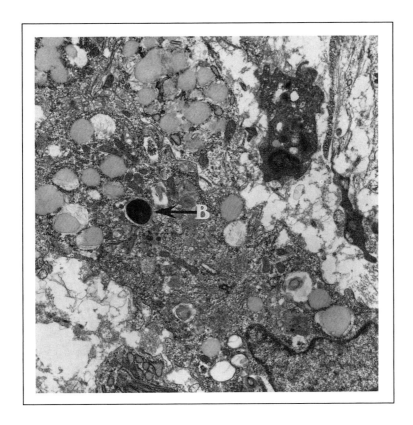

Introduction

Craig L. Levitz, BA
John L. Esterhai, Jr, MD

A wound can be defined as the disruption of the normal anatomic relationships of tissue secondary to injury. An understanding of the factors involved in wound healing is essential in orthopaedic surgery. The orthopaedic surgeon must deal with the wounds, which are frequently contaminated, that occur as a result of trauma, as well as the intentional wounds caused by surgical incision. In either case, the healing process begins immediately after wounding. Wound healing restores tissue strength, resistance to infection, and protection from the external environment.

Wound healing is characterized by three distinct phases: An initial acute inflammatory response, a proliferative phase involving the synthesis of collagen from fibroblasts and a gain in tensile strength, and a maturation or remodeling phase. Such factors as trauma, hematoma, blood supply, temperature, infection, surgical technique, and suture material are known to affect the healing process.[1,2] However, growth factors, agents that stimulate cells or promote cellular proliferation, have only recently been recognized to initiate or mediate many if not most aspects of wound healing.

The nonspecific inflammation is hypothesized to be initiated by blood coagulation and the activation of the coagulation and kinin systems. Platelets play a major role in the initial cascade through the release of their granules. Platelet granules contain platelet-derived growth factor (PDGF), transforming growth factor-beta (TGF-β), transforming growth factor-alpha (TGF-α),

and platelet factor 4, all of which exhibit some chemotactic stimulus for macrophages, fibroblasts, and neutrophils.

Shortly after injury, neutrophils are the predominant cell type entering injured tissue, but after the first 48 hours, macrophages become the predominant cell type. Macrophages have long been known to be involved in wound debridement. However, it was realized that macrophages have additional functions in wound healing when Leibovich and Ross[3] noted that wounds depleted of macrophages exhibited delayed fibroblast proliferation and wound fibrosis. This discovery led to a number of studies examining the growth factors elaborated by wound macrophages.

The first chapter of this section, by Moelleken, reviews the role of growth factors in wound healing. The chapter begins by defining the mechanism of action of growth factors and looks specifically at the effect of growth factors and lymphokines on fibroblasts. The author goes on to take an indepth look at each growth factor thought to be involved in wound healing—TGF-β, TGF-α, PDGF, fibroblast growth factor (FGF), epidermal growth factor (EGF), insulin-like growth factor-1 (IGF-1), monocyte-derived growth factor (MDGF), interleukin-1 and interleukin-2, bone morphogenic protein (BMP), osteogenin, granulocyte-monocyte colony stimulating factor (GM-CSF), and interleukin-6—and concludes each discussion with a simplified summary of each growth factor's overall role in the healing process.

Orthopaedic surgeons focus a great deal of their attention on the prevention of wound infections. By carefully preparing the skin with bactericidal agents, maintaining rigorous sterile technique, minimizing intraoperative tissue damage, administering prophylactic antibiotics, and applying appropriate dressings, we have been able to decrease the rate of wound infection continually since the days of Lister. Nonetheless, wound infections remain a major cause of prolonged hospitalization, morbidity, and the increased cost of orthopaedic care. If wound infections are to be eradicated, other approaches must be added.

Wound infection is intimately associated with wound healing. Wounds that do not heal adequately are at increased risk of infection, and infection increases the likelihood of inadequate wound healing. Thus interventions that prevent failures of wound healing will decrease wound infections, and vice versa.

It is presently known that oxygen is crucial for appropriate wound healing without infection. This phenomenon has been studied in the past in the general surgery population, but there is a paucity of literature examining the role of oxygen in the treatment of orthopaedic injuries. The second chapter of this section, by Hopf and Hunt, reviews in detail the basic mechanisms of wound repair with particular emphasis on the role of oxygen in resistance to infection. Measurements of oxygen tension may aid our efforts to further decrease the rate of wound infection. After discussing techniques for assessing the adequacy of oxygen supply to the wound, the authors conclude by commenting on the applicability to orthopaedic patients of data linking wound healing and resistance to infection with local tissue oxygen tension. It appears that bone is as susceptible as subcutaneous tissue to vasoconstriction and low tissue oxygen tension, and is thus at risk for the associated impaired host defenses and impaired collagen deposition.

Preoperative or postoperative depletion of any of a variety of nutritional factors impairs host defenses and wound repair. Malnourished patients are at a significantly greater risk of delayed wound healing than are nutritionally sound patients. In the past 15 years, the nutritional status of the hospitalized patient has been the subject of intense research. As many as 50% of hospitalized patients may have significant protein or protein-calorie malnutrition. Most of this research has focused on the nonorthopaedic population, which is unfortunate, because orthopaedic surgeons are often faced with malnourished patients. Two populations of orthopaedic patients deserve particular attention in this regard: Older patients undergoing hip procedures are likely to have chronic protein-calorie malnutrition, and multiply-injured trauma patients with long-bone fractures are at high risk of developing protein-calorie malnutrition as a result of the catabolic state that trauma induces.

The cost penalty of complications in orthopaedic patients is closely related to nutritional status. The penalty in a sample of 100 patients with long bone fracture was 16%. Though slightly higher, it approximates the malnutrition cost penalty (14%), thus reiterating the close relationship. The average length of hospital stay was 26.0 (SD=13) days in patients with an infection and 12.0 (SD=6) days in patients without an infection. Multiplying the national cost figure of $1.7 billion by the 16% cost penalty estimates the national yearly cost of infections at $271 million dollars (C. Puskarich, personal communication).

The importance of nutritional repletion in general surgical patients is well established, although controversy remains about timing and ideal formulations. Few studies have investigated the impact of nutritional repletion or supplementation on bone repair, wound healing and infection, or outcome in orthopaedic patients. Much of the general surgical literature likely applies to orthopaedic patients, but studies are needed to define the unique problems and ideal approaches in orthopaedic populations.

In the third chapter in this section, on wound repair and nutrition, Hopf and Hunt examine the roles of specific vitamins or minerals in wound repair and host defenses and the impairments of wound repair or host defenses that occur when patients are vitamin or mineral deficient. The more general topic of protein-calorie malnutrition is then examined. It is suggested that correcting deficits preoperatively and maintaining adequate nutrition perioperatively can prevent complications of surgery or reduce the severity of these complications. The authors briefly describe normal metabolism and then go on to review the literature on the prevalence of malnutrition. The efficacy of perioperative nutritional support is reviewed, and care is taken to note that nutritional support, whether enteral or parenteral, is not without risk. The literature provides growing evidence that nutritional repletion reduces surgical complications in certain populations of patients. The authors conclude by suggesting literature-supported guidelines for nutritional therapy.

The fourth chapter of this section deals specifically with nutritional status and outcome in orthopaedic patients. The authors, Nelson and Puskarich, having reviewed the literature on the poor nutritional status of the general surgery population, seek to examine nutritional status and its effect on patient outcome in the orthopaedic population. The limited number of studies that focus on the orthopaedic population are discussed. In order to conduct research on nutrition and patient outcome, it is necessary to be able to assess nutritional status accurately and reliably. A brief discussion of suggested nutritional status indicators, therefore, is presented before the discussion of specific orthopaedic studies. The authors conclude that a considerable number of orthopaedic patients may be defined as malnourished at the time of hospital admission. Patients defined as malnourished are hospitalized longer and are at increased risk of developing complications following surgery.

The wound is a unique environment clearly different from the peripheral circulation. Wounds arising from radiation necrosis, chronic infection, and poor perfusion are characterized by hypoxic, acidic conditions that could be expected to alter cell function. Several studies describe differences between neutrophils in the peripheral circulation and various wounds, but the difference between neutrophils of distinct wound types is largely unknown. Phillips and associates[4] concluded that in the diabetic patient population, the impairment of incisional wound healing is caused by fibro-blast abnormalities. A single dose of basic FGF reverses this impairment.[5] In acute hematogenous osteomyelitis, the failure of tissue-based phagocytes appears to be critical to the development of a significant infection.

Orthopaedic surgeons frequently use muscle flaps to cover wounds incurred as a result of trauma or surgical incision. Brown and Khouri[6] demonstrated in rats the effectiveness of osteogenin on the custom fabrication of vascularized bone grafts. Anthony and associates[7] studied the use of muscle flaps in patients with chronic leg osteomyelitis, and long-term follow-up revealed a cure rate of 96%.[5] Francel and associates[8] reported a limb salvage rate in lower extremity microvascular reconstruction that approached 95%.[6] Certain flaps demonstrate a greater resistance to bacterial inoculation, both in clinically infected wounds and experimentally.[9]

Failure to understand the pathophysiology has hampered our development of innovative medical and surgical therapy for osteomyelitis. It is now understood that ischemia is the inciting event responsible for inducing polymorphonuclear infiltrates in skin flaps. The survival of a skin graft is related to the absence of chemotactic activity.[10] Hardesty and associates[11] demonstrated that pre- and postoperative smoking markedly increased flap necrosis. Preoperative cessation of smoking decreases flap necrosis. Edwards and associates[12] showed that the biochemical alterations that occur during storage under hyperbaric oxygen therapy are correlated with the survival of replanted limbs. The mechanism has not been worked out but is believed to be related to preservation of high-energy phosphates and glycogen.

The efficacy of a local muscle flap in the treatment of musculoskeletal infections relates both to its ability to obliterate dead space and its ability to enhance the local blood supply during the healing process. Adequate blood supply is necessary to maintain physiologic pH. Neutrophils associated with well-oxygenated wound environments, with superior blood flow and physiologic pH, are associated with superior phagocytic function.[13]

Though neutrophils are critically important as a first line of defense against infection, they may be deleterious if improperly activated.[14] The efficacy of the neutrophil against bacteria is determined by its state of activation. The higher its state of activation, the greater is the release of granular products, superoxide radicals, and other products toxic to bacteria.[15,16] A clear understanding of leukocyte activation within specific wound environments is necessary if we are to modulate leukocyte function to obtain a desired clinical effect.

The authors of the fifth chapter of this section present a study carried out in their laboratory to evaluate the effect of different environments on wound activation. They examine a wound with two distinct environments: A well vascularized musculocutaneous flap and a poorly perfused random flap pattern. Neutrophils were analyzed by five different parameters. The authors concluded that a poorly vascularized wound adversely affects neutrophil function. It appears that the neutrophil is modulated by the wound environment it enters. Unphysiologic pH and Po_2 are cited as sufficient cause to explain the phenomena of premature activation and decreased phagocytosis observed in neutrophils in poorly perfused wounds. The poorer vascularity of the random flap suggests an explanation for its inferior clinical results.

The relationship between serum antibiotic concentrations and concentrations reaching the wound site are inconsistent in chronic osteomyelitis. The ability of antimicrobial agents to penetrate and distribute into ischemic infected bone is not clearly resolved.[17] Several methods examined for delivering antibiotics to infected bone have given mixed results. Conventional polymethylmethacrylate bone cement antibiotic implants, although widely used, have been associated with incomplete and poorly controlled release of antibiotic.[18]

The sixth chapter attempts to explain the pathophysiology of osteomyelitis and the pharmacokinetics of antibiotic agents in normal and infected bone. This section, written by Fitzgerald and associates, presents experiments performed to examine the abnormalities in the host defense mechanisms observed in acute hematogenous osteomyelitis. Bioassay techniques were used to determine the distribution of antibiotics in various tissue fluids. These techniques have not been previously applied to osseous tissue. The authors present data that demonstrate that specific antimicrobial agents can enter the interstitial fluid space of both normal and infected osseous tissue. The authors conclude with a discussion of the physiologic impact of a local muscle flap on osteomyelitic bone.

Although osteomyelitis is an old disease, there have been relatively few advances in our understanding of certain aspects of therapy. The apparent failure of antimicrobial agents to relieve chronic osteomyelitis is particularly disappointing in view of the success of these drugs in so many other infections. There is no credible evidence that the deep-seated infection of chronic osteomyelitis can be permanently cured without complete surgical debridement of involved biomaterials and necrotic bone and soft tissue, followed by systemic antimicrobial therapy. Surgical management alone cannot eradicate the pathogenic bacteria that may have disseminated, and reliance on chemotherapy alone fails because the devascularized material present serves as a continued focus for bacterial growth. A wide arsenal of antibiotics effective against gram-positive and gram-negative organisms is demanded by the evolving etiologies of musculoskeletal infection.

Clinical research has been difficult to perform because of the marked variability of the disease and the important role of surgical treatment. Studies establish that a three-week course of antibiotics is effective in acute osteomyelitis. This therapy may be oral or parenteral, so long as there are effective levels of antimicrobial agents in the serum, however, the optimal therapy for chronic osteomyelitis remains to be defined.[19,20]

The seventh chapter of this section, by Norden, analyzes the lessons learned from animal models and the clinical application of these lessons to the treatment of osteomyelitis with antibiotics. The author begins by reviewing the history of experimental osteomyelitis models. He then considers clinical issues in the treatment of osteomyelitis and discusses the role of serum bactericidal titers in the management of osteomyelitis. The author moves on to comment on the outpatient management of osteomyelitis and to support the use of oral antimicrobial therapy. There is clearly a need to examine the differences in efficacy of the different antimicrobial agents in the treatment of chronic osteomyelitis, and the author concludes by presenting criteria for calling a study a "well conducted trial."

The eighth chapter in this section concerns adult septic arthritis. The authors, Ruggiero and Esterhai, discuss the etiology, organisms, joint involvement, pathophysiology, differential diagnosis, treatment, and prognosis, emphasizing recent work on cytokines, interleukin-1, and the effect of nonsteroidal anti-inflammatories.

In the ninth chapter, Gentry extensively reviews the antibiotic therapy for osteomyelitis. This discussion focuses on the third generation cephalosporins, the newer beta-lactams, and the oral fluoroquinolones. A historical note is made concerning the past use of oral penicillins. Prospective, randomized comparisons of parenteral versus oral therapy are presented. The chapter concludes with reports of resistant organisms and a word in favor of the continued move toward oral therapy.

Antiseptics are used by every surgeon before surgery for hand washing and to prepare the skin. Some surgeons also use antiseptics on wounds and in body cavities. Although the antibacterial efficacy of antiseptics is well documented, their effects on wound healing and on living tissue are poorly understood. In the last chapter of this section, Mader and associates present information about each of the commonly used classes of antiseptics. Organic agents and soaps are also mentioned. A thorough discussion follows this information, and general conclusions are drawn where warranted.

Despite our wide array of antibiotics, the liberal use of antiseptics, and adherence to meticulous surgical technique, we have been unable to conquer biomaterial-localized infections. These infections persist until the biomaterial is removed. They are associated with resistance to antibiotics and host de-

fenses and frequently involve traumatized tissue and microbial adherence to biomaterial and compromised tissue. In such cases, the tissue inevitably fails to integrate with the implant.[21] Antibiotics have been added to polymethylmethacrylate to reduce the incidence of postsurgical infection. Recent work shows that antibiotic incorporation into polymethylmethacrylate does not inhibit microbial adherence or colonization over a 48–hour test period.[22] These findings suggest that there is an intrinsic resistance to antibiotic-impregnated polymethylmethacrylate. Other studies show antibiotic resistance appears to be associated with surface colonization and with the type of biomaterial substrata involved. Resistance to antibiotics appears to be greater on polymer-like polymethylmethacrylate than on metal surfaces,[21] perhaps because of the toxic effect of polymethylmethacrylate on macrophages. Horowitz and associates[23] have shown that macrophages exposed to polymethylmethacrylate are lethally damaged, as reflected by the subsequent release of intracellular lactate dehydrogenase.

A clearer understanding of the interactions that occur on the surface of the biomaterial is necessary if we are to eradicate these infections. Hook and associates[24] and others[25] have spent the last decade examining the molecular mechanisms of microbial adhesion. Cell adhesion is a critical factor in microbial life. Bacterial adherence to host tissues is often the first step in the development of infection. The adhesion of bacteria depends predominantly on proteins present at the surface of bacterial cells (adhesins) that recognize and bind specific ligands in host tissue. The importance of the adhesin-ligand interaction depends on the site of infection or stage of the disease. The process of bacteria adherence to host tissue is dynamic and can be modulated by the bacteria, environment, host defenses, and antibacterial therapy. Sets of adhesins that allow strains of Staphylococcus aureus to colonize normal skin are compared with other sets that allow the bacteria to infect bone and soft tissue.

In vitro studies have demonstrated that staphylococci and streptococci can bind fibronectin or can adhere to fibronectin that is adsorbed on glass or plastic or is present in plasma clots. A fibronectin-binding protein has been isolated from *S aureus*.[26] The gene has been cloned from *Escherichia coli* and the nucleotide sequence has been determined.[27] This fibronectin receptor exhibits all of the characteristics for a classical ligand-receptor interaction.[24] These studies suggest that fibronectin may serve as a substrate for the adhesion of staphylococcal cells and that bacterial adhesion is mediated by the fibronectin receptor. It has also been suggested that staphylococcal colonization of polymethylmethacrylate prosthetic implants in vivo is mediated by bacterial adhesion to fibronectin on the implanted material. Analogs to the fibronectin receptor have been shown to inhibit the adhesion of bacterial cells to these model substrates.[25] These substances may be used clinically to prevent infections by interfering with bacterial adherence. Adhesin analogs may also be important vaccine components, because the generation of antibodies can lead to immunologic recognition as well as prevent attachment to the host.

References

1. Peacock EE: *Wound Repair*. Philadelphia, WB Saunders, 1984.
2. Peacock EE: Wound healing and wound care: *Principles of Surgery*, ed 4. New York, McGraw-Hill, 1984.
3. Leibovich SJ, Ross R: The role of the macrophage in wound repair: A study with hydrocortisone and antimacrophage serum. *Am J Pathol* 1975;78:71–100.
4. Phillips LG, Geldner P, Brou J, et al: Correction of diabetic incisional healing impairment with basic fibroblast growth factor. *Surg Forum* 1990;41;602–603.
5. Morgan RF: Plastic surgery. *Am Coll Surg Bul* 1991;76:43–47.
6. Brown DM, Khouri RK: Custom fabrication of vascularized bone grafts using osteoinductive transforming factors. *Surg Forum* 1990;41:593–594.
7. Anthony JP, Mathes SJ, Alpert BS: The muscle flap in the treatment of chronic lower extremity osteomyelitis: Results in patients over five years post-treatment. Presented at the 69th Annual Meeting of the American Association of Plastic Surgeons, Hot Springs, VA, May 1990.
8. Francel TJ, Vander Kolk CA, Manson PN, et al: Long term functional results and timing of soft tissue coverage of open tibial fractures. Presented at the 69th Annual Meeting of the American Association of Plastic Surgeons, Hot Springs, VA, May 1990.
9. Mathes SJ, Nahai F: *Clinical Applications for Muscle and Musculocutaneous Flaps*. St. Louis, CV Mosby, 1982.
10. Rees RS, Punch JD, Cashmer BA, et al: Should dying flaps be converted to skin grafts? *Surg Forum* 1990;41:603–605.
11. Hardesty RA, West SS, Shmidt S: Preoperative cessation of smoking and its relationship to flap survival. Presented at the 35th Annual Meeting of the Plastic Surgery Research Council, Washington, DC, April 1990.
12. Edwards RJ, Im MJ, Hoopes JE: Biochemical effects of hyperbaric oxygen on the storage of amputated limbs in rats. *Surg Forum* 1990;41:659–661.
13. Eshima I, Mathes SJ, Paty P: Comparison of intracellular bacterial killing in leukocytes isolated from musculocutaneous and random flaps. *Plast Reconstr Surg* 1990;86:541–547.
14. Turner RA, Shumacher HR, Myers AR: Phagocytic function of polymorphonuclear leukocytes in rheumatic diseases. *J Clin Invest* 1973;52:1632–1635.
15. Knighton DR, Halliday B, Hunt TK: Oxygen as an antibiotic: The effect of inspired oxygen on infection. *Arch Surg* 1984;119:199–204.
16. Van Epps DE, Garcia ML: Enhancement of neutrophil function as a result of prior exposure to chemotactic factor. *J Clin Invest* 1980;66:167–175.
17. Budsberg SC, Gallo JM, Starliper CE, et al: Cortical bone and serum concentrations of clindamycin direct local infusion vs intravenous administration. *Trans Orthop Res Soc* 1991;16:15.
18. Weston M, Sampath S, Robinson D, et al: Comparative *in vitro* release of antibiotics from nonbiodegradable and biodegradable implants for osteomyelitis. *Trans Orthop Res Soc* 1991;16:16.
19. Dich VQ, Nelson JD, Haltalin KC: Osteomyelitis in infants and children: A review of 163 cases. *Am J Dis Child* 1975;129:1273–1278.
20. Black J, Hunt TL, Godley PJ, et al: Oral antimicrobial therapy for adults with osteomyelitis or septic arthritis. *J Infect Dis* 1987;155:968–972.

21. Naylor PT, Myrvik QN, Gristina A: Antibiotic resistance of biomaterial-adherent coagulase-negative and coagulase-positive *Staphylococci. Clin Orthop* 1990;261:126–133.

22. Siverhus DJ, Edmiston CE, Stiehl JB: Microbial adherence and colonization of antibiotic impregnated methylmethacrylate bone cement. *Trans Orthop Res Soc* 1991;16:13.

23. Horowitz SM, Gautsch TL, Fondoza CG, et al: Macrophage exposure to polymethylmethacrylate leads to mediator release and injury. *J Orthop Res* 1991;9:406–413.

24. Hook M, et al: Interactions of bacteria with extracellular matrix proteins. *Cell Differ* 1990;32:433–438.

25. Raja RH, Raucci G, Hook M: Peptide analogs to a fibronectin receptor inhibit attachment of *Staphylococcus aureus* to fibronectin-containing substrates. *Infect Immun* 1990;58:2593–2598.

26. Esperen F, Clemmensen I: Isolation of a fibronectin-binding protein from *Staphylococcus aureus. Infect Immun* 1982;37:526–531.

27. Signas C, et al: Nucleotide sequence of the gene for a fibronectin-binding protein from *Staphylococcal aureus*: Use of this peptide sequence in the synthesis of biologically active peptides. *Proc Natl Acad Sci USA* 1989;86:699–703.

Chapter 21

Growth Factors in Wound Healing

Brent R.W. Moelleken, MD

Introduction

Initially, wound healing is associated with a nonspecific inflammation that is probably initiated by blood coagulation and the activation of the coagulation and kinin systems. Platelets play a major role in the initial cascade. Platelet granules contain platelet-derived growth factor, transforming growth factor-β, eosinophilic chemotactic factor (=transforming growth factor-α), and platelet factor 4. These factors all exhibit some chemotactic stimulus for macrophages, fibroblasts, and neutrophils.

Neutrophils constitute the predominant cell type entering injured tissue during the first 24 to 48 hours after injury. Shortly thereafter, macrophages become the predominant type of cell in the wound. In 1975, researchers realized that macrophages provided functions in wound healing in addition to wound debridement, when they noted that a wound depleted of macrophages exhibited delayed fibroblast proliferation and wound fibrosis.[1] This predated a veritable explosion of information about the growth factors elaborated by wound macrophages. Growth factors are now recognized to initiate or mediate many, if not most, aspects of wound healing.

Growth Factors and Cytokines

A growth factor is an agent that stimulates cells or promotes cellular proliferation. Its actions with an external receptor lead to intracellular changes and subsequently to alterations in cellular division. Growth factors have been named for their origins (MDGF, macrophage-derived growth factor), their target-cell specificity (EGF, epidermal growth factor), or their activity in cell culture (TGF-β, transforming growth factor beta).[2]

Cell surface receptors on the target cells exhibit a high affinity for the growth factors. Growth factors have several signal transduction mechanisms that allow their membrane-growth factor interactions to be translated into cellular events. Tyrosine kinase stimulation and proto-oncogene transcription are two common intracellular pathways. When growth factors such as platelet-derived growth factor (PDGF), EGF, or insulin-like growth factor-I (IGF-I) interact with their surface receptors, an intracellular domain activates tyrosine kinase. Tyrosine residues on cytoplasmic proteins become phosphorylated and, hence, activated. Through a cascade of events, DNA synthesis and cellular division results. Growth factors can directly result in the transcription of proto-oncogenes. Much in the manner of thyroid-stimulating hormones (TSH), PDGF, fibroblast growth factor (FGF), and EGF induce the transcription of c-fos and c-myc, proto-oncogenes associated with increased rates of cellular proliferation (as well as mutagenesis and tumorigenesis).[3]

Growth factors alter their target cells by acting either as competence or as progression factors. A competence factor, such as PDGF, acts by bringing a cell to the growth arrest point (the competence point), which renders it vulnerable to other mitogenic factors. A progression factor, such as somatomedin C, propels a normal cell forward to DNA synthesis. These two mechanisms are strongly synergistic in inducing mitogenic activity.[4] It is becoming clear that growth factors can also induce the migration of fibroblasts, neutrophils, and macrophages, among other cells. Thus, in addition to being mitogens, they are also chemoattractants and draw fibroblasts and neutrophils into the wound environment.

Growth factors have different means of reaching their target tissues. IGF-I reaches the target cells via an endocrine pathway after being transported through the bloodstream on a high-molecular-weight carrier protein. PDGF reaches an adjacent cell in a paracrine fashion. Several autocrine loops have been described in which a cell produces a growth factor and is at the same time a receptor cell for that factor. Negative and positive feedback loops have been demonstrated in a number of growth factor systems, including fibroblast somatomedin (SM-C).[5]

Growth Factor and Lymphokine Effects on Fibroblasts

Fibroblasts play a critically important role in wound epithelialization, collagen deposition, and wound remodeling. A number of growth factors have been assayed for their effects on fibroblasts. Tumor necrosis factor-α (TNF-α) and PDGF consistently demonstrate stimulatory and mitogenic activity toward fibroblasts. Interleukin 1-α and β are able to enhance the replication of already proliferating cells. TNF-α and transforming growth factor-β (TGF-β) have actually inhibited the growth of fibroblasts. In high doses (500 ng/ml), TNF-α has caused cellular death. The deleterious effects of TNF-α on fibroblasts are probably mediated in part by prostaglandin E_2, because indomethacin, a known prostaglandin E_2 synthesis inhibitor, blocks cellular death under identical concentrations of TNF-α. TGF-β was inhibitory at concentrations above 100 ng/ml, an effect unrelated to the presence of pros-taglandin E_2.[6] The in vivo interrelationship of growth factors and their target cells is complex. A systematic investigation into the actions of growth factors in isolated environments is warranted.

Transforming Growth Factor-β (TGF-β)

TGF-β is a two-chain polypeptide with a molecular weight of 25,000. It is synthesized by a variety of cells, including macrophages, lym-phocytes, bone and kidney cells, and neoplastic cell lines. However, it is found in highest concentration in platelet α-granules, where con-centrations are 10– to 1,000–fold higher than in other nonmalignant tissues. TGF-β is released when platelets come in contact with throm-bin.[7,8] Its association with α-granules is based upon the release of TGF-β concomitantly with the α-granule marker β-thromboglobulin under certain experimental conditions.[9] There is evidence suggesting an as-sociation of TGF-β with a binding protein.[10] Of note, PDGF is also associated with platelet alpha-granules and is released upon injury. TGF-β alone has a high affinity for the TGF-β receptor. It was initially described as a substance that promoted loss of contact inhibition and anchorage-independent growth, two characteristics that are both prop-erties of malignant cells. The factor was not present in identical, un-transformed cell lines, which suggests that it may have a role in the transformation of chemically and virally transformed cells.[11] When its presence was detected in a variety of nontransformed cells, it became clear that TGF-β played a non-neoplastic role in wound healing. Ac-tivation of lymphocytes induces transcription of the TGF-β gene.[12]

TGF-β interacts with a number of other growth factors. It is capable of stimulating or reducing cellular proliferation of both malignant and nonmalignant cell lines, largely, it seems, because of its interactions with other growth factors. When coincubated with PDGF, TGF-β in-duces fibroblast proliferation. When exposed to EGF (epidermal growth factor) alone, however, TGF-β in identical concentrations in-hibits fibroblast growth. At identical concentrations, for example, it may stimulate fibroblast growth in the presence of PDGF or inhibit the same cells in the presence of EGF, presumably by interfering with mitogenesis.[13] Levels of TGF-β have been measured, and peak levels have not been found to correlate with times of maximal healing. There was no relation to the number of such specific cellular types (as po-lymorphonucleotides, lymphocytes, and macrophages) with the overall levels of TGF-β.[14] The seemingly contradictory functions of TGF-β in diverse environments attest to its complex role in vivo.

TGF-β plays an important role in bone healing and development. TGF-β appears to be identical to cartilage-inducing peptide, a factor thought to be important in endochondral bone formation.[15] Indeed, TGF-β seems to play a major role in osteogenesis and chondrogenesis.[16] Daily injections of subtype 1 or 2 of TGF-β into the subperiosteal region of newborn rat femurs resulted in local formation of intramembranous bone and cartilage. The cartilage was eventually replaced with endochondrally ossified bone. Gene expression of both types I and II collagen was noted to be increased. Moreover, injection under identical experimental circumstances of TGF-β2 induced the synthesis of TGF-β1, suggesting an autoregulatory role of TGF-β. Mesenchymal precursor cells in the periosteum can be stimulated to differentiate by TGF-β. TGF-β influences nearly all cell types involved in bone formation, including chondrocytes, osteoblasts, and osteoclasts.[17–20] It is present also during normal endochondral ossification.[21] Levels of TGF-β in bone are 100 times higher than they are in soft tissues.

Experimentally, TGF-β has been shown to have an important general role in the wound healing process. It appears to stimulate directly the production of collagen through activation of fibroblasts, protein, and nucleic acid in animal models when implanted subcutaneously or in wound cylinders.[22,23] It increases fibroblast proliferation and collagen deposition in Hunt-Schilling wound chambers,[22] and it reduces the deleterious effects of adriamycin on wound healing in a similar model. In this respect, it appears to be more effective than PDGF and EGF. The administration of all three growth factors together reversed 90% of the adriamycin-induced impairment in wound healing.[24] Administration of TGF-β induces development of granulation tissue in mice.[23] One study indicated that tensile strength of wounds is improved in wounds treated, at the time of wounding, with TGF-β.[25] Tensile strength was even temporarily increased above normal levels, as seen in healthy animals.[24] Interestingly, fetal incisional wounds, which normally heal scarlessly, can be induced to fibrose and scar with the administration of TGF-β.[26]

Matrix synthesis is influenced by TGF-β in vitro, an important link to its role in fibrosis. In fibroblastic cell lines, TGF-β promotes collagen fibronectin formation selectively.[23] It is likely that TGF-β has an important in vivo role in the synthesis and regulation of extracellular matrix proteins. In vitro studies using a rat kidney fibroblast model indicate that TGF-β is necessary for the proliferation of cells, and that it can be substituted for fibronectin with no disturbance in the three-dimensional array of cells, an indication of its role in anchorage-dependent cellular proliferation.[27]

Fibroplasia is clearly increased by TGF-β in most cell systems, although not in all. In some systems, TGF-β can replace PDGF and/or EGF, which suggests a more complex role for this growth factor in fibroblast regulation.[28] Many of the assays for assessing the role of TGF-β are confounded by the presence of human serum, which, in addition to TGF-β, contains several other growth factors.[29]

Overall, TGF-β seems to play a role in fibroplasia, collagen synthesis, neovascularization, and extracellular matrix synthesis in a variety of animal systems and possibly also in humans.

Transforming Growth Factor-α (TGF-α)

Structurally dissimilar from TGF-β, TGF-α is a peptide with a molecular weight of 5,700. Initial reports described a transforming growth factor that was synergistic with TGF-β in its effects on rat kidney fibroblasts. It was subsequently discovered that the two peptides were structurally dissimilar.[30-31] TGF-α binds into the EGF receptor (as does EGF). It is produced by macrophages, platelets and keratinocytes, and some virally transformed cells. Biologically, EGF and TGF-α seem to be identical.[9] TGF-α shares homology with EGF and with the vaccinia growth factor (VGF). In culture, TGF-α stimulates proliferation of epithelial cells, endothelial cells, and fibroblasts.[32] Because TGF-α induces the proliferation of keratinocytes and also is produced by them, an autocrine physiology is inferred. Elevated levels of TGF-α have been linked to psoriasis and to some squamous cell carcinomas.[33] This growth factor has been isolated from fetal tissues, but has not yet been isolated from normal adult tissues.[34]

Experimentally, topically applied TGF-α has been associated with faster epithelialization in a pig, partial thickness burn model,[35] in which it proved considerably more active than EGF.

Platelet-Derived Growth Factor (PDGF)

A polypeptide with a molecular weight of 31,000, PDGF is stored in the alpha granules of platelets and is released when the platelet is activated. After injury, hemorrhage occurs, and platelets are extravasated, form fibrin clots, and are activated. Platelet degranulation occurs when the platelet is exposed to thrombin or fibrillar collagen. PDGF has been divided into two active proteins, PDGF I and PDGF II, both of which are present in normal human serum. They appear to be functionally identical.[36] Indeed, it is possible that PDGF II is a degradation product of PDGF I. The sequence of PDGF-encoding regions and their chromosomal locations have been defined.[37] PDGF can be further broken down with reducing agents to an A and B chain, with loss of biologic activity.[38] PDGF binds tightly to specific receptors with a K_d of 1×10^{-9}. The ligand-receptor interaction produces a mitogenic signal that increases DNA synthesis.[39]

An interesting homology (93%) has been found between the gene encoding for PDGF and an oncogene, v-sis. The oncogene v-sis encodes for a transforming protein p28[v-sis], which in turn is derived from a fibrosarcoma-causing retrovirus (SSV) in the woolly monkey. Both p28[v-sis] and PDGF bind to the same receptor in fibroblasts and seem to elicit identical mitogenic and chemotactic responses from fibroblasts.[40] Just as with PDGF, an autocrine stimulation mechanism is postulated for the transformation of SSV cells by p28[v-sis]. A human osteosarcoma line, U-2 OS, also secretes a PDGF-like compound, as do endothelial cells after treatment with thrombin.[41,42] Cultured arterial smooth muscle cells from newborn rats and the intima from injured arteries secrete a homodimer of the A chain of PDGF.[43] Human peripheral blood monocytes release a PDGF-like compound after activation.[44] Excreted PDGF is rapidly cleared by the liver, with a half-life of two minutes.[45]

Several cell types in addition to platelets appear to synthesize PDGF, including macrophages, fibroblasts, smooth muscle cells, and vascular endothelium. It was first realized that serum was necessary for the growth of fibroblasts.[46] Later, this growth factor was localized to the alpha granules of platelets,[47] and subsequently to PDGF.[48] PDGF clearly serves as a powerful chemoattractant for smooth muscle cells, fibroblasts, and leukocytes.[49] Its mitogenic activity, however, depends on the presence of other growth factors. The proliferation of mesenchymal cells requires TGF-β or EGF.[50] PDGF is produced by endothelial cells, vascular smooth muscle cells, and platelets. Because these cells reside adjacent to one another, a paracrine response for PDGF has been postulated.[3] An autocrine component of the response may also exist, because smooth muscle cells produce PDGF.

PDGF may play a role in long-term connective tissue remodeling. PDGF seems to play a role in wound remodeling by stimulating collagenase secretion by fibroblasts.[51] It acts as a chemoattractant for fibroblasts as well as a co-mitogen, in conjunction with other growth factors, toward fibroblasts. The combination of these factors suggests a greater role for long-term tissue matrix remodeling. This theory is supported by experimental evidence. The breaking strength of wounds is augmented for up to seven weeks after a single dose of PDGF. The deleterious effects of diabetes are ameliorated (collagen deposition and cellularity in wounds). PDGF, when applied to incisional wounds in rats, induces an increase in collagen deposition and cellularity.[52] In addition to affecting fibroblasts, PDGF possesses powerful mitogenic properties for glial cells and smooth muscle cells.[53]

PDGF also appears to be chemotactic (probably through different regions of the polypeptide from those that stimulate mitogenesis)[54] for several cell types, including neutrophils and monocytes.[55] At higher concentrations than those necessary for chemotaxis, PDGF activates neutrophils and monocytes.[56] PDGF is chemotactic for smooth muscle cells and fibroblasts.[57]

PDGF is released when platelets clump and are activated. For this reason, it has been postulated that PDGF plays a role in atherogenesis at the point where endothelial injury occurs and platelet aggregation supervenes. PDGF may, therefore, act as a mitogen for smooth muscle cells, a prominent feature of the atherosclerotic plaque.[49]

Overall, PDGF exerts powerful mitogenic and chemoattractant stimuli on cells critical to wound healing. Its distribution is initiated by vascular injury and platelet-mediated fibrin clots. It directly recruits and activates neutrophils and monocytes, possibly in a concentration-gradient fashion. After initiation of this inflammatory phase of wound healing, it serves to activate mesenchymal cells necessary in the proliferative phase, including endothelial cells and smooth muscle cells. In the remodeling phases of wound healing, PDGF stimulates fibroblasts to secrete the collagenase and extracellular matrix that are important in wound remodeling.

Fibroblast Growth Factor (FGF)

FGF is one of a group of similar (or identical) growth factors, which share the ability to bind heparin. They induce angiogenesis and mitogenesis of endothelial cells. Two subtypes, acidic fibroblast growth factor (aFGF) and basic fibroblast growth factor (bFGF), which were initially isolated from brain and pituitary, respectively, have been recognized. Each appears to be derived from a single gene; differences in the multiple similar growth factors within the same class seem to be the result of differences in posttranslational processing.[58,59] These growth factors range in molecular weight from 17,000 to 25,000. The length of bFGF ranges from 146 to 155 amino acids; aFGF is 140 amino acids long. They share homology with a number of other growth factors. It has been suggested that the entire group be subclassified as heparin-binding growth factor (HBGF).

FGF was first described as a factor that had been isolated from bovine brain and pituitary tissue and that possessed mitogenic activity toward fibroblasts in culture and toward endothelial cells. A plethora of growth factors have been described that seem to be identical to FGF. These include hepatoma-derived growth factor, chondrosarcoma-derived growth factor, β-retina-derived growth factor, cartilage-derived growth factor, astroglial growth factor 2, eye-derived growth factor, cationic hypothalamus-derived growth factor, class 2 and β-heparin-binding growth factors.[60] Endothelial cell growth factors α and β (ECGF-A, ECGF-B) may be post-transcriptionally modified FGF.[61] Interleukin-1 has been noted to have a structure similar to that of bFGF.[62] All these compounds share a high degree of similarity to the structure of aFGF or bFGF, with differences in the length of the N-terminus.

The mechanism of action of FGF is still largely unknown. It appears to be released from granules, where it may be stored in a preformed state. Several cell types possess cellular receptors for FGF. It has been proposed that FGF and other heparin-binding growth factors are concentrated on the cellular surface, perhaps bound to heparin sulfate, the major glycosaminoglycan on the endothelial cell surface. This complex may influence angioneogenesis in vivo.[63] FGF seems to control the production of extracellular matrix components, including fibronectin and some collagen types.[64]

FGF appears to increase angiogenesis, fibroplasia, and collagen deposition. In nanogram quantities it induces the formation and growth of capillaries in the rabbit cornea,[65] in the chick embryo,[66] and in a rat model.[67]

bFGF, which is known to act as a mitogen, stimulates chondrocytes and endothelial cells, as well as other mesenchymally derived cells. Several authors have noted that it enhances the proliferation and life span of cells, and that it is necessary for the maintenance of cell lines in culture.[60] Fibroblasts are also stimulated in the presence of bFGF to produce collagen.[68] Collagen accumulation can be blocked by administering antiserum to bFGF.[69] Several studies have documented

317

an increase in wound organization, in the breaking strength of wounds, and in collagen deposition in incisional wounds and wound cylinders treated with bFGF. In a guinea pig model, FGF stimulated neovascularization and epithelialization.[70] In a polyvinyl alcohol sponge model in rats, bFGF (bovine cartilage-derived factor) accelerated wound healing by increasing collagen, protein, DNA synthesis, and cellular proliferation.[68] bFGF possesses mitogenic properties with respect to human epidermal keratinocytes and connective tissue cells. In one study, aFGF appeared to promote axonal regeneration through a matrix-filled tube.[71]

Overall, FGF and its associated heparin-binding growth factors appear to stimulate collagen synthesis, to possess powerful mitogenic and angiogenic properties toward mesenchymal cells, and, possibly, to modulate extracellular matrix synthesis.

Epidermal Growth Factor (EGF)

EGF is a small single-chain polypeptide of 6,000 daltons (53 amino acids). Remarkably stable, it can survive boiling or treatment with acid. The tertiary structure is maintained by six disulfide bonds. EGF may circulate in the plasma bound to a high-molecular-weight protein, much like IGF-I. Structurally, EGF resembles TGF-α and vaccinia virus growth factor (VVGF). TGF-α may in fact be a fetal form of EGF.[72] EGF, initially isolated in 1937 as a factor derived from human urine, inhibited the action of gastric acid.[73] It is currently isolated from mouse salivary glands, from human urine, from milk, and from Brunner's glands in the small intestine. The sequence for EGF has been localized to chromosome 4.[74] EGF resembles v-erb-B, a viral oncogene of the avian erythroblastosis virus.[75]

EGF binds to a surface receptor, and the receptor-ligand complex is internalized.[76] A tyrosine kinase cascade is initiated as the complex is internalized, the complex, as well as other cytoplasmic proteins,[77] is phosphorylated, and free intracellular Ca^{2+} rises. After the ligand-receptor complex has been internalized, cellular morphology changes markedly and cells grow and divide rapidly. Cells typically dedifferentiate during rapid growth and division until the influence of EGF is removed, at which time they resume their differentiated state as collagen-producing fibroblasts.[78]

EGF is best known for its ability to stimulate keratinization and epidermal growth. Its actions in vivo, thus far, are restricted to epithelial cells, although several other cell types, including fibroblasts, glial cells, chondrocytes, and smooth muscle cells,[79] respond to EGF. Largely mitogenic in action, EGF increases synthesis of DNA, RNA, protein, and hyaluronic acid (HA). It seems to affect such epidermal structures as hair follicles, sweat glands, and the arrector pili muscle, based on the assumption that the presence of EGF receptors indicates cells influenced by EGF.[80] Cellular growth is the major result of EGF stimulation of a target cell. EGF serves as a progression factor: cells that are competent to proceed with division do so under its influence.

EGF (urogastrone) has been used experimentally to reduce the degree of gastric ulceration and the subjective pain in patients with duodenal ulcers.[81] EGF has prevented the development of hyaline membrane disease in prematurely born sheep.[82] Experimentally, topically applied EGF has been shown to accelerate the healing of split-thickness skin graft donor sites in pigs[83] and the healing of burn wounds.[84] Fibroblasts possess EGF receptors and proliferate in response to EGF in vitro, with increases in collagen and DNA content observed.[85] Collagenase production is stimulated, indicating a possible role in wound remodeling.[86]

EGF may have important implications for bone healing. Proliferation of periosteal fibroblasts and DNA production by cultured osteoblasts are improved after incubation with EGF.[87] Rat calvaria take up EGF and grow in culture.[88] After topical administration of EGF, corneal epithelial healing is improved in rats, rabbits, and primates, and stromal healing is improved in rabbits and monkeys.[89] When administered in a wound chamber model, EGF clearly promotes collagen deposition and proliferation of fibroblasts,[85] as well as marked angiogenesis and an increase in fibroblast DNA content.[90] A single clinical trial in humans reports accelerated rates of healing of split-thickness skin graft donor sites when they are treated with EGF.[91]

Overall, EGF promotes fibroplasia, increased DNA content in mesenchymal cells, and improvement in wound healing in the eye, deep wounds, and skin wounds. It may hold considerable clinical promise in the treatment of ulcers and difficult bone or skin wounds. Its more widespread use awaits randomized clinical trials in humans for these and other specific indications.

Insulin-Like Growth Factor (IGF-I)

IGF-I and the somatomedins are polypeptide hormones that weigh 7,500 daltons. They are structurally similar to proinsulin, with which they share a 50% homology. They possess insulin-like activity. The somatomedins are recognized as being the mediators of the actions of growth hormone. Interestingly, they are present in large amounts in fetal tissue, and seem to be important in insuring adequate birth weight.[92] It is likely they function in an endocrine fashion, reaching their target cells through the bloodstream.

In general, somatomedins are anabolic hormones, which, like insulin, promote the synthesis of protein, glycogen, DNA, RNA, glycosaminoglycans, cellular replication, and the transport of glucose and amino acids across the cell membrane. Somatomedin stimulates collagen synthesis in fibroblasts in vitro. For maximal biologic response, fibroblast-synthesized somatomedin seems to require PDGF.[5]

Monocyte-Derived Growth Factor (MDGF)

This growth factor, which weighs 40,000 daltons, appears to be functionally distinct from other macrophage- or monocyte-derived growth factors, such as PDGF, TGF-β, bFGF, IGF-I and IL-1.[93] It may actually represent more than one growth factor. When animals were treated with hydrocortisone and antimacrophage serum, it was noted, in 1975, that fibroblast proliferation was inhibited. Subsequently, it was demonstrated that isolated macrophages secrete a factor that stimulates fibroblasts.[94] This factor is synthesized by macrophages and is secreted into the extracellular environment, probably in a constitutive fashion. It does not appear that any MDGF is stored within intracellular vesicles or granules. In this respect it differs from such growth factors as PDGF, which is stored within platelet alpha granules. Secretion of MDGF is enhanced if the macrophage is activated with one of a number of factors, including LPS, concanavalin A, fibronectin or phorbol esters.[95,96] MDGF, which functions largely as a mesenchymal stimulator, acts on fibroblasts, smooth muscle cells, endothelial cells, and other mesenchymal cells.[97]

Interleukin 1 (IL-1) and Interleukin 2 (IL-2)

IL-1, a macrophage product known to stimulate fibroblasts, is chemotactic for polymorphonucleotides. Its structure is similar to that of bFGF.[62] IL-1 stimulates collagenase and may play a role in cartilage resorption and bone remodeling. It may also play a regulatory role in fibroblast proliferation.[98] IL-1 was originally described as a macrophage-derived, T-cell growth factor, mitogenic both for T cells and fibroblasts, but not for other mesenchymal cells, such as arterial smooth muscle cells or vascular endothelial cells.[99]

IL-2 is synthesized by helper T lymphocytes. It is responsible indirectly for fibroblast proliferation through as yet poorly described immune mechanisms, although it does not seem to have any direct effect on fibroblast proliferation.[100]

Bone Morphogenetic Proteins (BMP) and Osteogenin

Bone initiation, the first step in new bone formation, is known to be regulated by osteogenin and bone morphogenetic proteins (BMP). These substances have recently been isolated, purified, and cloned. It appears that BMP and osteogenin act, in conjunction with PDGF, TGF-β isoforms, IGF-1 and -2, and FGF, to promote newly induced bone in cell culture and collagen ceramic composites.[101,102] Cartilage development in response to BMP has been observed. Occurrence of cartilage-specific proteoglycan H (PG-H) and type II collagen has been detected in an in vitro system with an implanted diffusion chamber.[103] In a rabbit model, placement of BMP and associated noncollagenous proteins induces adventitial and muscle connective-tissue derived cells to form a fibrous and chondro-osteoprogenetic pattern of bone development, which means that BMP can induce a change in differentiation of otherwise uncommitted cells.[104] Experimentally, BMP has been used to restore bone loss after osteomyelitis and ablative surgery[105,106] and to achieve union in experimental posterolateral spondylodesis procedures.[107] Ectopic periosteal bone formation can be induced experimentally when BMP is placed in a collagen matrix carrier and into the dorsal muscles in mice.[108] BMP has been shown to cause connective tissue outgrowths of neonatal muscle to differentiate into cartilage. BMP acted synergistically with other growth factors, especially IL-1, TGF-β and FGF, in inducing cartilage formation.[109,110]

Granulocyte-Macrophage Colony Stimulating Factor (GM-CSF) and Interleukin-6 (IL-6)

Colony-stimulating factors are glycoproteins. Their biologic specificity is defined by their ability to stimulate proliferation and differentiation of peripheral hemopoietic cells and their stem cell precursors. The family, which includes granulocyte-stimulating factor (G-CSF), GM-CSF, macrophage-stimulating factor (M-CSF), multi-CSF[111] and IL-1, -2 and -6, functions largely as hematopoietic agents and increases cellularity and leukocyte response in vivo.[112] The colony-stimulating factors stimulate stem cells to proliferate and activate mature peripheral cells, including neutrophils, macrophages, and lymphocytes. These factors have proven especially potent at activating peripheral neutrophils. GM-CSF has been cloned, and a recombinant form is available (rhM-CSF). GM-CSF is a small glycoprotein growth factor. GM-CSF gene expression may be influenced by other growth factors, such as tumor necrosis factor-cachectin or endotoxin, IL-1, and IL-6. Its receptor is characterized by a high affinity (Kd 2×10^{-8}) for GM-CSF and by sparse distribution. Two functional classes of receptor have been observed, one that specifically binds GM-CSF and another that competes with IL-3. Signal transduction involves a tyrosine kinase and probably a G-protein, which in turn stimulate a Na^+-H^+ exchange pump.[113]

GM-CSF is a potent hematopoietic growth factor both in vivo and in vitro. After stimulation, it is produced by several cell types, especially T cells and macrophages. Once activated, macrophages secrete GM-CSF, IL-1, and tumor necrosis factor, the latter two of which stimulate further GM-CSF production by endothelial and fibroblast cells. It is postulated that GM-CSF produced by endothelial cells and fibroblasts and even epithelial cells acts as a chemotactic factor for neutrophils, monocytes, and eosinophils in a paracrine fashion.[114,115]

There is limited experimental indication that GM-CSF and related substances may play a role in bone homeostasis, in particular resorption, especially in the presence of infection. Cultured osteoblasts from a mouse fracture callus system secrete M-CSF, GM-CSF, and IL-6 in response to lipopolysaccharides in vitro. Whole bone preparations appear to secrete IL-1, IL-6, M-CSF, and GM-CSF. Cells prepared from a fracture callus of a mouse fracture model secrete GM-CSF, IL-6, and IL-1. Osteoclasts are known to produce M-CSF, GM-CSF, and IL-6. IL-1 may play a role in bone resorption.[116]

GM-CSF has a limited potential to induce growth in a number of tumor specimens, including breast and lung. It produces a predictable growth response in bone marrow, and has been used for leukemic patients to induce hematopoiesis. It appears to increase the production of neutrophils, eosinophils, and monocytes, which makes it possible, in certain experimental settings, to use a higher dose of chemotherapeutic agents in treating patients with malignancies, AIDS, and bone marrow transplantation.[117,118] Side effects, when GM-CSF is administered intravenously, include myalgias, fever, fluid retention, and serosal effusions.[119]

Conclusion

Wound healing begins at the moment of injury. Platelet-contained factors are released that act directly on target cells, inducing them to proliferate, synthesize, and produce growth factors. Growth factors act through a complex set of autocrine, paracrine, and, occasionally, endocrine pathways to promote wound healing. The current literature is replete with new interrelationships between growth factors and their target cells. A review of the structure, mechanisms of action, and experimental and clinical studies of the most common growth factors involved in wound healing leads one to recognize that the paucity of understanding of their biological interrelationships necessitates continued experimental and clinical studies.

References

1. Leibovich SJ, Ross R: The role of the macrophage in wound repair: A study with hydrocortisone and antimacrophage serum. *Am J Pathol* 1975;78:71–100.
2. McGrath MH: Peptide growth factors and wound healing. *Clin Plast Surg* 1990;17:421–432.
3. Coughlin SR, Escobedo JA, Williams LT: Molecular mechanisms of platelet-derived growth factor action, in Barbul A, Pines E, Caldwell M, et al (eds): *Growth Factors and Other Aspects of Wound Healing: Biological and Clinical Implications.* New York, Alan R. Liss, 1988.
4. Nemeth GG, Bolander ME, Martin GR: Growth factors and their role in wound and fracture healing, in Barbul A, Pines E, Caldwell M, et al (eds): *Growth Factors and Other Aspects of Wound Healing: Biological and Clinical Implications.* New York, Alan R. Liss, 1988.
5. Clemmons DR, Shaw DS: Purification and biologic properties of fibroblast somatomedin. *J Biol Chem* 1986;261:10293–10298.
6. Thornton SC, Por SB, Walsh BJ, et al: Interaction of immune and connective tissue cells: I. The effect of lymphokines and monokines on fibroblast growth. *J Leukoc Biol* 1990;47:312–320.
7. Assoian RK, Komoriya A, Meyers CA, et al: Transforming growth factor-β in human platelets: Identification of a major storage site, purification, and characterization. *J Biol Chem* 1983;258:7155–7160.

8. Assoian RK, Sporn MB: Type β transforming growth factor in human platelets: Release during platelet degranulation and action on vascular smooth muscle cells. *J Cell Biol* 1986;102:1217–1223.

9. Sporn MB, Roberts AB, Wakefield, LM, et al: Transforming growth factor-beta: Biological function and chemical structure. *Science* 1986;233:532–534.

10. Pircher R, Jullien P, Lawrence DA: Beta-transforming growth factor is stored in human blood platelets as a latent high molecular weight complex. *Biochem Biophys Res Commun* 1986;136:30–37.

11. De Larco JE, Todaro GJ: Growth factors from murine sarcoma virus-transformed cells. *Proc Natl Acad Sci USA* 1978;75:4001–4005.

12. Kehrl JH, Wakefield LM, Roberts AB, et al: Production of transforming growth factor beta by human T lymphocytes and its potential role in the regulation of T cell growth. *J Exp Med* 1986;163:1037–1050.

13. Roberts AB, Anzano MA, Wakefield LM, et al: Type-β transforming growth factor: A bifunctional regulator of cellular growth. *Proc Natl Acad Sci USA* 1985;82:119–123.

14. Cromack DT, Sporn MB, Roberts AB, et al: Transforming growth factor β levels in rat wound chambers. *J Surg Res* 1987;42:622–628.

15. Seyedin SM, Thomson AY, Bentz H, et al: Cartilage-inducing factor A: Apparent identity to transforming growth factor-β. *J Biol Chem* 1986;261:5693–5695.

16. Joyce ME, Roberts AB, Sporn MB, et al: Transforming growth factor-β and the initiation of chondrogenesis and osteogenesis in the rat femur. *J Cell Biol* 1990;110:2195–2207.

17. Canalis E, McCarthy TL, Centrella M: Growth factors and the regulation of bone remodeling. *J Clin Invest* 1988;81:277–281.

18. Centrella M, McCarthy TL, Canalis E: Transforming growth factor β is a bifunctional regulator of replication and collagen synthesis in osteoblast-enriched cell cultures from fetal rat bone. *J Biol Chem* 1987;262:2869–2874.

19. Robey PG, Young MF, Flanders KC, et al: Osteoblasts synthesize and respond to transforming growth factor-type β (TGF-β) in vitro. *J Cell Biol* 1987;105:457–463.

20. Seyedin SM, Thomas TC, Thompson AY, et al: Purification and characterization of two cartilage-inducing factors from bovine demineralized bone. *Proc Natl Acad Sci USA* 1985;82:2267–2271.

21. Carrington JL, Roberts AB, Flanders KC, et al: Accumulation, localization, and compartmentation of transforming growth factor β during endochondral bone development. *J Cell Biol* 1988;107:1969–1975.

22. Sporn MB, Roberts AB, Shull JH, et al: Polypeptide transforming growth factors isolated from bovine sources and used for wound healing in vivo. *Science* 1983;219:1329–1331.

23. Roberts AB, Sporn MB, Assoian RK, et al: Transforming growth factor type β: Rapid induction of fibrosis and angiogenesis in vivo and stimulation of collagen formation in vitro. *Proc Natl Acad Sci USA* 1986;83:4167–4171.

24. Lawrence WT, Norton JA, Sporn MB, et al: The reversal of an Adriamycin induced healing impairment with chemoattractants and growth factors. *Ann Surg* 1986;203:142–147.

25. Mustoe TA, Pierce GF, Thomason A, et al: Accelerated healing of incisional wounds in rats induced by transforming growth factor β. *Science* 1987;237:1333–1336.

26. Krummel TM, Michna BA, Thomas BL, et al: Transforming growth factor β (TGF-beta) induces fibrosis in a fetal wound model. *J Pediatr Surg* 1988;23:647–652.

27. Ignotz RA, Massague J: Transforming growth factor-beta stimulates the expression of fibronectin and collagen and their incorporation into the extracellular matrix. *J Biol Chem* 1986;261:4337–4345.

28. Anzano MA, Roberts AB, Sporn MB: Anchorage-independent growth of primary rat embryo cells is induced by platelet-derived growth factor and inhibited by type-beta transforming growth factor. *J Cell Physiol* 1986;126:312–318.

29. Assoian RK: The role of growth factors in tissue repair IV. Type β-transforming growth factor and stimulation of fibrosis, in Clark RAF, Henson PM (eds): *The Molecular and Cellular Biology of Wound Repair.* New York, Plenum Press, 1988.

30. Marquardt H, Hunkapiller MW, Hood LE, et al: Transforming growth factors produced by retrovirus-transformed rodent fibroblasts and human melanoma cells: Amino acid sequence homology with epidermal growth factor. *Proc Natl Acad Sci USA* 1983;80:4684–4688.

31. Roberts AB, Frolik CA, Anzano MA, et al: Transforming growth factors from neoplastic and nonneoplastic tissues. *Fed Proc* 1983;42:2621–2626.

32. Madtes DK, Raines EW, Sakariassen KS, et al: Induction of transforming growth factor-alpha in activated human alveolar macrophages. *Cell* 1988;53:285–293.

33. Coffey RJ Jr, Derynck R, Wilcox JN, et al: Production and auto-induction of transforming growth factor-α in human keratinocytes. *Nature* 1987;328:817–820.

34. Nexo E, Hollenberg MD, Figueroa A, et al: Detection of epidermal growth factor-urogastrone and its receptor during fetal mouse development. *Proc Natl Acad Sci USA* 1980;77:2782–2785.

35. Schultz GS, White M, Mitchell R, et al: Epithelial wound healing enhanced by transforming growth factor-α and vaccinia growth factor. *Science* 1987;235;350–352.

36. Raines EW, Ross R: Platelet-derived growth factor: I. High yield purification and evidence for multiple forms. *J Biol Chem* 1982;257:5154–5160.

37. Doolittle RF, Hukapiller MW, Hood LE, et al: Simian sarcoma virus onc gene, v-sis, is derived from the gene (or genes) encoding a platelet-derived growth factor. *Science* 1983;221:275–277.

38. Betsholtz C, Johnsson A, Heldin CH, et al: cDNA sequence and chromosomal localization of human platelet-derived growth factor A-chain and its expression in tumour cell lines. *Nature* 1986;320:695–699.

39. Yarden Y, Escobedo JA, Kuang WJ, et al: Structure of the receptor for platelet-derived growth factor helps define a family of closely related growth factor receptors. *Nature* 1986;323:226–232.

40. Deuel TF, Huang JS: Platelet-derived growth factor: Purification, properties, and biologial activities. *Prog Hematol* 1983;13:201–221.

41. Huang JS, Huang SS: Role of growth factors in oncogenesis: Growth factor proto-oncogene pathways of mitogenesis, in *Growth Factors in Biology and Medicine.* (Ciba Foundation Symposium 116) London, Pitman, 1985, pp 46–65.

42. Bowen-Pope DF, Vogel A, Ross R: Production of platelet-derived growth factor-like molecules and reduced expression of platelet-derived growth factor receptors accompany transformation by a wide spectrum of agents. *Proc Natl Acad Sci USA* 1984;81:2396–2400.

43. Sejersen T, Betsholtz C, Sjolund M, et al: Rat skeletal myoblasts and arterial smooth muscle cells express the gene for the A chain but not the gene for the B chain (c-sis) of platelet-derived growth factor (PDGF) and produce a PDGF-like protein. *Proc Natl Acad Sci USA* 1986;83:6844–6848.

44. Martinet Y, Bitterman PB, Mornex JF, et al: Activated human monocytes express the c-sis proto-oncogene and release a mediator showing PDGF-like actvity. *Nature* 1986;319:158–160.

45. Bowen-Pope DF, Malpass TW, Foster DM, et al: Platelet-derived growth factor in vivo: Levels, activity, and rate of clearance. *Blood* 1984;64:458–469.

46. Kohler N, Lipton A: Platelets as a source of fibroblast growth-promoting activity. *Exp Cell Res* 1974;87:297–301.

47. Witte LD, Kaplan KL, Nossel HL, et al: Studies of the release from human platelets of the growth factor for cultured human arterial smooth muscle cells. *Circ Res* 1978;42:402–409.

48. Ross R, Vogel A: The platelet-derived growth factor. *Cell* 1978;14:203–210.

49. Grotendorst GR, Seppa HEJ, Kleinman HK, et al: Attachment of smooth muscle cells to collagen and their migration toward platelet-derived growth factor. *Proc Natl Acad Sci USA* 1981;78:3669–3672.

50. Grotendorst GR, Grotendorst CA, Gilman T: Production of growth factors (PDGF and TGF-β) at the site of tissue repair, in Barbul A, Pines E, Caldwell M, et al (eds): *Growth Factors and Other Aspects of Wound Healing: Biological and Clinical Implications*. New York, Alan R. Liss, 1988.

51. Bauer EA, Cooper TW, Huang JS, et al: Stimulation of in vitro human skin collagenase expression by platelet-derived growth factor. *Proc Natl Acad Sci USA* 1985;82:4132–4136.

52. Pierce GH, Mustoe TA, Deuel TF: Transforming growth factor-β induces increased directed cellular migration and tissue repair in rats, in Barbul A, Pines E, Caldwell M, et al (eds): *Growth Factors and Other Aspects of Wound Healing: Biological and Clinical Implications*. New York, Alan R. Liss, 1988.

53. Huang JS, Olsen TJ, Huang SS: The role of growth factors in tissue repair I: Platelet-derived growth factor, in Clark RAF, Henson PM, (eds): *The Molecular and Cellular Biology of Wound Repair*. New York, Plenum Press, 1988.

54. Williams LT, Antoniades HN, Goetzl EJ: Platelet-derived growth factor stimulates mouse 3T3 cell mitogenesis and leukocyte chemotaxis through different structural determinants. *J Clin Invest* 1983;72:1759–1763.

55. Deuel TF, Senior RM, Huang JS, et al: Chemotaxis of monocytes and neutrophils to platelet-derived growth factor. *J Clin Invest* 1982;69:1046–1049.

56. Tzeng DY, Deuel TF, Huang JS, et al: Platelet-derived growth factor promotes human peripheral monocyte activation. *Blood* 1985;66:179–183.

57. Grotendorst GR, Chang T, Seppa HEJ, et al: Platelet-derived growth factor is a chemoattractant for vascular smooth muscle cells. *J Cell Physiol* 1982;113:261–266.

58. Abraham JA, Mergia A, Whang JL, et al: Nucleotide sequence of a bovine clone encoding the angiogenic protein, basic fibroblast growth factor. *Science* 1986;233:545–548.

59. Abraham JA, Whang JL, Tumolo A, et al: Human basic fibroblast growth factor: Nucleotide sequence and genomic organization. *EMBO J* 1986;5:2523–2528.

60. Fox GM: The role of growth factors in tissue repair III: Fibroblast growth factor, in Clark RAF, Henson PM, (eds): *The Molecular and Cellular Biology of Wound Repair*. New York, Plenum Press, 1988.

61. Burgess WH, Mehlman T, Marshak DR, et al: Structural evidence that endothelial cell growth factor beta is the precursor of both endothelial cell growth factor alpha and acidic fibroblast growth factor. *Proc Natl Acad Sci USA* 1986;83:7216–7220.

62. Gimenez-Gallego G, Rodkey J, Bennett C, et al: Brain-derived acidic fibroblast growth factor: Complete amino acid sequence and homologies. *Science* 1985;230:1385–1388.

63. Shing Y, Folkman J, Sullivan R, et al: Heparin affinity: Purification of a tumor-derived capillary endothelial cell growth factor. *Science* 1984;223:1296–1299.

64. Gospodarowicz D: Localisation of a fibroblast growth factor and its effect alone and with hydrocortisone on 3T3 cell growth. *Nature* 1974;249:123–127.

65. Gospodarowicz D, Bialecki H, Thakral TK: The angiogenic activity of the fibroblast and epidermal growth factor. *Exp Eye Res* 1979;28:501–514.

66. Klagsbrun M, Shing Y: Heparin affinity of anionic and cationic capillary endothelial cell growth factors: Analysis of hypothalamus-derived growth factors and fibroblast growth factors. *Proc Natl Acad Sci USA* 1985;82:805–809.

67. Buntrock P, Jentzsch KD, Heder G: Stimulation of wound healing, using brain extract with fibroblast growth factor (FGF) activity: I. Quantitative and biochemical studies into formation of granulation tissue. *Exp Pathol* 1982;21:46–53.

68. Davidson JM, Klagsbrun M, Hill KE, et al: Accelerated wound repair, cell proliferation, and collagen accumulation are produced by a cartilage-derived growth factor. *J Cell Biol* 1985;100:1219–1227.

69. Davidson JM, Buckley A, Woodward S, et al: Mechanisms of accelerated wound repair using epidermal growth factor and basic fibroblast growth factor, in Barbul A, Pines E, Caldwell M, et al (eds): *Growth Factors and Other Aspects of Wound Healing: Biological and Clinical Implications.* New York, Alan R. Liss, 1988.

70. Fourtanier AY, Courty J, Muller E, et al: Eye-derived growth factor isolated from bovine retina and used for epidermal wound healing in vivo. *J Invest Dermatol* 1986;87:76–80.

71. Cordeiro PG, Seckel BR, Lipton SA, et al: Acidic fibroblast growth factor enhances peripheral nerve regeneration in vivo. *Plast Reconstr Surg* 1989;83:1013–1021.

72. Derynck R, Roberts AB, Winkler ME, et al: Human transforming growth factor-alpha: Precursor structure and expression in *Escherichia coli. Cell* 1984;38:287–297.

73. Gray JS, Wieczorowski E, Ivy AC: Inhibition of gastric secretion by extracts of normal male urine. *Science* 1939;89:489–490.

74. Zabel BU, Eddy RL, Lalley PA, et al: Chromosomal locations of the human and mouse genes for precursors of epidermal growth factor and the beta subunit of nerve growth factor. *Proc Natl Acad Sci USA* 1985;82:469–473.

75. Ullrich A, Coussens L, Hayflick JS, et al: Human epidermal growth factor receptor cDNA sequence and aberrant expression of the amplified gene in A431 epidermoid carcinoma cells. *Nature* 1984;309:418–425.

76. Gullick WJ, Downward J, Foulkes JG, et al: Antibodies to the ATP-binding site of the human epidermal growth factor (EGF) receptor as specific inhibitors of EGF-stimulated protein-tyrosine kinase activity. *Eur J Biochem* 1986;158:245–253.

77. Aoyagi T, Suya H, Umeda K, et al: Epidermal growth factor stimulates tyrosine phosphorylation of pig epidermal fibrous keratin. *J Invest Dermatol* 1985;84:118–121.

78. Banks AR: The role of growth factors in tissue repair II: Epidermal growth factor, in Clark RAF, Henson PM (eds): *The Molecular and Cellular Biology of Wound Repair.* New York, Plenum Press, 1988.

79. McAuslan BR, Bender V, Reilly W, et al: New functions of epidermal growth factor: Stimulation of capillary endothelial cell migration and matrix dependent proliferation. *Cell Biol Int Rep* 1985;9:175–182.

80. Nanney LB, Magid M, Stoscheck CM, et al: Comparison of epidermal growth factor binding and receptor distribution in normal human epidermis and epidermal appendages. *J Invest Dermatol* 1984;83:385–393.

81. Koffman CG, Elder JB, Ganguli PC, et al: Effect of urogastrone on gastric secretion and serum gastrin concentration in patients with duodenal ulceration. *Gut* 1982;23:951–956.

82. Sundell HW, Gray ME, Serenius FS, et al: Effects of epidermal growth factor on lung maturation in fetal lambs. *Am J Pathol* 1980;100:707–725.

83. Nanney LB: Epidermal growth factor-induced effects on wound healing, abstract. *Clin Res* 1987;35:706A.

84. Brown GL, Curtsinger L III, Brightwell JR, et al: Enhancement of epidermal regeneration by biosynthetic epidermal growth factor. *J Exp Med* 1986;163:1319–1324.

85. Laato M, Niinikoski J, Lebel L, et al: Stimulation of wound healing by epidermal growth factor: A dose-dependent effect. *Ann Surg* 1986;203:379–381.

86. Chua CC, Geiman DE, Keller GH, et al: Induction of collagenase secretion in human fibroblast cultures by growth promoting factors. *J Biol Chem* 1985;260:5213–5216.

87. Canalis E, Raisz LG: Effect of epidermal growth factor on bone formation in vitro. *Endocrinology* 1979;104:862–869.

88. Centrella M, Canalis E: Local regulators of skeletal growth: A perspective. *Endocr Rev* 1985;6:544–551.

89. Brightwell JR, Riddle SL, Eiferman RA, et al: Biosynthetic human EGF accelerates healing of Neodecadron-treated primate corneas. *Invest Ophthalmol Vis Sci* 1985;26:105–110.

90. Buckley A, Davidson JM, Kamerath CD, et al: Sustained release of epidermal growth factor accelerates wound repair. *Proc Natl Acad Sci USA* 1985;82:7340–7344.

91. Brown GL, Nanney LB, Griffen J, et al: Enhancement of wound healing by topical treatment with epidermal growth factor. *N Engl J Med* 1989;321:76–79.

92. Conover CA, Rosenfeld RG, Hintz RL: Hormonal control of the replication of human fetal fibroblasts: Role of somatomedin C/insulin-like growth factor I. *J Cell Physiol* 1986;128:47–54.

93. Singh JP, Bonin PD: Purification and biochemical properties of a human monocyte-derived growth factor. *Proc Natl Acad Sci USA* 1988;85:6374–6378.

94. Leibovich SJ, Ross R: A macrophage-dependent factor that stimulates the proliferation of fibroblasts in vitro. *Am J Pathol* 1976;84:501–514.

95. Glenn KC, Ross R: Human monocyte-derived growth factor(s) for mesenchymal cells: Activation of secretion by endotoxin and concanavalin A. *Cell* 1981;25:603–615.

96. Leslie CC, Musson RA, Henson PM: Production of growth factor activity for fibroblasts by human monocyte-derived macrophages. *J Leukocyte Biol* 1984;36:143–159.

97. Martin BM, Gimbrone MA Jr, Majeau GR, et al: Stimulation of human monocyte/macrophage-derived growth factor (MDGF) production by plasma fibronectin. *Am J Pathol* 1983;111:367–373.

98. Schmidt JA, Mizel SB, Cohen D, et al: Interleukin-1, a potential regulator of fibroblast proliferation. *J Immunol* 1982;128:2177–2182.

99. Libby P, Wyler DJ, Janicka MW, et al: Differential effects of human interleukin-1 on growth of human fibroblasts and vascular smooth muscle cells. *Arteriosclerosis* 1985;5:186–191.

100. Barbul A: Role of T cell-dependent immune system in wound healing, in Barbul A, Pines E, Caldwell M, et al (eds): *Growth Factors and Other Aspects of Wound Healing: Biological and Clinical Implications.* New York, Alan R. Liss, 1988.

101. Reddi AH, Cunningham NS: Bone induction by osteogenin and bone morphogenetic proteins. *Biomaterials* 1990;11:33–34.

102. Seyedin SM: Osteoinduction: A report on the discovery and research of unique protein growth factors mediating bone development. *Oral Surg Oral Med Oral Pathol* 1989;68:527–530.

103. Nogami H, Ono Y, Oohira A: Bioassay of chondrocyte differentiation by bone morphogenetic protein. *Clin Orthop* 1990;258:295–299.

104. Kubler N, Urist MR: Bone morphogenetic protein-mediated interaction of periosteum and diaphysis. Citric acid and other factors influencing the generation of periosteal bone. *Clin Orthop* 1990;258:279–294.

105. Johnson EE, Urist MR, Finerman GA: Distal metaphyseal tibial nonunion. Deformity and bone loss treated by open reduction, internal fixation, and human bone morphogenetic protein (LBMP). *Clin Orthop* 1990;250:234–240.

106. Johnson EE, Urist MR, Finerman GA: Repair of segmental defects of the tibia with cancellous bone grafts augmented with human bone morphogenetic protein: A preliminary report. *Clin Orthop* 1988;236:249–257.

107. Ragni PC, Lindholm TS: Bone formation and static changes in the thoracic spine at uni- or bilateral experimental spondylodesis with demineralized bone matrix (DBM). *Ital J Orthop Traumatol* 1989;15:237–252.

108. Nakahara H, Takaoka K, Koezuka M, et al: Periosteal bone formation elicited by partially purified bone morphogenetic protein. *Clin Orthop* 1989;239:299–305.

109. Kawamura M, Urist MR: Growth factors, mitogens, cytokines and bone morphogenetic protein in induced chondrogenesis in tissue culture. *Dev Biol* 1988;130:435–442.

110. Mahy PR, Urist MR: Experimental heterotopic bone formation induced by bone morphogenetic protein and recombinant human interleukin-1 B. *Clin Orthop* 1988;237:236–244.

111. Metcalf D: The induction and inhibition of differentiation in normal and leukaemic cells. *Philos Trans R Soc Lond [Biol]* 1990;327:99–109.

112. Gutterman J, Vadhan-Raj S, Logothetis C, et al: Effects of granulocyte-macrophage colony-stimulating factor in iatrogenic myelosuppression, bone marrow failure, and regulation of host defense. *Semin Hematol* 1990;27(suppl):15–24.

113. Griffin JD, Cannistra SA, Sullivan R, et al: The biology of GM-CSF: Regulation of production and interaction with its receptor. *Int J Cell Cloning* 1990;8(suppl 1):35–45.

114. Gasson JC, Fraser JK, Nimer SD: Human granulocyte-macrophage colony-stimulating factor (GM-CSF): Regulation of expression. *Prog Clin Biol Res* 1990;338:27–41.

115. Gasson JC, Baldwin GC, Sakamoto KM, et al: The biology of human granulocyte-macrophage colony-stimulating factor (GM-CSF). *Prog Clin Biol Res* 1990;352:375–384.

116. Horowitz M, Einhorn E: Effect of Endotoxin (LPS) on bone allograft incorporation, bone cell function and fracture repair. Presented at the Workshop of the American Academy of Orthopaedic Surgeons and National Institute of Arthritis and Musculoskeletal and Skin Diseases on Musculoskeletal Infection, Dallas-Fort Worth, TX, Nov 9, 1990.

117. Drings P, Fischer JR: Biology and clinical use of GM-CSF in lung cancer. *Lung* 1990;168(suppl):1059–1068.

118. Scadden DT: Granulocyte macrophage colony stimulating factor (GM-CSF) in AIDS. *Prog Clin Biol Res* 1990;338:163–176.

119. Ruef C, Coleman DL: Granulocyte-macrophage colony-stimulating factor: Pleiotropic cytokine with potential clinical usefulness. *Rev Infect Dis* 1990;12(1):41–62.

Chapter 22

The Role of Oxygen in Wound Repair and Wound Infection

Harriet Williams Hopf, MD
Thomas K. Hunt, MD

Introduction

The prevention of postoperative wound infections, including osteomyelitis, is the focus of a great deal of attention perioperatively. Careful preparation of the skin (both the patient's and the surgeon's) with bactericidal agents, rigorous attention to maintenance of sterile technique, minimizing tissue damage intraoperatively, prophylactic antibiotics, and appropriate dressing of the wound have all been shown to decrease the rate of wound infections. Nonetheless, infections remain a major cause of prolonged hospitalization, morbidity, and increased cost for orthopaedic patients. If wound infections are to be eradicated, other approaches must be added. It is now clear that oxygen is crucial for appropriate healing without infection, and we are currently investigating methods of improving oxygen delivery to wounded tissues.

Wounds that do not heal adequately are at increased risk for infection, and infection increases the likelihood of inadequate wound healing. Thus, any discussion of prevention of wound infections must include a discussion of methods of promoting wound healing.

This chapter reviews the basic mechanisms of wound repair, with particular emphasis on the role of oxygen in resistance to infection and techniques that assess the adequacy of the oxygen supply to the wound. Although specific applications of these data and techniques to orthopaedic patients are currently limited, they offer promise for the future.

Oxygen and Wound Healing

Creation of a wound, whether by surgical incision or trauma, disrupts the local vascular supply. The ensuing cascade of events (Fig. 1) causes polymorphonuclear leukocytes, lymphocytes, and, later, macrophages and fibroblasts to migrate to the site of injury. The disrupted blood vessels thrombose back to the nearest perfused capillary loop,

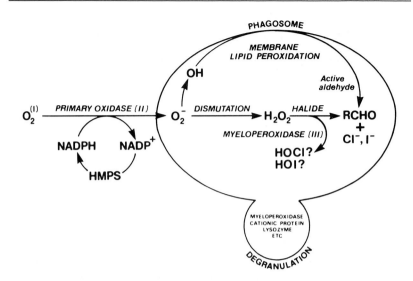

Fig. 1 *Schema of the oxidative bacteria-killing mechanism and its relationship to the non-oxidative mechanism. (Reproduced with permission from Hunt TK: Disorders of repair and their management, in Hunt TK, Dunphy JE (eds):* Fundamentals of Wound Management. *New York, Appleton-Century-Crofts, 1979, pp 68–168.)*

creating small areas of unperfused tissue 50 to 100 μ wide in subcutaneous tissue. The unperfused space becomes hypoxic (P_{O_2}, 0 to 30 torr), hypercarbic (P_{CO_2}, 50 to 80 torr), and acidotic (pH, 6.5 to 7.2) with lactate levels of as much as 15 mM. Although these conditions may interfere with host defenses and collagen deposition, macrophages in this hypoxic, high-lactate environment produce a factor that stimulates angiogenesis in adjacent, better-oxygenated tissue.[1-3] With progressive revascularization, oxygen tension in the wound increases.

Both in vitro and in vivo studies have shown that collagen hydroxylation, cross-linking, and deposition are proportional to P_{O_2}.[4-15] Goodson and Hunt[16] and Rabkin and associates[17] showed that wound healing can be assessed by measurement of collagen ingrowth into subcutaneously implanted expanded polytetrafluoroethylene tubes. Wound tensile strength is proportional to hydroxyproline deposition, a measure of collagen deposition, in rats (Wicke BC, Halliday B, Scheuenstul H, Foree B, Hunt TK, unpublished data). In animals, hydroxyproline deposition is proportion to arterial P_{O_2} (P_{aO_2}).[16] In surgical patients, hydroxyproline deposition in expanded polytetrafluoroethylene tubes left in place for seven days postoperatively is proportional to oxygen tension in subcutaneous tissues (P_{sqO_2}). This effect is evident even when P_{sqO_2} is higher than normal.[18]

Thus, with progressive revascularization of the subcutaneous tissue, oxygen tension in the wound increases, leading to greater collagen deposition by fibroblasts. When revascularization is inadequate or the newly formed vessels are constricted, hypoxia continues and wound healing cannot proceed normally.

Oxygen and Resistance to Infection

Host defenses against infection are also oxygen-dependent. Neutrophils are the first immune cell to appear in the wound. They gain access to the wound by demargination, diapedesis, and migration through connective tissue. Because neutrophils derive energy principally from anaerobic glycolysis, however, even severe hypoxia has little effect on migration and phagocytosis.[1-3]

Neutrophils kill phagocytosed bacteria in two ways. One, degranulation, is not oxygen-dependent. Phagocytosis of bacteria stimulates degranulation of leukocytic granules that contain bactericidal enzymes. The other, "oxidative killing," is oxygen-dependent. Neutrophils convert molecular oxygen to high-energy radicals (superoxide, hydroxyl radical, peroxides, aldehydes, hypochlorite, and hypoiodite), increasing oxygen consumption ten- to 20–fold. Oxidative killing is the primary mechanism by which those bacteria most commonly isolated from infected wounds are killed. These include *Staphylococcus aureus*, *Klebsiella*, *Proteus*, and *Serratia* organisms, and anaerobes.[19-23]

There is significant evidence linking oxygen and resistance to infection. Hohn[19] showed that the rate of killing of *S aureus* by neutrophils in vitro begins to decrease at an ambient Po_2 of about 30 torr and is reduced dramatically below 5 to 15 torr. Babior[24] measured an apparent K_m for oxygen of primary oxidase (which catalyzes superoxide production) of 8.5 torr. This allows the calculation that superoxide production by neutrophils is proportional to local oxygen tension between 0 and approximately 80 torr.

Oxygen tensions of less than 30 torr are common in wounds. Silver[25] demonstrated a steep Po_2 gradient in wound tissue. Near the wound capillary, oxygen tension in the tissue approaches that of arterial blood. Toward the healing edge of the wound, oxygen tension decreases, almost reaching 0 at 100 to 150 μ from the nearest functioning capillary. Hypovolemia causes vasoconstriction of the most distal capillaries, and the hypoxic area increases.

The importance of oxidative killing of certain bacteria (specifically those most often found in wound infections) is shown by comparing polymorphonuclear leukocytes in an anoxic environment with those from patients with chronic granulomatous disease, a genetic disorder in which the primary oxygenase is absent or deficient and oxygen radical production is seriously depressed. Normal neutrophils in an anoxic environment also cannot produce superoxide and kill bacteria at a rate equal to that of neutrophils from patients with chronic granulomatous disease.[19] In both cases, bacteria are killed only by degranulation. Bacteria that are most susceptible to oxidative killing frequently cause infections in patients with chronic granulomatous

SIZE OF SKIN LESION
AFTER INJECTION 10^7 E coli

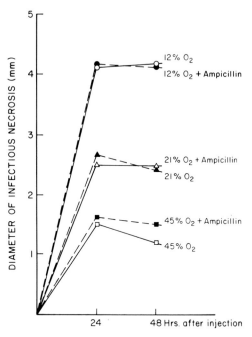

AMPICILLIN GIVEN 2 hr. POST INOCULATION

Fig. 2 *Effect of oxygen and/or antibiotic on lesion diameter after intradermal injection of bacteria into guinea pigs. (Reproduced with permission from Hunt TK, Knighton DR, Price DC, et al: Oxygen in the prevention and treatment of infection, in Root RK, Trunkey DD, Sande MA (eds):* New Surgical and Medical Approaches in Infectious Diseases. *New York, Churchill Livingstone, 1987, pp 1–16.)*

disease. Until the discovery of antibiotics, these patients died of infection during childhood.

In vivo studies have shown these findings to be of clinical importance. Knighton and associates[26] studied the development of lesions in guinea pig dermis after injection of *Escherichia coli*. When the guinea pigs were kept in an hypoxic environment (Fio_2, 0.12), the lesions all became necrotic. Addition of either ampicillin at the time of inoculation or supplemental oxygen even hours later decreased the number and size of necrotic lesions. The effects of oxygen and ampicillin are additive. An Fio_2 of 0.45 had almost the same effect as ampicillin (Fig. 2).

Gottrup and associates[27] and Chang and Mathews[28] created skin flaps in dogs in order to study the effect of local rather than systemic (inspired) oxygen tension. In these flaps, mean extracellular Po_2 ranged

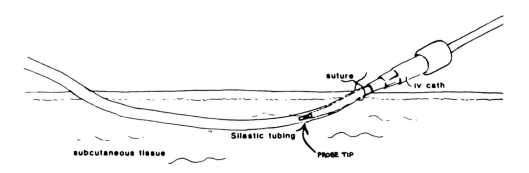

Fig. 3 *Schematic diagram of the subcutaneous oxygen tonometer. The fluorescent probe is inserted through the catheter hub.*

from 60 torr at the proximal end to 15 torr at the distal end. *S aureus* organisms were injected intradermally along the length of each flap. Invasive, necrotizing infections developed only in regions where tissue oxygen tension was less than about 40 torr at the time of injection. Varying Fio_2 and Pao_2 levels led to changes in infectability only as a reflection of changes in local Po_2.

Measurement of Subcutaneous Wound Tissue Oxygen Tension ($Psqo_2$)

In general, an adequate Po_2 in the healing tissue prevents infection and allows normal collagen deposition. In order to measure $Psqo_2$ in humans to verify the clinical importance of these data, Hunt and associates[29-33] developed a subcutaneously implanted tonometer (Fig. 3). When saline is placed within the tubing, the Po_2 of the saline equilibrates with that of the surrounding tissue. Measuring Po_2 within the tonometer yields a value for mean subcutaneous Po_2.

Oxygen measurements were originally made with a Clark electrode placed within the tonometer. The present measuring device employs a fluorescent probe. Fluorescence of the indicator is decreased in direct proportion to the concentration of oxygen. Because the reaction is temperature-dependent, temperature is measured at the tip of the probe.

This technique for measuring $Psqo_2$ verified the clinical importance of local tissue oxygen tension. In a recently completed study of 127 patients undergoing general surgery, largely through abdominal wounds (T.K. Hunt, unpublished data), $Psqo_2$ was measured on post-operative days 0, 1, and 2 while the patient breathed first room air and then 60% oxygen by face mask. The $Psqo_2$max (Po_2 at $Fio_2 = 0.6$ averaged over the three days of the study) was calculated for each patient. Mean $Psqo_2max$ for all subjects was 71 ± 19 torr. Only two of 56 patients (3.6%) with $Psqo_2max$ levels above 71 torr had wound infections, whereas wound infections developed in 15 of 71 patients (21%) with values below 71 torr. Length of operation, presence of significant systemic illness (three or more discharge diagnoses), site of operation (abdomen versus other), and degree of contamination of the wound—all equal risk factors according to the Study on the Effect of Nosocomial Infection Control (SENIC), which included 120,000 patients[34]—correlated with $Psqo_2max$. The $Psqo_2$, however, predicts wound infection regardless of preoperatively determined risk. "Low-risk" patients with low $Psqo_2$ values are at high risk for wound infection, whereas "high-risk" patients with high $Psqo_2$ values are at low risk.

The two patients in our study with $Psqo_2max$ values above 71 torr in whom wound infections developed had multiple severe risk factors for infection, including morbid obesity, malnutrition, contaminated wounds, and the need for postoperative ventilation. Apparently, then, a $Psqo_2$ value above 70 torr protects against wound infection but can be overwhelmed by other factors. Oxygen tension, however, seems to be the most important factor yet identified.

Peripheral Perfusion

The above data indicate that maintenance of an adequate $Psqo_2$ is crucial to healing without infection. Indeed, a supranormal $Psqo_2$ value is probably also beneficial, and may be an appropriate postoperative goal.

In fact, however, mean $Psqo_2max$ is lower in surgical patients (71 ± 19 torr) than in normal controls (117 ± 29 torr). A number of factors often present in the postoperative period have been shown to affect $Psqo_2$. Application of local heat over the tonometer significantly increases $Psqo_2$ in postoperative patients.[35] In normal volunteers, smoking causes a significant decrease in $Psqo_2$, from 65 ± 7 torr to 44 ± 3 torr, that lasts as long as an hour.[36] Infusion of epinephrine into normal volunteers causes a rapid and significant decrease in $Psqo_2$.[37] In some patients, breathing supplemental oxygen was not followed by an increase in $Psqo_2$.[31] In about one third of these patients, infusion of a fluid bolus did increase $Psqo_2max$, thereby implicating hypovolemia as a factor.

These observations led to the conclusion that $Psqo_2$ is determined largely by peripheral perfusion. When vasoconstriction is induced, $Psqo_2$ decreases; with vasodilation, $Psqo_2$ increases. The other major factors influencing $Psqo_2$ are arterial oxygen content and local oxygen consumption. The well-documented decrease in Pao_2 in postoperative patients[38–40] does not completely account for the decrease in $Psqo_2$, which must, therefore, result from peripheral vasoconstriction. The relative contribution of these two factors varies from patient to patient.

Using Fick's principle, a relative measure of subcutaneous perfusion

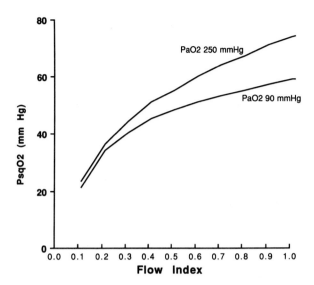

Fig. 4 *Calculated subcutaneous Po₂ for decreasing flow index for Pao₂ of 90 mmHg and 250 mmHg, assuming base excess to be 0 mEq/L, pH 7.40, and core temperature 37 C. (Adapted with permission from Hopf HW, Jensen JA, Hunt TK: Calculation of subcutaneous tissue blood flow.* Surg Forum 1988;39:33–36.)

(the flow index) can be calculated: FI = (F*subj* / F*nl*) = [Vsqo_2*subj* / (Cao_2 - Cvo_2*subj*) / Vsqo_2*nl* / (Cao_2 − Cvo_2*nl*)], where FI equals flow index; F*subj*, subcutaneous perfusion in the subject; F*nl*, normal subcutaneous perfusion; Vsqo_2, subcutaneous tissue oxygen consumption; Cao_2, subcutaneous arterial oxygen content; and Cvo_2, subcutaneous venous oxygen content (note that this is *not* mixed venous oxygen content—oxygen consumption by subcutaneous tissue is quite low). Because the subcutaneous tissue oxygen consumption is small (approximately 0.7 vol%[41]) and relatively constant for various Po_2 values, this equation can be simplified: flow index equals subcutaneous arterial oxygen content minus normal subcutaneous venous oxygen content divided by subcutaneous oxygen content minus the subject's subcutaneous venous oxygen content, or FI = (Cao_2 − Cvo_2*nl*) / (Cao_2 − Cvo_2*subj*). Gottrup and associates[27] extrapolated a relationship between $Psqo_2$ and subcutaneous Pvo_2: that is, subcutaneous Pvo_2 = $Psqo_2$ + 10 torr. Oxygen content therefore may be calculated from oxygen tension when hemoglobin, pH, and temperature are known.[42-45]

We have calculated that oxygen extraction by subcutaneous tissue (Cao_2 − Cvo_2) in normal volunteers is about 0.7 vol%.[42] Assuming that the flow index equals 1.0 for normal subjects, this agrees with measurements of subcutaneous tissue oxygen consumption by Evans and Naylor.[41] Theoretical curves generated from the flow index (Fig. 4) predict a rapid decrease in $Psqo_2$ as subcutaneous blood flow decreases to 50% or less of normal (flow index, 0.5). In actual practice, we have seen flow index values as high as 5 (marked vasodilation) and as low as 0.1 to 0.2 (severe vasoconstriction).

The postoperative decrease in $Psqo_2max$ represents a reduction in peripheral perfusion, with a flow index of about 0.7. Flow index in surgical patients may be as low as 0.1 to 0.2 with severe vasoconstriction, and rarely reaches 1.0, or normal flow. A number of factors—inadequate replacement of perioperative fluid losses, anxiety, pain, the stress of anesthesia and surgery, and cold—impair peripheral perfusion perioperatively. All these factors act through a common pathway, the sympathetic nervous system.[37,46,47] Stimulation of the sympathetic nervous system leads to catecholamine release and peripheral vasoconstriction.

The stress response, which is beneficial in the absence of medical care, seems to be counterproductive in the surgical setting. Interventions that prevent peripheral vasoconstriction should enhance $Psqo_2$ and, therefore, decrease the rate of wound complications. The effects of pain control (with epidural analgesia), intraoperative temperature maintenance, and pharmacologic sympathetic blockade on the rate of wound infections and complications are currently being investigated.

Application to Orthopaedic Patients

Although few studies on tissue oxygenation include orthopaedic patients, the data linking wound healing and resistance to infection with local tissue oxygen tension apply. Interventions that decrease wound complications in general surgery should work equally well in orthopaedic surgery.

There is further evidence that perfusion of bone is sacrificed early by the sympathetic nervous system. In one study of progressive, acute blood volume depletion (as much as 65% of initial volume) in dogs,[48] microspheres were used to measure blood flow to different organs. $Psqo_2$ was measured continuously. Although kidney perfusion was fairly well maintained until blood volume was reduced by 30% to 40%, subcutaneous perfusion diminished rapidly even when blood loss was less than 10%. Similarly, bone showed an early, rapid decrease in blood flow during hemorrhage, implying that bone is as susceptible as subcutaneous tissue to vasoconstriction and low oxygen tension, with the associated impaired host defenses and collagen deposition. Measurement of $Psqo_2$ in orthopaedic patients, therefore, may provide information on the adequacy of the oxygen supply not only to the incision but also to the injured bone.

Conclusion

The data linking wound tissue oxygen tension and appropriate healing without infection are very strong. The present challenge is to use these data to improve outcome in surgical patients. While data from general surgery patients on the benefits of sympathetic blockade, epidural analgesia, and temperature maintenance will certainly apply to orthopaedic patients, studies specifically in orthopaedic populations also should prove valuable. For example, the benefits of supplemental oxygen, including hyperbaric oxygen, are limited by the adequacy of local flow. Measurement of Psqo$_2$ in patients with osteomyelitis may allow assessment of the probability of benefit to each individual patient, and guide interventions aimed at improving perfusion. Studies are needed to determine the role of Psqo$_2$ monitoring in improving outcome in different subpopulations of orthopaedic patients. Finally, while Psqo$_2$ reflects adequacy of bone perfusion, techniques to measure bone tissue oxygen tension should be developed. The subcutaneous tonometer likely can be adapted for this use.

In sum, measurements of oxygen tension provide a promising means of decreasing still further the rate of wound infections and complications in orthopaedic patients. Further development of the technology, with modification for measurements in bone, should be pursued.

References

1. Knighton DR, Hunt TK: The defenses of the wound, in Howard RJ, Simmons RL (eds): *Surgical Infectious Diseases*, ed 2. Norwalk, CT, Appleton & Lange, 1988, pp 188–193.
2. Niinikoski J, Jussila P, Vihersaari T: Radical mastectomy wound as a model for studies of human wound metabolism. *Am J Surg* 1973;126:53–58.
3. Hunt TK: Physiology of wound healing, in Clowes GHA Jr (ed): *Trauma, Sepsis, and Shock: The Physiological Basis of Therapy*. New York, Marcel Dekker, 1988, pp 443–471.
4. Niinikoski J: Oxygen and wound healing. *Clin Plast Surg* 1977;4:361–374.
5. Chvapil M, Hurych J, Ehrlichová E: The influence of various oxygen tensions upon proline hydroxylation and the metabolism of collagenous and non-collagenous proteins in skin slices. *Hoppe Seyler Z Physiol Chem* 1968;349:211–217.
6. Hunt TK, Pai MP: The effect of varying ambient oxygen tensions on wound metabolism and collagen synthesis. *Surg Gynecol Obstet* 1972;135:561–567.
7. Kivisaari J, Vihersaari T, Renvall S, et al: Energy metabolism of experimental wounds at various oxygen environments. *Ann Surg* 1975;181:823–828.
8. Niinikoski J: Effect of oxygen supply on wound healing and formation of experimental granulation tissue. *Acta Physiol Scand* 1969;334(suppl):1–72.
9. Prockop D, Kaplan A, Udenfriend S: Oxygen-18 studies on the conversion of proline to hydroxyproline. *Biochem Biophys Res Commun* 1962;9:162–166.
10. Uitto J, Prockop DJ: Synthesis and secretion of under-hydroxylated procollagen at various temperatures by cells subject to temporary anoxia. *Biochem Biophys Res Commun* 1974;60:414–423.
11. Prockop DJ, Kivirikko KI, Tuderman L, et al: The biosynthesis of collagen and its disorders (first of two parts). *N Engl J Med* 1979;301:13–23.
12. Pietilä K, Jaakkola O: Effect of hypoxia on the synthesis of glycosaminoglycans and collagen by rabbit aortic smooth muscle cells in culture. *Atherosclerosis* 1984;50:183–190.

13. Knighton DR, Hunt TK, Scheuenstuhl H, et al: Oxygen tension regulates the expression of angiogenesis factor by macrophages. *Science* 1983;221;1283–1285.

14. Knighton DR, Silver IA, Hunt TK: Regulation of wound-healing angiogenesis: Effect of oxygen gradients and inspired oxygen concentration. *Surgery* 1981;90:262–270.

15. Forrester JC, Zederfeldt BH, Hayes TL, et al: Tape-closed and sutured wounds: A comparison by tensiometry and scanning electron microscopy. *Br J Surg* 1970;57:729–737.

16. Goodson WH III, Hunt TK: Development of a new miniature method for the study of wound healing in human subjects. *J Surg Res* 1982;33:394–401.

17. Rabkin JM, Hunt TK, von Smitten K, et al: Wound healing assessment by radioisotope incubation of tissue samples in PTFE tubes. *Surg Forum* 1986;37:592–594.

18. Jönsson K, Jensen JA, Goodson WH III, et al: Wound healing in subcutaneous tissue of surgical patients in relation to oxygen availability. *Surg Forum* 1986;37:86–88.

19. Hohn DC, MacKay RD, Halliday B, et al: Effect of O_2 tension on microbicidal function of leukocytes in wounds and in vitro. *Surg Forum* 1976;27:18–20.

20. Mandell GL: Bactericidal activity of aerobic and anaerobic polymorphonuclear neutrophils. *Infect Immun* 1974;9:337–341.

21. McRipley RJ, Sbarra AJ: Role of the phagocyte in host-parasite interactions: XII. Hydrogen peroxide-myeloperoxidase bactericidal system in the phagocyte. *J Bacteriol* 1967;94:1425–1430.

22. Selvaraj RJ, Sbarra AJ: Relationship of glycolytic and oxidative metabolism to particle entry and destruction in phagocytosing cells. *Nature* 1966;211:1272–1276.

23. Klebanoff SJ: Oxygen metabolism and the toxic properties of phagocytes. *Ann Intern Med* 1980;93:480–489.

24. Babior BM: Oxygen-dependent microbial killing by phagocytes (first of two parts). *N Engl J Med* 1978;298:659–668.

25. Silver IA: The measurement of oxygen tension in healing tissue. *Prog Resp Res* 1969;3:124–135.

26. Knighton DR, Halliday B, Hunt TK: Oxygen as an antibiotic: The effect of inspired oxygen on infection. *Arch Surg* 1984;119:199–204.

27. Gottrup F, Firmin R, Hunt TK, et al: The dynamic properties of tissue oxygen in healing flaps. *Surgery* 1984;95:527–536.

28. Chang N, Mathes SJ: Comparison of the effect of bacterial inoculation in musculocutaneous and random-pattern flaps. *Plast Reconstr Surg* 1982;70:1–10.

29. Niinikoski J, Heughan C, Hunt TK: Oxygen tensions in human wounds. *J Surg Res* 1972;12:77–82.

30. Niinikoski J, Hunt TK: Measurement of wound oxygen with implanted Silastic tube. *Surgery* 1972;71:22–26.

31. Chang N, Goodson WH III, Gottrup F, et al: Direct measurement of tissue oxygen tension in postoperative patients. *Surg Forum* 1982;33:52–54.

32. Hunt TK, Rabkin J, Jensen JA, et al: Tissue oximetry: An interim report. *World J Surg* 1987;11:126–132.

33. Gottrup F, Firmin R, Rabkin J, et al: Directly measured tissue oxygen tension and arterial oxygen tension assess tissue perfusion. *Crit Care Med* 1987;15:1030–1036.

34. Haley RW, Culver DH, Morgan WM, et al: Identifying patients at high risk of surgical wound infection: A simple multivariate index of patient susceptibility and wound contamination. *Am J Epidemiol* 1985;121:206–215.

35. Rabkin JM, Hunt TK: Local heat increases blood flow and oxygen tension in wounds. *Arch Surg* 1987;122:221–225.

36. Jensen JA, Goodson WH, Hopf HW, et al: Cigarette smoking decreases tissue oxygen. *Arch Surg* 1991, in press.

37. Jensen JA, Jonsson K, Goodson WH III, et al: Epinephrine lowers subcutaneous wound oxygen tension. *Curr Surg* 1985;42:472–474.

38. Craig DB: Postoperative recovery of pulmonary function. *Anesth Analg* 1981;60:46–52.

39. Ford GT, Whitelaw WA, Rosenal TW, et al: Diaphragm function after upper abdominal surgery in humans. *Am Rev Respir Dis* 1983;127:431–436.

40. Simonneau G, Vivien A, Sartene R, et al: Diaphragm dysfunction induced by upper abdominal surgery: Role of postoperative pain. *Am Rev Respir Dis* 1983;128:899–903.

41. Evans NTS, Naylor PFD: The dynamics of changes in dermal oxygen tension. *Resp Physiol* 1966;2:61–72.

42. Hopf HW, Jensen JA, Hunt TK: Calculation of subcutaneous tissue blood flow. *Surg Forum* 1988;39:33–36.

43. Kelman GR, Nunn JF: *Computer-Produced Physiological Tables for Calculations Involving the Relationships Between Blood Oxygen Tension and Content.* London, Butterworths, 1968.

44. Kelman GR: Digital computer subroutine for the conversion of oxygen tension into saturation. *J Appl Physiol* 1966;21:1375–1376.

45. Severinghaus JW: Simple, accurate equations for human blood O_2 dissociation computations. *J Appl Physiol* 1979;46:599–602.

46. Derbyshire DR, Smith G: Sympathoadrenal responses to anaesthesia and surgery. *Br J Anaesth* 1984;56:725–739.

47. Halter JB, Pflug AE, Porte D Jr: Mechanism of plasma catecholamine increases during surgical stress in man. *J Clin Endocrinol Metab* 1977;45:936–944.

48. Gosain A, Rabkin J, Reymond JP, et al: Tissue oxygen tension and other indicators of blood loss or organ perfusion during graded hemorrhage. *Surgery* 1991;109:523–532.

Chapter 23

Wound Repair and Nutrition

Harriet Williams Hopf, MD
Thomas K. Hunt, MD

Introduction

Preoperative or postoperative depletion of a variety of nutritional factors impairs host defenses and wound repair. Deficiencies of specific vitamins or minerals may lead to specific impairment of wound repair or host defenses. Some effects of this depletion are well-described, while others are less clear. Up to 50% of hospitalized patients may have significant protein or protein-calorie malnutrition. Moreover, trauma induces a catabolic state that may lead rapidly to protein-calorie malnutrition. Two populations of orthopaedic patients deserve particular attention in this regard: older patients undergoing hip procedures are likely to have chronic protein-calorie malnutrition, and multiply-injured trauma patients with long-bone fractures are at high risk of developing protein-calorie malnutrition.

The importance of nutritional repletion in general surgical patients is well established, although controversy remains about timing and ideal formulations. A direct link between protein-calorie malnutrition and impaired host defenses, with increased risk of wound infection, is less well-established but likely. Few studies have investigated the impact in orthopaedic patients of nutritional repletion or supplementation on bone repair, wound healing and infection, or outcome. Although much of the general surgical literature is probably applicable to orthopaedic patients, studies are needed to define the unique problems and ideal approaches in orthopaedic populations.

Role of Vitamins

Vitamin C Adequate vitamin C (ascorbic acid) is essential for normal healing; however, wound healing is impaired only after about six months of dietary vitamin C deficiency. Vitamin C is required for the hydroxylation of the amino acids proline and lysine during the postsynthetic modification of collagen. Inadequate dietary vitamin C leads to increased capillary permeability and fragility, with frequent rupture and hemorrhage. Formation of new capillaries is decreased or absent in the healing wound. These abnormalities reflect inadequate production of basement membrane collagen. Tensile strength of the wound is diminished because of inadequate collagen deposition, as well as deposition of abnormal collagen.[1,2]

Wound remodeling is a continuous process in which collagen lysis and deposition are in equilibrium. With vitamin C deficiency, collagen lysis proceeds normally, but collagen deposition is decreased. Thus, mature, well-healed wounds frequently break down in patients with scurvy.[3]

Normal, uninjured humans require about 20 to 30 mg of vitamin C daily to prevent the development of scurvy; however, daily vitamin C requirements are increased in the burned or trauma patient. After trauma, plasma levels of vitamin C fall immediately and in proportion to the severity of the injury. It is not clear whether this is a result of increased vitamin C metabolism, accumulation of vitamin C at the site of the injury, or both. Supplementation with vitamin C (100 to 2,000 mg/day, depending on the severity of the injury) prevents development of the changes seen with ascorbic acid deficiency.[1]

In addition, vitamin C evidently is required for the reduction of oxygen to superoxide.[1,2] The production of free radicals, including superoxide, is involved in "oxidative killing," an important mechanism by which neutrophils kill certain bacteria. Thus, vitamin C deficiency may also impair resistance to infection in wounded tissue.

B Vitamins Several B vitamins contribute to normal healing. Vitamin B_1 (thiamine) is a cofactor for lysyl oxidase, an enzyme that catalyzes the formation of lysine-lysine bonds, which increase the strength of collagen. Deficiency in vitamin B_1 can also decrease amounts of collagen, particularly type III.[3]

Vitamin B_5 (pantothenic acid) appears to play a role in cell replication. Deficiency of the vitamin impairs wound strength, and histological examination of wound sections in rats reveals a decreased density of fibroblasts.[3]

Open skin wounds heal abnormally in rats fed diets deficient in vitamin B_6 (pyridoxine) and vitamin B_2 (riboflavin) for five weeks before injury. The healing tissue shows increased vascularity and cellularity with decreased collagen matrix deposition. Biotin-deficient rats show similar changes but to a very mild degree.[1]

Fracture healing is abnormal in rats fed a diet deficient in vitamin B_6 for 21 days prior to injury. Deficiency of vitamin B_6 decreases periosteal glucose-6–phosphate dehydrogenase activity and appears to create an imbalance between osteoblastic and osteoclastic activity. Callus size and new bone production are significantly decreased. Some regions of the bone may appear osteoporotic.[4]

Megaloblastic anemia resulting from folate or vitamin B_{12} (cyanocobalamin) deficiency is not uncommon in surgical patients. Anemia, however, unless it is severe (hematocrit less than 17%), does not impair wound repair.[5] Severe anemia would be corrected perioperatively in any case.

Rats deficient in vitamin B_5, vitamin B_6, and folic acid produce fewer antibody-forming cells and, thus, less antibody in response to an antigenic stimulus. B vitamin deficiency may also impair bacterial killing.[1]

Traumatic injury and sepsis lead to a decrease in total body levels of the B vitamins, particularly B_1, B_2, and nicotinamide.[1] Therefore, it is recommended that severely injured patients receive 5 to 10 times the usual daily requirement of B vitamins.

Vitamin A   Although the mechanisms are poorly understood, vitamin A clearly plays a significant role in wound healing. Known processes in which vitamin A is required include: epithelial growth, synthesis of glycoproteins and proteoglycans, labilizing lysosomal membranes, cellular immunity, reproduction, and vision.[1] The inflammatory response is dependent on the presence of adequate vitamin A. Vitamin A also opposes the anti-inflammatory effects of steroids, and can correct wound healing impairment in patients receiving long-term steroid therapy.[1-3]

In vitamin A-deficient animals, epithelization, collagen synthesis, wound contraction, prolyl hydroxylase activity, and collagen cross-linking are all impaired. In humans, isolated vitamin A deficiency is uncommon. It is associated with epithelial metaplasia, increased infection, delayed wound healing, and diminished stress tolerance.[1]

Vitamin A may become depleted during prolonged stress or infection as a result of increased urinary excretion. Large doses of corticosteroids also rapidly deplete liver stores of vitamin A. Daily supplementation with 25,000 international units (IU) of vitamin A (five times the recommended daily dose) should be adequate to avoid impaired wound healing even in severely injured or ill patients.[1,3]

In orthopaedic patients, vitamin A may accelerate fracture healing. It has been shown to promote cell proliferation and matrix formation. Vitamin A deficiency causes thinning of cortical bone, increasing the risk of fracture.[6]

Prolonged large doses of vitamin A (over 50,000 IU/day) can be toxic. Symptoms of vitamin A toxicity include excessive inflammatory response, visual disturbances, coma, and pseudotumor cerebri.[1,3]

Vitamin D   Vitamin D plays an essential part in regulating calcium metabolism and, therefore, is critical in fracture repair. Vitamin D is first converted to 25–hydroxycholecalciferol in the liver, and then to the active form, 1,25–dihydroxycholecalciferol, in the kidney. The active form is required for synthesis of the protein that binds and then transfers calcium and phosphorus from intestinal epithelial cells to the portal circulation. Vitamin D helps regulate urinary excretion of calcium and phosphorus and promotes calcium mobilization from bone by increasing citrate production.[1,3,6]

In vitamin D-deficient patients, fractures heal poorly. Repletion of vitamin D may return fracture repair to normal. Trauma patients should receive one to two times the recommended daily dose (400 IU) to prevent depletion as a result of increased loss.[1]

Patients receiving phenytoin are susceptible to osteomalacia and fractures. Administration of vitamin D and calcium may prevent these complications of anticonvulsant therapy.[1]

Vitamin E   Vitamin E stabilizes membranes. There are few studies of its role in wound healing, but these indicate that vitamin E retards fibrosis and healing. The anti-inflammatory properties of vitamin E, which are similar to those of steroids, may stem in part from stabilization of macrophage membranes.[1-3] Vitamin E also has antioxidant properties, which may in fact decrease damage to the wound induced by oxygen radicals released by leukocytes.[3]

Vitamin K   Vitamin K is required for the post-translational carboxylation of glutamate in factors II, VII, IX, and X. Vitamin K deficiency leads to deficient coagulation, which may impair wound healing, as wound hematomas predispose to infection and poor tissue repair.[1,3]

More recent evidence indicates that vitamin K may also be required for bone repair. Osteocalcin, a vitamin K dependent, calcium-binding protein synthesized by osteoblasts, is chemotactic for osteoclast precursors and monocytes and, thus, appears to be involved in bone remodeling. Some studies have demonstrated impaired histologic fracture healing in dicoumarol-treated rats. Einhorn and associates[7] found no difference in mechanical or histologic measurements in rats fed a vitamin K-deficient diet. The effects of chronic vitamin K deficiency (dietary or warfarin induced) have not been evaluated.

Role of Minerals

Macrominerals   Because calcium is one of the main components of bone, its metabolism and maintenance are clearly crucial in wound healing. During early fracture-healing, however, dietary calcium is less important than mobilization of calcium from other bones. Callus formation progresses normally even in the presence of calcium deficiency. Later stages of bone healing and ultimate mechanical strength are more susceptible to dietary insufficiency when bones' stores are no longer being mobilized for calcium.[8]

Magnesium is essential for wound repair, because it is a cofactor for a large number of the enzymes involved in protein synthesis.[1] Magnesium deficiency, which is usually related to alcoholism and malabsorption, induces depression, muscular weakness, dizziness, potential seizures, and metabolic acidosis.[1]

Trace Minerals   Copper, manganese, and zinc are also essential cofactors for many enzymes involved in protein synthesis. Copper, for example, is required for the function of lysyl oxidase, clearly an important enzyme for wound repair.[1,3] Manganese is a cofactor for superoxide dismutase; therefore, bacterial killing may be impaired by a deficiency of this mineral.[1]

Zinc is a cofactor for RNA and DNA polymerase. Inadequate serum zinc (<100 μg/100 ml) is associated with poor wound healing and impaired immune function. Repletion to normal levels returns the healing to normal but excess zinc does not improve wound healing beyond normal. Serum and total body zinc levels may decrease rapidly after trauma.[1-3] Long-term steroid therapy will decrease serum zinc levels. Patients who are receiving steroids and have impaired wound healing should receive both supplemental vitamin A and zinc to restore healing.[3]

Inadequate iron (Fe^{2+}) impairs collagen deposition and wound healing, because iron is required for the hydroxylation of proline and lysine. This effect is most marked in immature animals. Iron deficiency is quite common and may result from prolonged or severe blood loss, infection, or inadequate dietary intake. Iron deficiency is easily detected and treated. Treatment should be aggressive.[1,6]

Molybdenum, cobalt, chromium, selenium, vanadium, and tin are all essential, although at very low levels. The role of these elements in wound healing is largely unknown. Because selenium, acting with vitamin E, stabilizes membranes, excessive replacement of selenium may impair wound healing.[1]

Protein-Calorie Malnutrition

Malnutrition, whether chronic or acute, impairs wound healing and host defenses. Vitamin and mineral deficits seldom occur in surgical patients in the absence of protein-calorie malnutrition. Correction of deficits before surgery and maintenance of adequate nutrition (enterally or parenterally) afterwards may prevent complications or reduce their severity. Adequate and timely assessment of nutritional status is, therefore, critical in surgical and trauma patients.

Normal Metabolism   Energy requirements in humans are met by the metabolism of carbohydrates, proteins, and fats. Carbohydrates and proteins provide about 4 kcal/g; fats provide about 9 kcal/g.[9]

Carbohydrates are stored mainly in the liver and muscle as glycogen. These stores are sufficient to supply basal calorie requirements for less than one day. Even during starvation, however, glycogen stores remain largely intact because most tissues preferentially use fat and protein. Only the brain, red blood cells, and leukocytes are glycogen dependent.[9,10] In hypoxic areas, such as the leading edge of a wound or a fracture site, anaerobic metabolism requires glucose as a substrate.[11]

Body protein makes up a large potential energy source that can be converted to glucose in the liver through gluconeogenesis. All proteins in the body, however, serve a function. Therefore, metabolism of protein to glucose leads to a negative nitrogen balance, with the loss of muscle, plasma proteins, and enzymes. Structural proteins, such as tendon and bone, however, are relatively spared.[9,10]

Excess protein in the diet is converted to fat for storage. Under normal circumstances, the majority of calories are supplied by fat metabolism. After several days of starvation, the brain begins to use ketones (derived from fat) as an alternate energy source.[9,10]

Protein-calorie malnutrition, with its resultant loss of essential proteins, leads to inadequate wound and fracture healing and impaired host defenses. Protein depletion appears to affect cellular more than humoral immunity. Thus, malnourished patients show decreased T-cell numbers, decreased response to mitogen stimulation, and loss of delayed hypersensitivity reactions. Phagocytic cell function and complement levels may also be impaired.[12,13]

Prevalence of Malnutrition Surgery, trauma, and infection result in a catabolic state with a negative nitrogen balance. Glucagon, glucocorticoid, and catecholamine levels remain elevated, while insulin levels remain depressed. In the presence of this ongoing stress response, the administration of glucose does not prevent protein catabolism as it does in pure starvation. The degree of catabolism is proportional to the severity of injury. Long bone fractures induce a 20% to 30% increase in basal energy expenditure, multiple trauma and sepsis a 50% to 80% increase, and extensive thermal injury up to a 100% to 150% increase.[9,11] In patients who are unable to take in adequate protein and calories to meet the increased demand, the negative nitrogen balance will increase and be prolonged. Even provision of maximal enteral or parenteral nutrition cannot restore an anabolic state until physiologic stresses and the resultant high levels of stress hormones resolve.[14]

A significant proportion of elective surgery patients have long-standing malnutrition resulting from chronically reduced intake. Warnold and Lundholm[15] found evidence of preoperative malnutrition in 12% of 215 Swedish noncancer patients. About 50% of both medical and surgical patients at an urban Boston hospital showed evidence of malnutrition.[16] Muller and associates[14] found severe malnutrition in 12% of German patients scheduled for major gastrointestinal surgery. In a New Zealand hospital, 43% of inpatients awaiting surgery had evidence of impaired nutrition, although malnutrition was evident in only 5% of patients scheduled for routine elective surgery.[10] In a study of 129 orthopaedic patients in Houston, 42% showed evidence of malnutrition. These included 29% of patients presenting for total hip arthroplasty and 57% of multiple trauma patients five days postinjury.[11]

Effects of Malnutrition on Outcome Interventions to improve the nutritional status of surgical patients are indicated only if they clearly improve outcome in these patients. The identification of predictive markers that are easily and inexpensively measured in a clinical setting is crucial. Hill and associates[10] measured total body water, total body protein, and total body fat using tritiated water dilution and in vivo neutron activation analysis. Their results have uncovered inaccuracies in several commonly used markers for malnutrition. Total body water increases (as extracellular fluid accumulates) at about the same rate that total body protein decreases. Thus, measurements of weight loss may be misleading in acute malnutrition. Anthropometric measurements (eg, triceps skin fold) underestimate total body fat by about 19%. Changes in total body water with ongoing nutritional depletion also render anthropometric measurements inadequate.

Although their use in total body analysis provides accurate and precise information, tritiated water dilution and in vivo neutron activation analysis are not widely available. Other assessments that have been used as predictive markers include weight loss and weight as a percentage of ideal body weight, anthropometric measurements, creatinine/height index, serum proteins including albumin and transferrin, total iron-binding capacity, total lymphocyte count, tests of anergy/delayed hypersensitivity, and urinary nitrogen measurements for estimates of nitrogen balance. Of these, serum albumin and total lymphocyte count appear to be the most useful.[10,11,15,17-25] Serum albumin and total lymphocyte count are also markers for sepsis or infection; however, unrecognized infection will impair wound healing even in the absence of malnutrition,[20] and, in any case, infection will likely induce a catabolic state.

Pettigrew and Hill[20] evaluated the adequacy of nutritional assessment in 218 patients scheduled for abdominal surgery. Anthropometric measurements did not identify a subset of patients at high risk of complications. "Global assessment" by the surgeon also did not accurately identify a subset of high-risk patients. On the other hand, 33% of patients with a serum albumin lower than 3.3 g/dL developed major complications. Moreover, a careful history (including dietary history) and physical examination identified 17% of the patients as "high risk." Of these, 32% developed major complications.

In a study of 263 surgical patients at a suburban New Jersey hospital, a 4.6–fold increase in complications occurred in patients with a serum albumin lower than 3.5 g/dL.[18] In a study of patients undergoing abdominal surgery, complications occurred in 31% and death in 39% of those with serum albumin lower than 3.5 g/dL and total lymphocyte count lower than 1500/µL. Complications occurred in 40% and death in 20% of patients with decreased total lymphocyte count alone. Complications occurred in 21% and death in 7% of patients with decreased serum albumin alone. When patients' albumin was lower than 2.8 g/dL, complications occurred in 55% and death in 55%.[26] Among orthopaedic patients, complications developed in 37% with decreased serum albumin and/or total lymphocyte count. Seventy-two percent of multiple trauma patients with low serum albumin developed complications. Of the patients in this study who developed a complication, 59% had a low serum albumin and/or total lymphocyte count.[11] Among 23 patients undergoing a Syme amputation, all of whom met Wagner's criteria, the wound healed in six out of seven who had a normal serum albumin and total lymphocyte count and one out of one who had a low total lymphocyte count. However, the wound healed in only one out of four with a low serum albumin and two out of 11 with both a low total lymphocyte count and a low serum albumin.[23]

Although more than 10% weight loss is frequently cited as increasing the risk of postoperative complications,[15] Windsor and Hill[21] found weight loss to be predictive of increased complications only if it was associated with clear physical impairment, such as fatigue, weakness, shortness of breath, mood changes, unhealed or infected wounds, and/ or serum albumin lower than 3.2 g/dL. In patients with more than 10% weight loss without physical impairment, total body protein and fat were no different than in controls, but were significantly diminished in patients with impairment.

Nitrogen balance may also be an inappropriate marker for adequacy of nutritional replacement. In a study comparing two TPN formulations in rats, Barbul and associates[27] found that rats in the group with more negative nitrogen balance in fact showed improvement in wound healing and immune function variables.

Efficacy of Perioperative Nutritional Support

Clearly, perioperative malnutrition impairs wound healing and resistance to infection. There is no evidence, however, that nutritional support in excess of calculated requirements is beneficial. In malnourished dogs, decreased serum IgG and complement, total lymphocyte count, and neutrophil chemotaxis all correct with nutritional repletion.[28] Early postoperative TPN in previously normally nourished rats leads to weight gain, improved wound tensile strength, and increased anastomotic bursting pressure.[25] Fracture-healing is impaired in rats fed diets deficient in either protein or mineral postoperatively; however, diets containing protein or minerals in excess of calculated requirements do not affect fracture-healing.[8]

Nutritional support, whether enteral or parenteral, however, is not without risk. Aspiration and diarrhea are common with feeding tubes, and central line placement may be complicated by pneumothorax, hemothorax, subclavian vein thrombosis, and catheter sepsis.[10] The decision to implement perioperative nutritional supplementation or repletion, therefore, requires the surgeon to weigh the benefits (improved healing and resistance to infection) against the risks. Careful outcome studies of different methods of nutritional repletion are required to allow for informed decisions. There is strong and growing evidence that nutritional repletion reduces surgical complications, at least in certain populations of patients. The data are somewhat conflicting, and further studies are clearly needed.

In 167 malnourished patients scheduled for surgery for gastrointestinal cancer, ten days of preoperative total parenteral nutrition (TPN) with glucose and protein resulted in a 2–kg weight gain, improvement in serum protein levels and measures of immunocompetence, and a reduction in wound complications and mortality when compared with patients who received a regular hospital diet for ten days.[14] The severity, but not the incidence, of infectious complications was decreased. Patients who received 50% of their nonprotein calories as lipid had a significantly higher mortality than either of the other groups, and this arm of the study was discontinued early on. The reasons for this increase in mortality are unclear.

In a cooperative Veterans Administration (VA) study, patients received either seven to 15 days of preoperative TPN and at least three days of postoperative TPN, or no TPN until at least three days after surgery. All patients who received TPN had an increased risk of infection (including pneumonia and wound infections). In patients with mild malnutrition, there was no decrease in noninfectious complications. In patients with moderate malnutrition, there was a decrease in noninfectious complications (generally wound complications), but this was offset by the increase in infectious complications. In severely malnourished patients, the significant decrease in wound complications was much greater than the slight increase in infectious complications.[29]

TPN administered for at least seven days preoperatively in 50 of 145 severely malnourished surgical patients decreased the incidence of complications 59%, of sepsis 60%, and of death 81%.[24] Of 70 patients with gastric carcinoma in a randomized study, those who received seven to ten days of preoperative TPN had a significantly lower rate of wound infection.[30] In 26 patients with gastric carcinoma with a weight loss of more than 10 lbs, there was no difference in complication rate between those who received 48 hours of preoperative and ten days of postoperative TPN and those who received no TPN.[31]

Haydock and Hill[19,32] evaluated wound healing in 36 normally nourished, 21 mildly malnourished, and nine moderately malnourished surgical patients by measuring hydroxyproline (collagen) deposition in subcutaneously implanted expanded polytetrafluoroethylene (ePTFE) tubes. They found that even in mildly malnourished patients, or patients in whom inadequate dietary intake was of short duration, hydroxyproline content was about half of normal.[19] Collagen deposition was increased in 47 malnourished patients after only one week of TPN, even in the absence of improvement in serum malnutrition.[30]

In a more recent study by the same group, immediate postoperative total enteral nutrition (TEN) was evaluated in 32 general surgery patients without existing malnutrition. They found that hydroxyproline deposition in ePTFE tubes was significantly greater in the enterally fed than in the control patients, who received only 5% dextrose solutions intravenously until clinically able to tolerate oral intake.[33]

There is growing evidence that enteral nutrition is superior to parenteral nutrition. In a study of immediate (12–18 hours postinjury) TEN in major abdominal trauma patients, Moore and associates found a 69% decrease in septic complications.[34] In a followup study comparing TEN with TPN, there were 117% more infectious complications and 600% more major septic complications (abdominal abscess, pneumonia) in the TPN than the TEN group.[35] Infection rates in the TEN groups were similar in the two studies.

Guidelines for Nutritional Therapy

The data on the efficacy of perioperative nutritional support are somewhat conflicting. Parenteral nutrition is indicated only when the risks of that support are less than the risk inherent in the patient's nutritional state. Enteral nutrition is preferable to parenteral if feasible, because it maintains gut integrity and may decrease bacterial translocation.[36] In patients with severe malnutrition who are scheduled for major surgery, delay of surgery for TPN is probably indicated. The length of delay is again controversial, but probably should be at least seven to ten days. With mild or moderate malnutrition, delay for TPN is probably contraindicated. However, postoperative nutritional support should be considered, particularly if the patient may remain without oral intake for a prolonged period.

In patients in whom surgery is delayed for other reasons, TPN should be instituted if severe malnutrition exists. If mild to moderate malnutrition is present and the patient is expected to be without oral intake or to receive limited calories for five to seven days, TPN should be initiated early. Three liters of 5% dextrose supplies only 600 calories, so patients undergoing multiple tests for which they remain without oral intake for much of the day may in effect be starved.[10,22,32]

Nutritional support should be started early in trauma patients who are expected not to take adequate oral nutrition for three to four days. These patients are stressed and, thus, will progress to significant protein depletion more rapidly than other patients.[32]

The ideal formulation for TPN remains controversial. In general, it is recommended that patients receive 1.5 to 3 g protein/kg/day. There is some evidence, however, that low-protein diets may improve survival in sepsis.[37,38] There is also evidence for the use of specific amino acids. For example, branched-chain amino acids may slow muscle protein catabolism. Glutamine may help maintain gut mucosal function and integrity.[13]

Arginine has many beneficial effects, including decreasing urinary nitrogen excretion, enhancing collagen synthesis, increasing total lymphocyte count, and enhancing T-cell function.[39] Arginine-deficient rats show impaired wound strength and collagen deposition, while arginine supplementation improves these variables even in the absence of preexisting arginine deficiency.[40] Oral arginine supplementation improved collagen deposition in ePTFE tubes implanted subcutaneously in nonoperated normal volunteers.[41,42] Lymphocyte function was also improved in these subjects. The beneficial effects of arginine probably stem in part from its nutritional role as a precursor for proline. Arginine is also a secretagogue for both growth hormone and somatomedin, which may mediate its effects on wound healing.[43]

Total calories should be about 30 to 40 kcal/kg/day.[1,10,14,22,29] In recent years, recommendations are for fewer calories than in the past. Measurement or estimation of basal energy expenditure can help guide caloric content. The increase in basal energy expenditure with fever, trauma, sepsis, and other states must be taken into account.

The relative contribution of lipids to caloric content is also controversial. There is some evidence that excess lipids may be detrimental.[14] Limiting lipid administration to one to two days a week is probably advisable.

Conclusion

Many orthopaedic and trauma patients are at high risk of developing protein-calorie malnutrition, potentially in association with one or more vitamin or mineral deficiencies. While it is clear that appropriate nutritional support will benefit the malnourished patient, it is not yet clear what is the ideal treatment for malnutrition in the surgical setting. The best protocols for repleting patients are being sought in general surgery. However, little has been done to apply these concepts to orthopaedic patients. Elucidation of the roles of vitamin D, calcium, and phosphorus in normal metabolism requires further study, particularly given the enormous role of these factors in bone healing. Further investigation into the optimal replacement of these factors during trauma, sepsis, and operation is needed. Finally, development of techniques that rapidly, accurately, and inexpensively assess nutritional status is crucial for providing guidelines for therapy.

References

1. Levenson SM, Seifter E, Van Winkle W: *Fundamentals of wound management in surgery: Nutrition.* New Jersey, Chirurgecom, Inc, 1977.
2. Orgill D, Demling RH: Current concepts and approaches to wound healing. *Crit Care Med* 1988;16:899–908.
3. Goodson WH III, Hunt TK: Wound healing and nutrition, in Kinney JM, Jeejeebhoy KN, Kill GL, et al (eds): *Nutrition and Metabolism in Patient Care.* Philadelphia, WB Saunders, 1988, pp 635–642.
4. Dodds RA, Catterall A, Bitensky A, et al: Abnormalities in fracture healing induced by vitamin B6–deficiency in rats. *Bone* 1986;7:489–495.
5. Hunt TK, Rabkin J, von Smitten K: Effects of edema and anemia on wound healing and infection. *Curr Stud Hematol Blood Transfus* 1986;53:101–111.
6. Heppenstall RB: Fracture and Cartilage Repair, in Deveney CW, Dunphy JE, Heppenstall RB, et al (eds): *Fundamentals of Wound Management in Surgery: Selected Tissues.* New Jersey, Chirurgecom, Inc, 1977, pp 1–35.
7. Einhorn TA, Gundberg CM, Devlin VJ, et al: Fracture healing and osteocalcin metabolism in vitamin K deficiency. *Clin Orthop* 1988;237:219–223.
8. Einhorn TA, Bonnarens F, Burstein AH: The contributions of dietary protein and mineral to the healing of experimental fractures: A biomechanical study. *J Bone Joint Surg* 1986;68A:1389–1395.
9. Schwartz SI (ed): *Principles of Surgery.* New York, McGraw-Hill, 1984, pp 68–78.
10. Streat SJ, Hill GL: Nutritional support in the management of critically ill patients in surgical intensive care. *World J Surg* 1987;11:194–201.
11. Jensen JE, Jensen TG, Smith TK, et al: Nutrition in orthopaedic surgery. *J Bone Joint Surg* 1982;64A:1263–1272.
12. Christou N: Perioperative nutritional support: Immunologic defects. *JPEN* 1990;14:186S-192S.
13. Daly JM, Reynold J, Sigal RK, et al: Effect of dietary protein and amino acids on immune function. *Crit Care Med* 1990;18:S86–S93.
14. Muller JM, Keller HW, Brenner J, et al: Indications and effects of preoperative parenteral nutrition. *World J Surg* 1986;10:53–63.
15. Warnold I, Lundholm K: Clinical significance of preoperative nutritional status in 215 noncancer patients. *Ann Surg* 1984;199:299–305.

16. Bistrian BR, Blackburn GL, Hallowell E, et al: Protein status of general surgical patients. *JAMA* 1974;230:858–860;

17. Blackburn GL, Bistrian BR, Maini BS, et al: Nutritional and metabolic assessment of the hospitalized patient. *JPEN* 1977;1:11–22.

18. Seltzer MH, Bastidas JA, Cooper DM, et al: Instant nutritional assessment. *JPEN* 1979;3:157–159.

19. Haydock DA, Hill GL: Impaired wound healing in surgical patients with varying degrees of malnutrition. *JPEN* 1986;10:550–554.

20. Pettigrew RA, Hill GL: Indicators of surgical risk and clinical judgement. *Br J Surg* 1988;73:47–51.

21. Windsor JA, Hill GL: Weight loss with physiologic impairment. *Ann Surg* 1988;207:209–296.

22. Smith TK: Prevention of complications in orthopedic surgery secondary to nutritional depletion. *Clin Orthop* 1987;222:91–97.

23. Dickhaut SC, DeLee JC, Page CP: Nutritional Status: Importance in predicting wound-healing after amputation. *J Bone Joint Surg* 1984;66A:71–75.

24. Mullen JL, Buzby GP, Matthews DC, et al: Reduction of operative morbidity and mortality by combined preoperative and postoperative nutritional support. *Ann Surg* 1980;192:604–613.

25. Delany HM, Demetriou AA, Teh E, et al: Effect of early postoperative nutritional support on skin wound and colon anastomosis healing. *JPEN* 1990;14:357–361.

26. Freed BA, Corliss RD, Bergman RS, et al: Serum albumin level and total lymphocyte count as predictors of morbidity and mortality in patients undergoing abdominal surgery. *JPEN* 1982;6:584.

27. Barbul A, Fishel RS, Shimazu S, et al: Intravenous hyperalimentation with high arginine levels improves wound healing and immune function. *J Surg Res* 1985;38:328–334.

28. Dionigi R, Zonta A, Dominioni L, et al: The effects of total parenteral nutrition on immunodepression caused by malnutrition. *Ann Surg* 1977;185:467–474.

29. Buzby GP: Perioperative nutritional support. *JPEN* 1990;14:197S–199S.

30. Williams RH, Heatley RV, Lewis MH, et al: A randomized controlled trial of preoperative intravenous nutrition in patients with stomach cancer. *Br J Surg* 1976;6:667.

31. Holter AR, Rosen HM, Fischer JE: The effects of hyperalimentation on major surgery in patients with malignant disease. *Acta Chir Scand* 1976;466:86–97.

32. Haydock DA, Hill GL: Improved wound healing response in surgical patients receiving intravenous nutrition. *Br J Surg* 1987;74:320–323.

33. Schroeder D, Gillanders L, Mahr K, et al: Effects of immediate postoperative enteral nutrition on body composition, muscle function, and wound healing. *JPEN* 1991;15:376–383.

34. Moore EE, Jones TN: Benefits of immediate jejunostomy feeding after major abdominal trauma: A prospective, randomized study. *J Trauma* 1986;26:874–881.

35. Moore FA, Moore EE, Jones TN, et al: TEN versus TPN following major abdominal trauma—reduced septic morbidity. *J Trauma* 1989;29:916–923.

36. Saito H, Trocki O, Alexander JW, et al: The effect of route of nutrient administration on the nutritional state, catabolic hormone secretion, and gut mucosal integrity after burn injury. *JPEN* 1987;11:1–7.

37. Alexander JW, Gonce SJ, Miskell PW, et al: A new model for studying nutrition in peritonitis. *Ann Surg* 1989;209:334–340.

38. Peck MD, Alexander JW, Gonce SJ, et al: Low protein diets improve survival from peritonitis in guinea pigs. *Ann Surg* 1989;209:448–454

39. Kirk SJ, Barbul A: Role of arginine in trauma, sepsis, and immunity. *JPEN* 1990;14:226S-229S.

40. Seifter E, Rettura G, Barbul A, et al: Arginine: An essential amino acid for injured rats. *Surgery* 1978;84:224–230.

41. Barbul A, Lazarou SA, Efron DT, et al: Arginine enhances wound healing and lymphocyte immune responses in humans. *Surgery* 1990;108:331–337.

42. Barbul A, Sisto DA, Wassserkrug HL, et al: Arginine stimulates lymphocyte immune response in healthy human beings. *Surgery* 1981;90:244–251.

43. Barbul A, Rettura G, Levenson SM, et al: Wound healing and thymotropic effects of arginine: A pituitary mechanism of action. *Am J Clin Nutr* 1983;37:786–794.

Chapter 24

Nutritional Status and Outcome in Orthopaedic Patients

Carl L. Nelson, MD
Cheryl L. Puskarich, PhD

Introduction

The nutritional status of hospitalized patients has been investigated intensely during the last 15 years. Much of this research has focused on nonorthopaedic patient populations. Published reports have indicated that 29% to 97% of hospitalized patients can be defined as malnourished at the time of admission.[1-17] The Nutritional Care Management Institute estimates that each year 10 to 15 million patients may be protein-calorie depleted at the time of hospital admission.[18] The reported consequences of nutritional depletion include lengthened hospital stay and an increased rate of complication. Patients defined as malnourished may be hospitalized up to 100% longer[6,7,15,19-21] and experience two to 20 times higher complication and death rates[5,10,11,16,22,23] than well-nourished patients. Investigations of wound healing in general surgery patients have revealed an association between nutritional status and delayed wound healing.[23-25] Malnourished patients are at significantly greater risk of delayed wound healing than are nutritionally sound patients.

The ability of nutritional supplementation to alter length of hospitalization and rate of complication also has been investigated in nonorthopaedic patient groups.[11,26-32] A reduction of 8% to 37% in average length of hospital stay has been reported in malnourished patients who received nutritional support.[21,27,33-35] Furthermore, several reports have suggested that nutritional supplementation can reduce the incidence of malnutrition-associated complications, such as wound infection and major sepsis, by 40% to 80%.[29,30,32,36] The single most important factor found to be correlated with failures in the effectiveness of supplemental support is delay in nutritional intervention.[18] Early detection is critical.

Obvious consequences of reducing length of hospital stay and rate of complication are improved quality of patient care and economic savings. Smith and Smith[18] have reported that malnourished patients may account for $100 billion in total hospital costs. The following cost savings per patient have been attributed to providing nutritional care to patients with protein-calorie malnutrition: major abdominal trauma, $3,356[37]; burns, $6,400[21]; intractable diarrhea, $14,750[35]; and bone marrow transplant, $1,436.[34]

Compared with the wealth of information thus far obtained from other surgery patient populations, relatively few studies have focused on orthopaedic patients. Our knowledge of nutritional status and its effect on outcome in orthopaedic patients is limited. A summary of these studies and their findings follows. An important component of conducting nutrition and patient outcome research is the ability to assess nutritional status. A brief discussion of suggested nutritional status indicators will therefore precede our discussion of specific orthopaedic studies.

Nutritional Assessment

Nutritional assessment is used to identify those patients who are admitted in a malnourished state, as well as to monitor patients while hospitalized. A variety of indicators have been proposed to identify or define the malnourished patient. The most commonly used are anthropometric (arm muscle circumference, triceps skinfold thickness, and weight for height), immunologic (total lymphocyte count, skin antigen testing), and biochemical (serum albumin, transferrin, and prealbumin levels).[18] Other indicators proposed include hematocrit and hemoglobin levels, percent weight loss, total iron-binding capacity, nitrogen balance, and hand-grip strength. Unfortunately, no generally accepted standard for identifying the nutritionally depleted patient exists at present. Consequently, agreement on which and how many of these indicators are necessary to accurately assess a patient's nutritional status is lacking.

Smith and Smith[18] proposed defining a patient as nutritionally depleted if levels for at least two (any two) indicators are below normal. Other research groups, through the use of multivariate statistical approaches, have developed formulae which incorporate several indicators to identify the nutritionally depleted patient. Mullen and associates,[31] for example, derived the prognostic nutritional index by statistically comparing a series of nutritional indicators in intra-abdominal and intrathoracic surgery patients with and without postoperative complications. The indicators incorporated in the prognostic nutritional index were serum albumin, triceps skinfold thickness, serum transferrin, and cutaneous delayed hypersensitivity reactivity. More recently, Rainey-Macdonald and associates[38] developed the nutritional index by comparing eight nutritional indicators in 55 surgical and critically ill patients with respect to the incidence of major septic complication. The nutritional index with the best power of prediction incorporated only serum albumin and transferrin levels. In their sample of patients, this index correctly classified outcome in 88% of the patients investigated.

As early as 1927, Cuthbertson[39] acknowledged that weight loss and negative nitrogen balance in long-bone fracture patients resulted from the trauma sustained. Howard and associates[40] confirmed these findings and demonstrated that negative nitrogen balance could be corrected through adjustments in diet. Until the early 1980s, however, few comparable studies in other orthopaedic patient samples were conducted.

In 1981 Pratt and associates[41] investigated the use of arm muscle circumference measurements to identify orthopaedic surgery patients (n = 106) at increased risk of developing a complication, specifically wound infection, following surgery. Patients who developed wound infections had a significantly smaller arm muscle circumference than those who did not develop a wound infection postoperatively. Pratt and associates also concluded that patients defined as malnourished, based on arm muscle circumference, who had undergone two or more previous operations in the past ten years were at increased risk of developing a postoperative complication. More specifically, a 42% rate of postoperative complication was reported for nutritionally depleted patients with multiple previous surgeries. Pratt and associates did, however, investigate a very diverse group of orthopaedic procedures. Patients undergoing total hip and knee arthroplasties, hand surgeries, foot surgeries, amputations, hip nailing, major joint fusions, implant removal, and open reduction in the lower extremity were investigated. Eleven of their patients had undergone incision and drainage of infections and were, therefore, infected before being included in the study. Only three patients developed a new infection postoperatively.

Studies

Nutritional status before and after surgery was investigated in 36 total hip replacement patients by Jensen and associates.[42] Anthropometric measurements and biochemical testing, as well as recall skin antigen testing, were conducted two days preoperatively, two and seven days postoperatively, and every ten days thereafter until the patient was discharged from the hospital. As expected, the prevalence of malnutrition before surgery varied depending on the nutritional indicator used. For example, a 24.2% rate of malnutrition was determined using creatinine/height index, while a 2.8% rate was calculated based on serum albumin values of less than 3.0 g/dl. In comparison with 36 randomly selected general orthopaedic patients, the nutritional parameters investigated were higher in total joint reconstruction patients, suggesting that these patients had been better nourished before their surgery. Results of nutritional assessments made two days after surgery indicated that serum albumin and transferrin values were significantly lower than the levels obtained before surgery, suggesting that total hip replacement surgery depressed visceral protein status. In these patients, serum transferrin and albumin levels improved somewhat, but were still lower on postoperative day seven.

A 22% (8/36) rate of postoperative infection (6 pulmonary infections and 2 wound infections) was reported by Jensen and associates.[42] No significant relationship between incidence of infection and any of the nutritional status indicators could be demonstrated. However, 70% of the patients who developed complications had abnormal serum transferrin and albumin values, total lymphocyte counts, and skin test indurations.

In a similar study, Jensen and associates[20] investigated nutritional status and patient outcome in two orthopaedic patient groups; elective and nonelective surgery patients. Group I (n=74), elective surgery patients, were nutritionally assessed as described in the previously discussed study.[42] Group II (n=55) consisted of multiple trauma and major long-bone fracture patients who required surgery. These patients were nutritionally assessed using the same indicators at five days following injury and every ten days thereafter until the patient returned to nutritionally sound status or was discharged from the hospital. The average prevalence of malnutrition two days prior to surgery in the elective surgery group was 35.3%. During hospitalization, twelve complications were observed in nine hip replacement patients. Although apparently not a statistically significant association, arm muscle circumference appeared to be the best single predictor of patients who developed complications. The average rate of malnutrition reported for nonelective surgery patients on the fifth day after injury was 57.2%. Of nonelective surgery patients who developed complications, 72% and 41% were determined to have severe or moderate depletion, respectively, in at least one of four visceral protein indices on the fifth day following injury. Although the amount of trauma sustained was not quantified, Jensen and associates[20] concluded that "additional trauma causes an additive or so-called dose-related increase in the risk of infection."

Dreblow, Anderson, and Moxness[43] investigated nutritional status at the time of admission and length of hospital stay in 82 patients hospitalized for orthopaedic reasons. Patients undergoing a wide variety of orthopaedic procedures were investigated. Nutritional assessments were made on the basis of body weight, triceps skinfold thickness, arm muscle circumference, serum albumin levels, and total serum iron-binding capacity. Of their patients, 48% were defined as suffering from protein-calorie malnutrition at the time of admission. A patient was defined as malnourished if one or more of the nutritional indicator values was deemed abnormal. Length of hospital stay was significantly longer in patients with serum albumin levels less than 3.5 g/dl and in those patients with abnormally low values for three or more of the indicators investigated.

Using anthropometric measurements, Bastow and associates[44] identified three general groups of elderly women with femoral neck fractures. Patients were categorized as well-nourished, thin, or very thin. Group assignment for the 744 patients included in their investigation was made on the basis of triceps skinfold thickness and arm muscle circumference. Approximately one-fifth (20%) of their patients were defined as thin or very thin. The mortality rates for the well-nourished, thin, and very thin elderly women were 4.4%, 8%, and 18%, respectively.

In a second study, Bastow and associates[45] investigated the effect of overnight nutritional supplementation on mortality rate and rehabilitation time. A total of 122 thin and very thin patients were randomized into two groups. Patients in group I received only the normal hospital ward diet. Patients in group II, in addition to receiving the normal ward diet, were tube fed overnight. Tube feeding began within five days of surgery. In order to determine if overnight supplementation altered patient appetite during the day, a daily calorie count of foods ingested orally was obtained. Rehabilitation time was measured as time to weightbearing and time to independent mobility.

The voluntary oral daily intake of tube-fed thin patients was significantly reduced compared with controls. No significant difference, however, in oral daily intake was found for very thin patients who received overnight tube feeding. Very thin patients who were tube fed had a significantly reduced hospital stay and a significantly shorter time to independent mobility. No significant differences in length of hospital stay or rehabilitation time were found within the thin patient group. Although mortality rate was lower in very thin tube-fed patients, the difference from controls was not statistically significant.

In a more recent study, Foster and associates[46] also investigated nutritional status in hip fracture patients. A series of 12 nutritional indicators were obtained preoperatively in 40 patients with a fracture of the hip. The relationship between the 12 indicators of nutritional status and mortality was examined. Albumin was the only nutritional indicator that was significantly associated with mortality. The mortality rate in patients with albumin values less than 3.0 g/dl was 70% compared with an 18% mortality rate in patients with albumin values equal to or greater than 3.0 g/dl. Although the prevalence of malnutrition was not specifically reported by Foster and associates, 12 of 34 (35%) patients, for whom albumin values were available, had albumin levels of less than 3.0 g/dl.

The relationship of nutritional status and wound healing in patients undergoing amputation has been investigated by Dickhaut and associates[24] and Kay and associates.[47] Dickhaut and associates retrospectively investigated preoperative serum albumin and total lymphocyte count levels in 23 patients with adult onset diabetes who had undergone a two-stage Syme amputation.[24] Patients with preoperative albumin levels of less than 3.5 g/dl and/or total lymphocyte count levels less than 1500/mm[3] were defined as malnourished. Using these criteria, 16 of their patients (70%) were defined as malnourished. Normal healing was observed in six of seven (86%) nutritionally sound patients and in three of 16 (19%) malnourished patients.

Similar results were obtained by Kay and associates[47] in an investigation of 41 consecutive patients with lower extremity amputations proximal to the Symes level. All patients were similarly nutritionally assessed using serum albumin and total lymphocyte count values obtained within one week of surgery. A total of 43 amputations were performed. Of these, 35 were below-knee and eight were above-knee amputations.

Of the 41 patients, 25 (61%) had abnormal albumin or total lymphocyte count values and were defined as malnourished. Amputations in approximately 94% (15/16) of the well-nourished patients healed uneventfully. In the malnourished group, however, 11 of 25 patients (44%) suffered local or systemic complications following surgery. Compared with the complication rate in nutritionally sound patients (6%), the complication rate in the malnourished group was significantly higher.

Similar results were obtained by Mandelbaum and associates,[37] in a nutritional study of 37 patients undergoing staged anterior and posterior spinal reconstructive surgery. The patients investigated represented a wide age range (5 to 74 years). All patients were nutritionally evaluated before, during, and after surgery using serum albumin and total lymphocyte count, which were retrospectively obtained. Malnourished patients were defined as those having a serum albumin level of less than 3.5 g/dl and total lymphocyte count level of less than 2000/mm^3. It should be noted, however, that the standard cutoff level for total lymphocyte count in most nutritional studies is 1500/mm^3. Mandelbaum and associates[37] reported that 31 of their patients (84%) were considered malnourished at some point during hospitalization. Preoperative total lymphocyte count and serum albumin levels were not significantly different from those obtained following the second surgery. Length of hospital stay after the second procedure was significantly greater in patients defined as malnourished following the procedure (16.2 days versus 12.4 days). The incidence of urinary tract infections was 40% in patients preoperatively defined as nutritionally depleted and 0% in nutritionally sound patients. The statistical significance of this difference was not tested.

Using the nutritional index of Rainey-Macdonald and associates,[38] (calculated as 1.2 times serum albumin plus 0.013 times serum transferrin minus 6.43), nutritional status at the time of admission and postoperative complications were investigated in 100 long-bone fracture patients by Nusbickel and associates.[13] Of their patients, 28 had negative nutritional index values and were defined as malnourished. Compared with the 72 patients defined as nutritionally sound (positive index values), the malnourished group was hospitalized 36% longer (19 days versus 12 days) and had a six times greater rate of postoperative complication (36% versus 6%). These differences were statistically significant (p < 0.05). All postoperative complications were infections. Fourteen patients (14%) developed an infection (five urinary tract infections, eight wound infections, and one osteomyelitis). Of these, ten (71%) occurred in patients defined as malnourished.

To investigate the relationship between trauma severity and preoperative serum transferrin and albumin levels, Nusbickel and associates[13] retrospectively obtained several measures of injury severity, namely trauma score,[48] injury severity score,[49] and abbreviated injury severity score.[49] Trauma severity measures were obtained for only 52% of the patient sample. A significant difference (p < 0.05) in all three trauma severity measures was found when nutritionally sound and depleted groups were compared. Malnourished patients, in this sample, experienced more extensive physiologic and organ system involvement than those patients defined as nutritionally sound. These results are in agreement with the earlier results of Cuthbertson[39] and Howard and associates,[40] which also demonstrated a relationship between nutritional status and the amount of trauma sustained. However, because of the limited trauma severity data obtained, the results of Nusbickel and associates should be verified in another sample of long bone fracture patients.

Nusbickel and associates[13] also investigated the effect of enteral nutritional supplementation on length of hospital stay and rate of complication. The 28 long-bone fracture patients defined as nutritionally depleted at the time of admission were prospectively randomized into two groups. Patients in the nonsupplemented group received the standard hospital diet, while patients in the supplemented group received an enteral nutritional supplement in addition to the normal hospital diet. A comparison of supplemented and nonsupplemented groups showed no significant differences (p > 0.10) in either length of hospital stay or rate of complication. The authors could not, however, make a definitive conclusion concerning the effect of supplementation, given the small sample of patients analyzed.

Puskarich and associates,[50] employing the same sample of 100 patients as Nusbickel and associates,[13] investigated the validity of not only the nutritional index, but also total lymphocyte count in identifying patients who did and did not develop postoperative infections. Nutritional index results (+ or − results only) were obtained as described above. Total lymphocyte count values, at the time of admission, were calculated as the total number of white blood cells times percent lymphocytes in the differential (measured per mm³). Patients with total lymphocyte count values equal to or greater than 1500/mm³ were defined as nutritionally sound. Those with total lymphocyte count values of less than 1500/mm³ were defined as malnourished.

Accuracy, sensitivity, specificity, and positive and negative predictive values were calculated for the nutritional index as well as for total lymphocyte count results. The following results were obtained for the nutritional index: accuracy, 78.0%; sensitivity, 79.1%; specificity, 71.4%; positive predictive value, 35.7%; negative predictive value, 94.4%. Because of the potentially mechanical nature of urinary tract infections, measures of validity were also calculated for wound infections only.[50] The following results were obtained: accuracy, 76.0%; sensitivity, 75.0%; specificity, 76.1%; positive predictive value, 25.0%; negative predictive value, 97.2%. Validity results obtained for total lymphocyte count values were as follows: accuracy, 50.6%; sensitivity, 50.0%; specificity, 54.5%; positive predictive value, 14.6%; negative predictive value, 87.5%.

Conclusions

Based on these results, the authors concluded that the nutritional index result was a better predictor of patient outcome (infection) than was the total lymphocyte count.[50] In addition, based on specifically positive predictive value results, the authors concluded that neither indicator used alone could adequately identify those patients that would develop an infection postoperatively. This should not, however, be interpreted to suggest that the nutritional index should not be used for nutritional evaluation of patients. Rather, the authors suggested that the ability of the nutritional index to predict patient outcome may improve if it is used in combination with other parameters.

In response to the lack of available data indicating the economic costs of malnutrition in orthopaedic patient populations, Puskarich and Nelson,[51] employing length of hospital stay data, calculated a malnutrition cost estimate for the 100 long-bone fracture patients discussed above. The economic costs due to malnutrition were estimated by converting average length of stay differences into a malnutrition cost penalty. These estimates included only hospital inpatient service and drug costs. The average daily cost of hospital inpatient service and drugs was $894 per patient. The difference in average length of stay between the nutritionally sound (12 days) and malnourished (19 days) groups was 7.0 days. From these data, a malnutrition cost penalty of 14% was calculated. This meant that it cost 14% more to treat the malnourished patient. The authors then applied the 14% cost penalty to national cost data reported by Grazier and associates[52] for a similar orthopaedic patient group. The annual national cost of malnutrition was estimated to be $232 million. Due to the exclusion of physician and indirect costs from their calculations, as well as the absence of other complications (such as delayed wound healing), the estimate presented was an underestimate of the cost due to malnutrition. Their data, despite being an underestimate, illustrated the potential magnitude of the financial problem of malnutrition in orthopaedic patients.

These authors also investigated the ability of nutritional index values and measures of trauma severity to identify patients who did or did not develop a postoperative complication.[51] Trauma score,[48] injury severity score,[49] and abbreviated injury severity score[49] were investigated. In their sample of 100 long-bone fractures, 14 patients (14%) developed an infection postoperatively. No statistically significant differences in trauma score, injury severity score, or abbreviated injury severity score were found when the 52 patients with and without complications were compared. Using discriminant function analysis, nutritional index values correctly classified 67% of the patients who developed a postoperative infection. The highest discriminatory power, 51%, for trauma severity measures was obtained when trauma, injury severity, and abbreviated injury severity scores were analyzed collectively. Despite their apparent influence on nutritional status, measures of trauma severity were less accurate than nutritional index values in predicting patient outcome.

From these studies, which focused on orthopaedic patient populations, it is clear that a considerable number of orthopaedic patients may be malnourished at the time of hospital admission. These patients are hospitalized longer and are at increased risk of developing complications following surgery. Although underestimated, the financial impact of malnutrition in at least one orthopaedic patient group has been presented.[51] The true magnitude of this financial impact has, however, yet to be illustrated.

Despite these investigations, our knowledge of nutritional status and outcome in orthopaedic patient populations is still limited. A series of important questions remain unanswered. Is the risk of malnutrition, before and after surgery, similar in all orthopaedic patients, regardless of the procedure performed? Can patient groups at increased risk of postoperative morbidity and mortality be identified? Can nutritional intervention, before and/or after surgery have a positive impact on patient outcome? Can we identify those patients who will and will not benefit from nutritional supplementation? Are there regional and/or institutional differences in rates of malnutrition and to what do we attribute these differences? What are the nutritional requirements of our patients and what supplements and protocols best meet these needs? What are the true financial costs of malnutrition in orthopaedic patients?

In order to effectively answer these questions, we should use research designs analogous to those used in epidemiological studies. Ideally, such studies should be prospective in nature and should give special attention to the indicators used to nutritionally evaluate patients. In several of the studies discussed, the prevalence of malnutrition varied considerably with the nutritional indicator used. Given that the parameters investigated reflect different metabolic functions and/or responses from different components of the body, this is not surprising. However, if nutritional status is assessed consistently, the results of different studies can be compared. Cross-study comparisons may also be facilitated by the use of well-defined measures of postoperative outcome. Consequently, validity can be tested and the issue of generalizability or how accurate the results are when applied to other similar patient groups can be addressed.

Other important research design considerations include (1) the use of statistical randomization (to determine, for example, whether a patient is to be supplemented or not supplemented); (2) the construction of a research design that controls for other suggested risk factors (such as age, socioeconomic status, or trauma severity); and (3) the use of sample sizes sufficiently large to maintain statistical validity. Small samples may not be representative of the larger populations from which they were drawn. This reduces, if not eliminates, the potential applicability of the results obtained. Unfortunately, many of the orthopaedic studies investigated very small samples of patients. Therefore, their results may not be reproducible. One possible solution to this problem would be to conduct multicenter studies. Not only would the problems of sample size be reduced, but, if chosen correctly, the study centers could also represent a range of geographic regions, which would increase the usefulness of the results obtained.

Epidemiologically sound research conducted in the area of nutritional status and outcome in orthopaedic patient populations may provide the answers to the questions discussed above. This information could improve the quality of patient care and reduce costs. Given the anticipated growth in orthopaedic patient populations, it is important that we increase our knowledge of nutrition and its effect upon outcome.

References

1. Bistrian BR, Blackburn GL, Hallowell E, et al: Protein status of general surgical patients. *JAMA* 1974;230:858–860.
2. Bistrian BR, Blackburn GL, Vitale J, et al: Prevalence of malnutrition in general medical patients. *JAMA* 1976;235:1567–1570.
3. Bollet AJ, Owens S: Evaluation of nutritional status of selected hospitalized patients. *Am J Clin Nutr* 1973;26:931–938.
4. Butterworth CE: Iatrogenic malnutrition: The skeleton in the hospital closet. *Nutr Today* 1974;9:4–8.
5. Buzby GP, Mullen JL, Mathews DC, et al: Prognostic nutritional index in gastrointestinal surgery. *Am J Surg* 1980;139:160–167.
6. Christensen KS: Hospitalwide screening increases revenue under prospective payment system. *J Am Diet Assoc* 1986;86:1234–1235.
7. Christensen KS, Gstundtner KM: Hospital-wide screening improves basis for nutrition intervention. *J Am Diet Assoc* 1985;85:704–706.
8. Hill GL, Blackett RL, Pickford I, et al: Malnutrition in surgical patients: An unrecognised problem. *Lancet* 1977;1:689–692.
9. Kamath SK, Lawler M, Smith AE, et al: Hospital malnutrition: A 33–hospital screening study. *J Am Diet Assoc* 1986;86:203–206.
10. Klidjian AM, Archer TJ, Foster KJ, et al: Detection of dangerous malnutrition. *JPEN* 1982;6:119–121.
11. Mullen JL, Gertner MH, Buzby GP, et al: Implications of malnutrition in the surgical patient. *Arch Surg* 1979;114:121–125.
12. Nelson S. Bottsford JE Jr, Long JM III: Finding malnourished patients in a community hospital: Development of a nutritional assessment service. *J SC Med Assoc* 1983;79:9–13.
13. Nusbickel FR, Nelson CL, Puskarich CL: Perioperative nutritional evaluation of orthopaedic trauma patients. Presented at the 56th Annual Meeting of the American Academy of Orthopaedic Surgeons, Las Vegas, NV, Feb 9–14, 1989.
14. Pinchcofsky-Devin GD, Kaminski MV Jr: Correlation of pressure sores and nutritional status. *J Am Geriatr Soc* 1986;34:435–440.
15. Seltzer MH, Bastidas JA, Cooper DM, et al: Instant nutritional assessment. *JPEN* 1979;3:157–159.
16. Warnold I, Lundholm K: Clinical significance of preoperative nutritional status in 215 noncancer patients. *Ann Surg* 1984;199:299–305.
17. Willard MD, Gilsdorf RB, Price RA: Protein-calorie malnutrition in a community hospital. *JAMA* 1980;243:1720–1722.
18. Smith A, Smith P: *Superior Nutritional Care Cuts Hospital Costs.* Chicago, Nutritional Care Management Institute, 1988.
19. Anderson MD, Collins G, Davis G, et al: Malnutrition and length of stay—a relationship? *Henry Ford Hosp Med J* 1985;33:190–193.
20. Jensen JE, Jensen TG, Smith TK, et al: Nutrition in orthopaedic surgery. *J Bone Joint Surg* 1982;64A:1263–1272.

21. Weinsier RL, Heimburger DC, Samples CM, et al: Cost containment: A contribution of aggressive nutritional support in burn patients, abstract. *Am J Clin Nutr* 1984;39:673.

22. Hickman DM, Miller RA, Rombeau JL, et al: Serum albumin and body weight as predictors of postoperative course in colorectal cancer. *JPEN* 1980;4:314–316.

23. Lewis RT, Klein H: Risk factors in postoperative sepsis: Significance of preoperative lymphocytopenia. *J Surg Res* 1979;26:365–371.

24. Dickhaut SC, DeLee JC, Page CP: Nutritional status: Importance in predicting wound-healing after amputation. *J Bone Joint Surg* 1984;66A:71–75.

25. Maillet JO: Evaluating your assessment program. *Nutr Supp Serv* 1982;4:19.

26. Askanazi J, Hensle TW, Starker PM, et al: Effect of immediate postoperative nutritional support on length of hospitalization. *Ann Surg* 1986;203:236–239.

27. Collins JP, Oxby CB, Hill GL: Intravenous aminoacids and intravenous hyperalimentation as protein-sparing therapy after major surgery: A controlled clinical trial. *Lancet* 1978;1:788–791.

28. Dietel M: Nutritional management of external small bowel fistulas. *Can J Surg* 1976;19:505.

29. Grimes CJ, Younathan MT, Lee WC: The effect of preoperative total parenteral nutrition on surgery outcomes. *J Am Diet Assoc* 1987;87:1202–1206.

30. Heatley RV, Williams RHP, Lewis MH: Pre-operative intravenous feeding: A controlled trial. *Postgrad Med J* 1979;55:541–545.

31. Mullen JL, Buzby GP, Waldman MT, et al: Prediction of operative morbidity and mortality by preoperative nutritional assessment. *Surg Forum* 1979;30:80–82.

32. Smale BF, Mullen JL, Buzby GP, et al: The efficacy of nutritional assssment and support in cancer surgery. *Cancer* 1981;47:2375–2381.

33. Moore EE, Jones TN: Benefits of immediate jejunostomy feeding after major abdominal trauma: A prospective, randomized study. *J Trauma* 1986;26:874–881.

34. Szeluga DJ, Stuart RK, Brookmeyer R, et al: Nutritional support of bone marrow transplant recipients: A prospective, randomized clinical trial comparing total parenteral nutrition to an enteral feeding program. *Cancer Res* 1987;47:3309–3316.

35. Smith AE, Powers CA, Cooper-Meyer RA, et al: Improved nutritional management reduces length of hospitalization in intractable diarrhea. *JPEN* 1986;10:479–481.

36. Mullen JL, Buzby GP, Mathews DC, et al: Reduction of operative morbidity and mortality by combined preoperative and postoperative nutritional support. *Ann Surg* 1980;192:604–613.

37. Mandelbaum BR, Tolo VT, McAfee PC, et al: Nutritional deficiencies after staged anterior and posterior spinal reconstructive surgery. *Clin Orthop* 1988;234:5–11.

38. Rainey-Macdonald CG, Holliday RL, Wells GA, et al: Validity of a two-variable nutritional index for use in selecting candidates for nutritional support. *JPEN* 1983;7:15–20.

39. Cuthbertson DP: The disturbance of metabolism produced by bony and nonbony injury, with notes on certain abnormal conditions of bone. *Biochem J* 1930;24:1244–1263.

40. Howard JE, Parson W, Stein KE, et al: Studies on fracture convalescence: I. Nitrogen metabolism after fracture and skeletal operations in healthy males. *Bull Johns Hopkins Hosp* 1944;75:156–168.

41. Pratt WB, Veitch JM, McRoberts RL: Nutritional status of orthopedic patients with surgical complications. *Clin Orthop* 1981;155:81–84.

42. Jensen JE, Smith TK, Jensen TG, et al: The Frank Stinchfield Award paper: Nutritional assessment of orthopaedic patients undergoing total hip replacement surgery, in Salvati EA (ed): *The Hip: Proceedings of the Ninth Open Scientific Meeting of The Hip Society.* St. Louis, CV Mosby, 1988, pp 123–135.

43. Dreblow DM, Anderson CF, Moxness K: Nutritional assessment of orthopedic patients. *Mayo Clinic Proc* 1981;56:51–54.

44. Bastow MD, Rawlings J, Allison SP: Undernutrition, hypothermia, and injury in elderly women with fractured femur: An injury response to altered metabolism? *Lancet* 1983;1:143–146.

45. Bastow MD, Rawlings J, Allison SP: Benefits of supplementary tube feeding after fractured neck of femur: A randomised controlled trial. *Br Med J* 1983;287:1589–1592.

46. Foster MR, Heppenstall RB, Friedenberg ZB, et al: A prospective assessment of nutritional status and complications in patients with fractures of the hip. *J Orthop Trauma* 1990;4:49–57.

47. Kay SP, Moreland JR, Schmitter E: Nutritional status and wound healing in lower extremity amputations. *Clin Orthop* 1987;217:253–256.

48. Champion HR, Sacco WJ, Carnazzo AJ, et al: Trauma score. *Crit Care Med* 1981;9:672–676.

49. Greenspan L, McLellan BA, Greig H: Abbreviated Injury Scale and Injury Severity Score: A scoring chart. *J Trauma* 1985;25:60–64.

50. Puskarich CL, Nelson CL, Nusbickel FR, et al: The use of two nutritional indicators in identifying long bone fracture patients who do and do not develop infections. *J Orthop Res* 1990;8:799–803.

51. Puskarich CL, Nelson CL: Economic costs due to malnutrition and the ensuing secondary complications that occur in orthopaedic fracture patients. Presented at the 58th Annual Meeting of the American Academy of Orthopaedic Surgeons, Anaheim, CA, March 7–11, 1991.

52. Grazier KL, Holbrook TL, Kelsey JL, et al: *The Frequency of Occurrence, Impact, and Cost of Musculoskeletal Conditions in the United States.* Chicago, American Academy of Orthopaedic Surgeons, 1984.

Chapter 25

A Poorly Vascularized Wound Adversely Affects Neutrophil Function

Brent R.W. Moelleken, MD
Stephen J. Mathes, MD
Thomas K. Hunt, MD

Introduction

Wounds arising from radiation necrosis, chronic infection, and poor perfusion are characterized by hypoxic, acidic conditions. A series of experiments was undertaken to elucidate the characteristics of neutrophils isolated from such an adverse wound environment and to compare their phagocytic and protein synthetic abilities with those of neutrophils isolated from a well-perfused and oxygenated milieu, the so-called favorable wound. An animal model was used to provide these two distinct wound environments.

Several studies describe the differences between neutrophils in the peripheral circulation and in various wounds, but the differences between neutrophils of distinct wound types are still largely unknown. This study defines and tests a model providing two distinct wound environments and studies leukocyte function within each.

Certain flap types have demonstrated a greater resistance to bacterial inoculation, both in clinically infected wounds and experimentally.[1] Neutrophils associated with well oxygenated wound environments, with superior blood flow and physiologic pH, are associated with superior phagocytic function.[2]

However, the same free radicals and powerful oxidants that aid in killing bacteria in an infected wound can also damage tissue through reperfusion injury associated with the no-reflow phenomenon. Neutrophils appear to mediate undesirable release of toxic products, as in the bloodstream of patients with ARDS (adult respiratory distress syndrome),[3] in heart muscle following reperfusion, and in microsurgical flaps after release of clamps.[4,5] The same neutrophil products that provide the first line of defense against infection can also be deleterious if improperly discharged.[6] The efficacy of the neutrophil against bacteria is determined by its state of activation; the higher the state of activation, the greater the release of granular products, superoxide radicals, and other products toxic to bacteria.[7,8] A clear understanding of leukocyte activation within specific wound environments is necessary if we are to modulate leukocyte function to obtain a desired clinical effect.

Concurrently with activation, neutrophils express the Mac-1 receptor (C3bi receptor, CD11b/CD18, Mo1, CR3) on their surface, increasing its mobilization from the intracellular storage granules to the cell surface. In addition to being a sensitive and specific marker for activation state, Mac-1 is an important membrane glycoprotein of the membrane integrin family. Its numerous functions include leukocyte adhesion and aggregation (probably by using extracellular matrix components as ligands), which enable the neutrophil to escape from the circulation through diapedesis and enter the wound. Patients with an inherited defect in CD18 (including Mac-1) synthesis have a condition called leukocyte adhesion disease (LAD). In the face of infection, they may mount white blood cell counts in excess of 100,000, but the neutrophils are unable to reach the wound.

Methods

Overview

A single stainless steel mesh wound cylinder was enclosed within the deep surfaces of a latissimus dorsi musculocutaneous flap and the contralateral random pattern flap of 30 six- to eight-week-old Yucatan miniature swine. The vascular anatomy of these models has been confirmed by barium latex, anatomic, and radiolabeled Xenon flow studies (Fig. 1). Wound fluid from each cylinder and peripheral blood were aspirated at three and again at seven days after implantation, at which time neutrophil kinetics demonstrated maximal diapedesis into the wound cylinders (Fig. 2). The neutrophils were isolated from the wound fluid and analyzed.

Wound Cylinders

Cylindrical stainless steel wound cylinders measuring 4 cm in length and 1 cm in diameter were surrounded by a latissimus dorsi musculocutaneous flap on the left side of six- to eight-week-old Yucatan miniature swine, and by an identically sized random pattern counterpart on the right side of the animal. The flaps, which were twice as long as they were wide, provided significantly different vascular milieux. Flaps of this sort, followed for 14 days in preliminary animals, were documented to survive completely. Wound fluid was aspirated with a 20–gauge needle at three and seven days after implantation, times chosen because large numbers of neutrophils collect within this period. The wound fluid is completely aspirated at three days, so that subsequent neutrophils collecting in the chambers are comprised predominantly of new cells.[9] The wound fluid that collects is transudative in nature and has a white blood cell count of approximately 1 to 2 × 10^6 polymorphonuclear neutrophils per cubic centimeter of wound fluid.

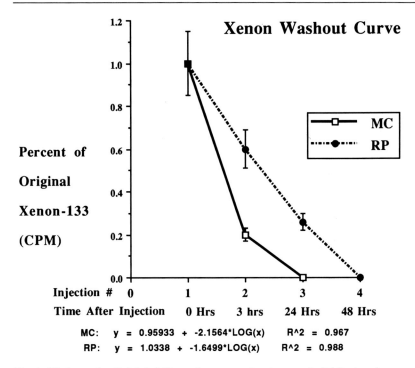

Fig. 1 *Washout of radiolabeled Xenon from musculocutaneous (solid line) and random pattern (broken line) wound cylinders. Note more rapid washout from musculocutaneous cylinders. Rates of washout were similar in two similar trials, one with intradermal injection into flaps overlying cylinders, the other directly into wound cylinders. In each case, washout of tracer from cylinders paralleled washout of tracer from the overlying tissue.*

Wound Model and Flap Design

Dissections were carried out on Yucatan miniature swine to confirm the presence of a thoracodorsal artery and vein on the musculocutaneous side and musculocutaneous perforators on the contralateral, random pattern side. The flap on the musculocutaneous side measured 6.5 cm × 13 cm and was elevated on the thoracodorsal artery. The flap on the random pattern side, which also measured 6.5 cm × 13 cm, was a mirror-image of the flap on the contralateral musculocutaneous side. In its evaluation, the latissimus dorsi muscle was left adherent to the chest wall, and the musculocutaneous perforators were divided as they entered the overlying skin and subcutaneous tissue of the random pattern flap. Both flaps survived the entire experiment without necrosis of their distal tips. Barium latex injections confirmed a typical musculocutaneous anatomic type, similar to that found in humans. Radiolabeled Xenon injections confirmed that blood flow in the skin overlying the wound cylinders and in the wound surrounding them was similar (Fig. 1).

369

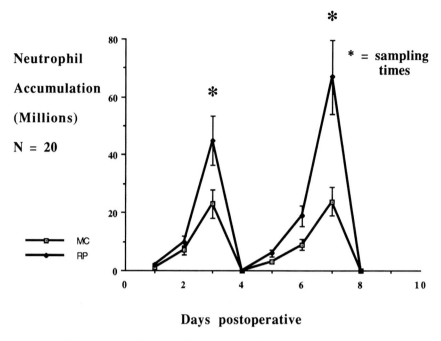

Fig. 2 *Neutrophil accumulation in musculocutaneous and random pattern wound environments expressed as millions of cells. Note that wound cylinders are completely aspirated at each timepoint (indicated with asterisks), so that at any given timepoint the majority of neutrophils sampled represent freshly diapedesed neutrophils. Note more rapid accumulation of neutrophils in random pattern environment.*

Studies

Radiographic Studies

Barium latex was injected into the femoral artery and magnification-grade radiography was used to confirm the similarity of the vascular anatomy of each type of flap to that found in the human.

Xenon Flow Studies

[133]Xenon was injected into wound cylinders and, in separate trials, into the dermis of the musculocutaneous and random pattern flaps, and its disappearance was monitored on a gamma counter. This study measured Xenon washout and provided a comparison between flow in the flap dermis and the underlying cylinder.

Neutrophil Isolation

Neutrophil isolation was performed by using a dextran T-500 (4% in 0.85% saline) sedimentation and discontinuous Percoll gradient by a modified method of Zimmerli and associates, modification by Zimmerli.[10] This procedure allowed isolation of more than 97% neutrophils with 97% viability by the trypan blue nuclear exclusion technique.[1] Neutrophils were isolated at 4 C to prevent spurious activation.[11] The limulus assay confirmed reagents free of endotoxin. Trials were conducted both with and without stimulation with phorbol myristate acetate.

Luminol Technique for Chemiluminescence

Luminol-mediated chemiluminescence, caused by neutrophil superoxide radical production, was measured by a previously described technique.[12] Cell concentration was adjusted to 2×10^4 neutrophils/ml. Luminol was added to scintillation vials both with and without phorbol myristate acetate.

Lactoferrin ELISA Assay for Monitoring Specific Granules

Lactoferrin was measured with an enzyme-linked immunosorbent assay (ELISA).[12] A 96–well plate was coated with antilactoferrin antibody. Neutrophil samples were maximally stimulated with phorbol myristate acetate and the cells induced to express their lactoferrin maximally. The supernatant was collected and placed on the antilactoferrin-containing plate. When treated with an antilactoferrin conjugated with peroxidase, the samples were quantitated on an ELISA reader.

Mac-1 Expression: Surface and Total Cellular

The isolated neutrophils were stained with OKM1, a monoclonal antibody directed at the Mac-1 receptor, and an ELISA assay was performed to allow calculation of the Mac-1 receptor present on the leukocyte surface.[13] We have developed and reported a new ELISA assay capable of measuring Mac-1 both on whole cells (surface Mac-1) and lysed cells (total cellular Mac-1).[14] Positive and negative controls included cell suspension alone, peroxidase-conjugated cell suspension alone, and nonspecific antibody not directed against Mac-1.

For whole-cellular assays, live cells were placed directly onto ELISA plates and were treated with glutaraldehyde. For lysed cellular assays, cells were frozen and thawed three times before being applied to plates in concentrations equivalent to whole-cellular assay. Cells were placed in equal concentrations onto 96–well plates (5×10^4 cells/well) and were treated with 2% glutaraldehyde in phosphate-buffered saline to fix cells to the ELISA plate. The plates were then treated with 0.5% bis-trimethylsilylacetamide for 30 minutes at room temperature (or overnight in refrigerator) to bind unoccupied glutaraldehyde moieties. Cells were washed four times with a phosphate-buffered saline and Tween solution (PBS/Tween).

Plates were treated with monoclonal antibody at a concentration of 35 mg/ml for one hour at 37 C. Hybridoma OKM1 monoclonal antibody was used at a concentration of 200 µl OKM1 per well. Wells were washed four times with PBS/Tween and were then incubated for 90 minutes with peroxidase-conjugated F(ab')$_2$ fragments of goat antimouse immunoglobulin G. Cells were again washed four times with PBS/Tween. Peroxidase substrate (0.1 ml) was added and incubated for 15 minutes. The reaction was stopped with 0.025 ml 8 N H_2SO_4 and the optical density read in an ELISA reader at an optical density of 450 nm, using blank well to blank instrument. Controls included HeLa cells (negative) and P388 macrophage cell line expressing Mac-1 constitutively (positive). For immunoprecipitation reactions, cellular isolates were radioiodinated and the membranes extracted with OKM1 anti-Mac-1 monoclonal antibody bound to Sepharose beads. Gel electrophoresis and autoradiography demonstrated characteristic 95 and 195 kd bands of Mac-1, which are very similar to those found in humans.

[35]S-Methionine Incorporation To Measure Protein Synthesis

Neutrophils isolated from wound fluid or blood were incubated for 24 hours in a methionine-poor medium, were radioiodinated, and the membrane- and granule-associated Mac-1 was extracted with OKM1 bound to Sepharose beads. The resultant isolates were subjected to autoradiography, allowing a semiquantitative assessment of the amount of protein synthesis. This method has been described elsewhere.[12] In both this and the previous assay, positive and negative controls were performed with cells known to be lacking in and to contain Mac-1 (HeLa and P-388 cells, respectively). Relative contributions to the CD11b and CD18 components were noted.

Phagocytosis Assay and Oxygen Determinations

A pan-sensitive strain of *Staphylococcus aureus* was cultured in tryptose-phosphate broth at 35 C for 18 hours with 10 μCi/ml ^{3}H glycine. The bacteria were centrifuged and washed in phosphate-buffered saline twice and were then resuspended in 5 ml of phosphate-buffered saline. A 1:20 dilution of this suspension was read at 500 nm in the ultraviolet-visual information storage spectrophotometer and standardized. Serum (5 ml) was added to the suspension, and it was incubated at 37 C for 30 minutes to opsonize the bacterial cells. Aliquots of 100 μl were counted to determine disintegrations per minute per colony-forming unit. Pig peripheral or wound polymorphonuclear neutrophils were diluted to 1×10^6 cells/ml and were placed into crimp-seal roller culture tubes. The tubes were sealed and gassed for 10 minutes under continuous flow at various oxygen concentrations. The liquid layer was mixed periodically to obtain the maximum gas interaction. Bacterial suspension (200 μl) was injected into each tube, and the tubes were incubated at 37 C for 60 minutes. The tubes were then agitated and decapped, and the contents were aliquoted into 1.0 ml microfuge tubes. Lysostaphin (100 μl at a concentration of 100 u/ml) was added to each tube, and the tubes were incubated at 37 C to digest non-ingested bacteria. The tubes were centrifuged in the microfuge, the supernatants aspirated, and 0.5 ml of 0.1% sodium dodecyl sulfate was added to dissolve polymorphonuclear neutrophil/bacterial complexes.

Table 1 Variables that influence wound healing

Sample Tested	Variables Measured					
	pH	Po_2	Lactiferrin*	pH	Po_2	Lactiferrin*
		(3 days)			(7 days)	
Musculocutaneous	7.33	120	8.42	7.32	117	4.03
Random pattern	7.17	38	5.98	7.05	21	2.97
Peripheral blood	7.40	160	6.71	7.38	154	6.70

*N = 6 cases

After 30 minutes at room temperature, the aliquots were transferred to liquid scintillation counting tubes and counted in the scintillation counter. Notably, although exhaust Po_2 from sealed gas-impermeable chamber read 0, fluid Po_2 values were as high as 110 mm Hg. Therefore, the Po_2 was confirmed by measuring the fluid in a calibrated blood gas analyzer.

Immunoprecipitation for Detection of Mac-1

Crossreactivity of monoclonal antibodies with pig Mac-1 was confirmed with standard immunoprecipitation reactions.[15,16]

Results

Wound Model

Anatomic dissections performed on the Yucatan miniature swine latissimus dorsi muscle and overlying skin revealed a musculocutaneous anatomy with a single thoracodorsal artery supplying the latissimus muscle from the axilla. On the contralateral side, an identical dissection was carried out except that a dissection plane between the subcutaneous fat and latissimus muscle was chosen. Multiple musculocutaneous perforators were encountered and divided, with flap circulation provided by proximal vascular connections with the subdermal plexus.

Barium latex anatomic studies in miniature swine confirmed the presence of a thoracodorsal artery and musculocutaneous perforators in the miniature swine latissimus dorsi musculocutaneous flap. On the contralateral side (random pattern flap), no central perforator was present; instead, transsected randomly distributed musculocutaneous perforators predominated. Thus, the miniature swine possessed a musculocutaneous pattern similar to that seen in human cadavers.[14] Measurements of pH and Po_2 (performed with standard arterial blood gas machine) on wound fluid immediately upon aspiration support findings of a hypoxic environment in random pattern flap cylinders and near systemic values in the musculocutaneous environment (Table 1). Animals were inspiring 40% O_2 by face mask at time of determinations.

Cylinder Blood Flow

At 3-, 5-, and 7-day timepoints, radiolabeled Xenon washout was observed to be greater on the musculocutaneous side than on the random pattern side, confirming the similarities of human and porcine musculocutaneous anatomy with respect to blood flow (Fig. 1). The differences are noticeable as early as 45 minutes after injection and achieve statistical significance at 3-, 24-, and 48-hour timepoints.

Neutrophil Accumulation

Neutrophil accumulation within wound cylinders (Fig. 2) allowed two aspiration timepoints consisting mainly of newly arrived neutrophils. More neutrophils accumulated under random pattern flaps than under musculocutaneous flaps.

Chemiluminescence Assay

Neutrophils from musculocutaneous and random pattern wound environments and peripheral blood were compared with respect to their baseline production of superoxide radical and their maximally stimulated (with phorbol myristate acetate) output, both at three and at seven days (Fig. 3). At the three-day timepoint, random pattern cells exhibited marginally higher baseline or stimulated superoxide radical production than musculocutaneous cells. However, at the seven-day timepoint, musculocutaneous cells had greater superoxide radical production ($p < 0.05$) than did random pattern-associated cells. Musculocutaneous cells exhibited an increase in responsiveness to phorbol myristate acetate three times as great as that of cells from the random pattern wound cylinder ($p < 0.02$).

Lactoferrin Assay

At the three-day sampling point, neutrophils from the hypoxic, acidic, random-pattern wound had lower levels of lactoferrin ($p < 0.02$) than did musculocutaneous cells; more lactoferrin had been degranulated from random pattern neutrophils as they became progressively activated. This trend was also noted for the seven-day samples ($p < 0.05$), where random pattern neutrophils exhibited lower remaining levels of lactoferrin. These data support the chemiluminescence data and indicate that the timing of activation random pattern neutrophils was unfavorable compared to that of the musculocutaneous cells (Table 1).

Mac-1 Surface Expression

Results from surface Mac-1 assays on six Yucatan miniature swine using the newly developed ELISA Mac-1 assay are reported (Table 2). Means values are indicated in tabular form and graphically. At the three-day sampling, random pattern cells exhibited higher Mac-1 levels than did musculocutaneous neutrophils ($p < 0.05$), indicating greater

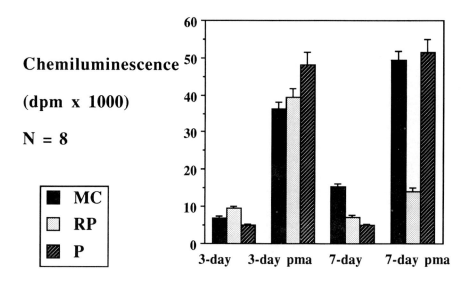

Fig. 3 *Diagram of chemiluminescence of polymorphonuclear neutrophils isolated from musculocutaneous (MC) and random pattern (RP) wound environments and peripheral blood. In each case, cells were maximally stimulated with phorbol ester phorbol myristate acetate to assess maximal reserves of the polymorphonuclear neutrophils. At the three-day day timepoint, RP cells exhibit a small (p = NS) increase in baseline and stimulated superoxide radical production over MC cells. However, at the 7-day timepoint, MC cells have higher baseline production of superoxide radical (p < 0.05) and much greater stimulated production of superoxide radical (p < 0.02). RP-associated cells activated prematurely and had minimal reserves remaining when maximally stimulated. By comparison, MC-associated neutrophils were very capable of mounting a response to a maximal stimulus.*

activation state of the random pattern cells. In response to a maximal stimulus, each recruited equal amounts from granular Mac-1 stores.

At the seven-day sampling, random pattern surface Mac-1 was again higher than musculocutaneous Mac-1. However, stimulated Mac-1 was significantly higher in the musculocutaneous group than the random pattern group. These differences appear to be related to the ability of musculocutaneous cells to synthesize the protein subunits which become incorporated into Mac-1 (see total cellular Mac-1 data in Table 2).

Bacterial Phagocytosis of Musculocutaneous and Random Pattern Flap Neutrophils

Neutrophils isolated from musculocutaneous wounds demonstrated superior bacterial phagocytosis of tritiated bacteria (N=6, p < 0.02) (Fig. 4).

Table 2 Mac-1 levels

Sample Tested	Surface Expression				Total Cellular Expression			
	3-day	3-day pma	7-day	7-day pma	3-day	3-day pma	7-day	7-day pma
Musculocutaneous	0.630	1.001	0.655	1.067	1.375	1.404	1.456	1.461
Random pattern	0.755	0.974	0.771	0.912	1.101	1.200	1.198	1.205
Peripheral blood	0.615	1.023	0.600	1.062	1.202	1.244	1.201	1.250

pma = phorbol myristate acetate

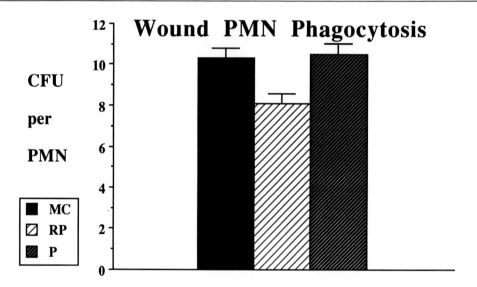

Fig. 4 *Phagocytosis of tritiated bacteria by polymorphonuclear neutrophils from two wound environments, musculocutaneous (MC) and random pattern (RP). Note superior phagocytosis by MC polymorphonuclear neutrophils of tritiated bacteria than by RP polymorphonuclear neutrophils. Results expressed as organisms ingested per polymorphonuclear neutrophil.*

Results: Studies on Peripheral (Control) Neutrophils

Bacterial Phagocytosis—Prestimulation

Peripheral (control) neutrophils were tested to evaluate the effect of prestimulation (Fig. 5). Prestimulated neutrophils were decidedly hampered in their ability to phagocytose bacteria (N=6, p < 0.05) by 15 minutes after administration of phorbol myristate acetate at a concentration of 10^{-8}M, a stimulus we determined by dose-response curves to be a maximal biologic stimulus. This decrement progressed until one hour, when neutrophils demonstrated severe decrements in function (N=6, p < 0.02).

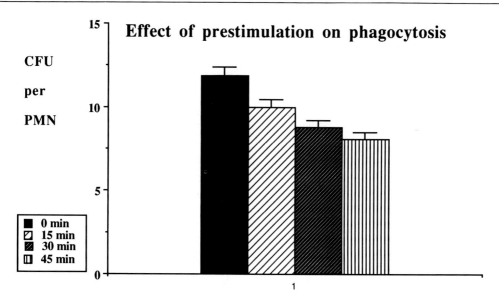

Fig. 5 *Effect of prestimulation on phagocytosis of tritiated bacteria by peripheral neutrophils. Note deleterious effect on number of organisms ingested per polymorphonuclear neutrophil as a function of time after maximal stimulation with $10^{-8}M$ phorbol myristate acetate.*

Bacterial Phagocytosis—pH Effect

Peripheral circulating (control) neutrophils were assayed for phagocytosis of tritiated bacteria (Fig. 6). They were placed in RPMI medium at different pH. Phagocytic function is adversely affected by a pH outside the physiologic range. The pH usually encountered in wound fluid associated with the musculocutaneous wound and random pattern wounds is denoted with boxes (N=6; p < 0.01 at pH of 7.0 vs 7.4 by Student's t-test).

Bacterial Phagocytosis—Po_2 Effect

Peripheral circulating (control) neutrophils in RPMI medium with controlled Po_2 demonstrated no decrement in phagocytic function until the Po_2 dropped to 39 mm Hg, at which point phagocytosis was reduced (N=6, p < 0.02 compared with Po_2 of 107.3) (Fig. 7).

Discussion

Several cell types participate in the early inflammatory reaction and defense against foreign microorganisms seen in wound infections. It is felt that neutrophils mediate in large part the initial antibacterial properties, possibly through increased neutrophil oxidative product

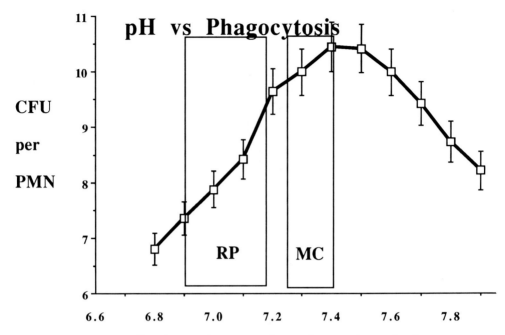

Fig. 6 *Effect of pH on phagocytosis of tritiated bacteria by peripheral polymorphonuclear neutrophils. Note how unphysiologic pH values have a deleterious effect on phagocytosis. Bracketed areas indicate pH ranges of respective flap wound cylinders. Numbers on the horizontal axis indicate pH.*

elaboration. Musculocutaneous flaps have demonstrated a greater resistance to bacterial inoculation in clinical and experimental settings.[1,2] Neutrophils in well oxygenated wound environments, with superior blood flow and physiologic pH, are associated with superior phagocytic function.

These data led us to believe that the anti-infective properties of the musculocutaneous flap may be mediated by individual neutrophils acting at vastly different levels of bactericidal efficiency, a phenomenon that may be linked to the superior blood flow and oxygenation of the muscle flap.[17,18]

Musculocutaneous flaps have considerable clinical utility because of their ability to heal and cover complex chronically infected, previously unsalvageable wounds[12,19] caused by osteomyelitis, radiation necrosis, and pressure ulcers.[18] It has been suggested that muscle-containing flaps activate neutrophils to greater bactericidal efficiency.[2] Musculocutaneous flaps have markedly better blood supply and oxygen delivery than conventional random pattern flaps.[1,12,18–21] The intracellular killing of bacteria in the presence of muscle may, therefore, be greater at the individual neutrophil level.[2,22]

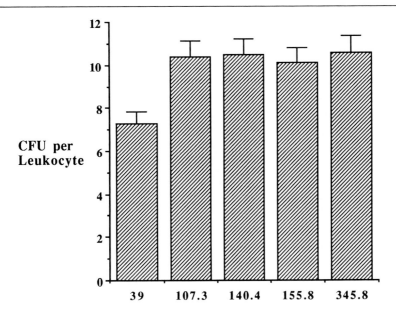

Fig. 7 *Effect of Po$_2$ on phagocytosis of tritiated bacteria by peripheral polymorphonuclear neutrophils. No detrimental effect was noted until Po$_2$ was lowered below 40 mm Hg. Results expressed as colony-forming unit ingested per polymorphonuclear neutrophils. Numbers on the horizontal axis indicate media Po$_2$.*

Cylinder Blood Flow

Data from our laboratory have shown that musculocutaneous flaps have superior dermal blood flow by the second and continuing through the fifteenth postoperative days.

The data presented here suggest that a hollow stainless steel cylinder surrounded by tissue is similar to the adjacent vascular milieu, because cylinder blood flow is similar to dermal blood flow. Because it is in equilibrium with the overlying tissue, it does not mimic an abscess (Fig. 1).

It is likely that the oxidative products released by random pattern neutrophils contribute to local tissue damage and potentiate the acidic conditions that characterize the random pattern flap, accounting for even more striking differences at the seven-day timepoint than at the three-day timepoint (see pH and Po$_2$ values for three- and seven-day timepoints). It is known that two weeks are required in a similar model before the delay phenomenon returns the random pattern flap to the level of the musculocutaneous flap,[22] so that the effects of oxidative tissue damage caused by degranulated neutrophils may exceed the restorative effects of capillary ingrowth at the seven-day timepoint tested in this study.

Neutrophil Isolation

Spurious activation of neutrophils occurs when they are subjected to experimental conditions found routinely in accepted isolation techniques.[11] Three precautions were taken to prevent this. Neutrophils were isolated at 0 C, a temperature at which neutrophil activation is temporarily halted, but the neutrophil remains undamaged. Only endotoxin-free solutions were used, as determined by the limulus assay for the presence of endotoxin, because endotoxin, a frequent contaminant of laboratory reagents, is a potent stimulant of neutrophils. All experiments requiring live neutrophils were performed expeditiously, as a permanent fall-off of neutrophil effectiveness is seen after five to six hours, in spite of unaffected Mac-1 levels. Larger numbers of neutrophils collect within random pattern cylinders than in the musculocutaneous cylinders. Similar findings have been noted in tumors, where poorly oxygenated regions of a mouse mammary adenocarcinoma are associated with larger numbers of polymorphonuclear neutrophils and other neutrophils as determined by FACS scanning techniques.[23] Neutrophils have been observed to accumulate in larger numbers in adverse wounds in heart muscle, a leukotriene-dependent function.[24] Both of these studies support our finding that increased numbers of neutrophils infiltrate a hypoxic wound.

Phorbol Myristate Acetate Stimulation

Control and phorbol myristate acetate-stimulated neutrophils were used to quantitate the reserve of the neutrophil. Stimulation with phorbol myristate acetate is a maximal leukocyte stimulus, and is believed to be analogous to maximal physiologic stimulation. The question may arise as to whether intracellular calcium measurements should be made in cells under various conditions. This is not of primary interest to this project, because the presence of intracellular calcium has been well-established as an important mediator of formyl-methionyleucyl-phenylalanine receptors and binding,[25,26] but not after stimulation with phorbol myristate acetate, which has been shown to be independent of free cytosolic calcium. Either stimulus elicits a potent activation response and upregulation of Mac-1. In our hands, the response exceeded that of formyl-methionyleucylphenylalanine, calcium ionophore, and c5a.

Chemiluminescence Data

The chemiluminescence data indicate that neutrophils appear to activate upon entry into a poorly vascularized wound. Random pattern cells activate and exhaust their reserves. Neutrophils from the well-perfused wound maintain their ability to release superoxide and lactoferrin until subsequently stimulated. It has recently been demonstrated that the partial pressure of O_2 influences in a dose-dependent fashion the myeloperoxidase pathway in neutrophils.[27] Hexose monophosphate shunt activity, hydrogen peroxide production, and hydroxyl radical production were all directly affected by the P_{O_2}. Products of the myeloperoxidase pathway, including hypochlorous acid and the so-called stable oxidants,[28,29] were inversely related to O_2 content, probably as a result of depletion of these substances at higher Po_2. Neutrophils were observed to exhibit a dramatic decrease in oxidative function at tension less than 10 torr. Areas of Po_2 in that range are encountered in many wounds.

Lactoferrin Expression

The chemiluminescence data corroborate the lactoferrin trials. More lactoferrin is expressed immediately upon entry into the wound of random pattern cells than it is for musculocutaneous-associated neutrophils, with resultant rapid depletion of random pattern lactoferrin stores.

Mac-1 (CD11b/CD18) Expression

The cell surface expression of Mac-1 receptors, complement receptors, and a newly-recognized member of the integrin family[30] are sensitive and specific indicators of the state of activation/adaptation of the neutrophil. In this study, they were assayed by monoclonal antibodies directed against antigens in the receptor. The Mac-1 receptor is also known as the C3bi receptor, the CR-3 receptor, Mo1 and (perhaps most accurately) as CD11b/CD18. The Mac-1 receptor in humans is composed of an alpha subunit (170 kd)-CD11b, which is unique to this integrin, and a beta subunit (95 kd)-CD18, which it shares with two other integrins in the same subfamily (LFA-1, gp 150/95).[31,32]

Functionally, the Mac-1 serves primarily as a complement receptor that binds to endothelial cell layers (hence its earlier name, complement receptor 3, or CR-3). Recently, it has been realized that another vital function of the Mac-1 may be to help the neutrophil adhere to such substances as fibronectin,[33] collagen, and fibrin. Mac-1 serves as an accurate indicator of neutrophil state of activation: As the neutrophil becomes successively activated, Mac-1 located within intracellular gelatinase-containing granules—or perhaps on the membranes of lactoferrin-containing (specific) granules, a source of debate—translocates by means of the cytoskeleton to the cell surface, where it can be measured with surface Mac-1 assays.

We have determined that M1–70 monoclonal antibody, which has previously been shown to be a blocking antibody for C3bi-mediated red blood cell rosetting, is actually a blocking antibody for Mac-1 adherence as well (unpublished data). It is, therefore, probable that M1–70 binds to a functional epitope on the Mac-1 glycoprotein complex. The data from the surface Mac-1 studies corroborate the findings that neutrophils activate upon entry into an adverse environment (random pattern cells) but not into a physiologic environment (musculocutaneous neutrophils). In the seven-day maximally stimulated group, more Mac-1 was present on the surface of musculocutaneous cells (p < 0.05). This finding either indicates greater loss of Mac-1 at the surface of random pattern cells or increased production of receptor by musculocutaneous cells. Protein synthesis—at least of the CD11b component of the Mac-1 glycoprotein—occurs in greater amounts in neutrophils exposed to a favorable wound environment (musculocutaneous cells) than neutrophils exposed to an unfavorable environment (random pattern).

Mac-1 Synthesis

Musculocutaneous neutrophils actually synthesize more Mac-1 than do cells in an unfavorable wound environment. This was suggested by our previous data, which reported differences in surface Mac-1[5] that were demonstrated directly in the total Mac-1 expression and in the radioactive sulfur incorporation assays. Two independent methods showed an increase in synthesis of Mac-1 of 16% to 20% in neutrophils in a well oxygenated environment. This suggests an additional advantage of the neutrophil from a favorable wound environment: an increase in the overall synthesis of Mac-1. Only synthesis of the CD11b subunit is increased; CD18 appears to be stored constitutively in large quantities, perhaps because it is shared by the other integrins CD11a/CD18 and CD11c/CD18 of the same integrin subfamily. This synthesis of Mac-1 may reflect a generally improved biosynthetic capability as a result of improved wound conditions (improved oxygen, nutrient delivery, lower acidity) or a specific ability to synthesize proteins that are later incorporated into Mac-1. It is clear, however, that cells isolated from a favorable wound milieu were more capable of synthesizing this Mac-1 subunit than were cells from a hypoxic, acidic environment (random pattern cells).

It is known that intracellular granules, possibly specific (lactoferrin-containing) granules, and possibly gelatinase-containing organelles,[34] house Mac-1 receptors.[35] With activation, these stores of receptor are translocated to the cell surface for subsequent expression on the cell surface.[36] This mechanism is not dependent on new protein synthesis (not actinomycin-D inhibitable), but is dependent on energy and an intact cytoskeleton. The kinetics of this phenomenon in different wound environments have not been well described. It has generally been assumed that all wounds are identical with respect to the behavior of their associated neutrophils, a finding this study refutes.

It has also generally been accepted that no Mac-1 is synthesized after a neutrophil is activated, but that Mac-1 is expressed from existing intracellular granules. Recently, however, it has been found that peripheral neutrophils synthesize Mac-1, together with a number of other proteins, including FcR, MHC Class I, actin, etc.,[37] and that, in general, primed, and then stimulated, neutrophils produce and express more proteins.[38] In our experiments, we have noted [35]S (sulfur-35) uptake in peripheral neutrophils when they are incubated overnight, which later becomes incorporated to some degree in Mac-1. The levels of Mac-1 measured in total cellular Mac-1 assays derived from lysed cells indicate that 20% more Mac-1 is produced in musculocutaneous-associated neutrophils than is produced by their random pattern counterparts.

Priming

A number of curious and sometimes paradoxical patterns of neutrophil function have been observed. Some studies have indicated that neutrophils can be primed, which means that prior exposure to a stimulus results in a synergistic increase in neutrophil product expression once the neutrophil is again stimulated.[39,40] This is in contrast to the modest output from a previously unstimulated neutrophil. This phenomenon has been shown to occur in wounds, in peritoneal exudate, and in peripheral neutrophils of burn and trauma patients. Neutrophils exhibit varying degrees of activation, deactivation (chemotactic deactivation), and adaptation when appropriately stimulated, but no explanation on the biochemical level adequately accounts for these widely varied and seemingly paradoxical responses.[41]

These data correlate well with data published by Paty and associates,[39] in which neutrophils that enter the wound environment exhibit the phenomenon of priming, or an improved ability to respond to subsequent stimulus. In that particular study, the rabbit was used as an experimental animal. The rabbit differs from the human in that it possesses a well-developed paniculus carnosus nourished by large axial perforators. In essence the paniculus carnosus, which is not present in humans, has its own blood supply from large axial perforators rather than from musculocutaneous sources. The rabbit skin, which has a high percentage of muscle and a separate blood supply, may function as a musculocutaneous flap. It is possible that priming reflects increased biosynthesis, which would explain the observed increase in killing capability of a mildly prestimulated neutrophil.

In Vitro pH and Po_2 Modulations

Leukocyte phagocytotic ability is decreased in unphysiologic pH and Po_2 environments. These deleterious effects of unphysiologic pH, Po_2, and prestimulation on phagocytosis have been observed in vitro and are in the same order of magnitude as that observed in neutrophils isolated from different wounds. This suggests that altered pH, Po_2, or prestimulation alone could account for the differences in phagocytotic ability observed between musculocutaneous and random pattern flap neutrophils.

Increased oxidative product release has been observed in reperfusion models where tissue is rendered hypoxic and then reperfused.[42] Oxidative product release and, therefore, depletion of granular stores, has shown to be reduced at very low Po_2[27] and is generally believed to be reduced in a dose-dependent fashion with decreasing oxygen tension. Low pH has been associated with other polymorphonuclear neutrophil defects, such as decreased migration.[43] These findings are all consistent with our findings of the defects in polymorphonuclear neutrophil function in adverse wound environments, and the greater accumulation of neutrophils in the adverse wound environment.

Conclusions

Chronic wounds are characterized by a low pH and Po_2. The wound model presented in this study collects a transudative fluid rich in neutrophils.

Whole cellular Mac-1 expression (and increased Mac-1 synthesis as determined by radioactive sulphur incorporation and total cellular Mac-1 determinations) occurred in musculocutaneous-associated cells. This correlates with our previous findings that superoxide anion expression, lactoferrin expression, and surface Mac-1 expression were altered in cells from an unfavorable wound environment (the random pattern wounds), which exhibited premature (and inappropriate) activation and degranulation, compared to neutrophils from a physiologic musculocutaneous wound environment.

Peripheral (control) neutrophils, when individually subjected to the variables of low pH, low Po_2, and prestimulation with phorbol myristate acetate, all exhibit decreases in phagocytic function similar in magnitude to those found in the poorly perfused random pattern wound environment. This suggests that unphysiologic pH, Po_2, or prestimulation alone can account for the differences in phagocytic function observed in vivo in the adverse wound.

It appears that the neutrophil is not predestined to degranulate in a formulaic manner, but is modulated in its behavior by the wound environment it enters. A poorly perfused wound is associated with activated neutrophils that have impaired bactericidal killing reserves, phagocytic function, and protein synthesis. Control peripheral cells subjected in vitro to hypoxia, acidity, or prestimulation all demonstrate decrements in phagocytic function similar in magnitude to those observed in vivo. Unphysiologic pH and po_2 are sufficient to explain the phenomena of premature activation and decreased phagocytosis observed in neutrophils of poorly perfused wounds.

Acknowledgment

Funding for this study was provided through the Marion-Surgical Infection Society prize and the Paralyzed Veterans of America.

References

1. Mathes SJ, Nahai F (eds): *Clinical Applications for Muscle and Musculocutaneous Flaps.* St. Louis, CV Mosby, 1982.
2. Eshima I, Mathes SJ, Paty P: Comparison of the intracellular bacterial killing activity of leukocytes in musculocutaneous and random-pattern flaps. *Plast Reconstr Surg* 1990;86:541–547.
3. Davis JM, Dineen P, Gallin JI: Neutrophil degranulation and abnormal chemotaxis after thermal injury. *J Immunol* 1980;124:1467–1471.
4. Douglas B, Weinberg H, Song Y, et al: Beneficial effects of ibuprofen on experimental microvascular free flaps: Pharmacologic alteration of the noreflow phenomenon. *Plast Reconstr Surg* 1987;79:366–374.
5. May JW Jr, Chait LA, O'Brien BM, et al: The no-reflow phenomenon in experimental free flaps. *Plast Reconstr Surg* 1978;61:256–267.

6. Turner RA, Schumacher R, Myers AR: Phagocytic function of polymorphonuclear leukocytes in rheumatic diseases. *J Clin Invest* 1973;52:1632–1635.

7. Knighton DR, Halliday B, Hunt TK: Oxygen as an antibiotic: The effect of inspired oxygen on infection. *Arch Surg* 1984;119:199–204.

8. Van Epps DE, Garcia ML: Enhancement of neutrophils function as a result of prior exposure to chemotactic factor. *J Clin Invest* 1980;66:167–175.

9. Moelleken BRW, Amerhauser A, Mathes SJ, et al: Adverse wound environments activate leukocytes prematurely. Presented at the 10th Annual Meeting of the Surgical Infection Society, Cincinnati, OH, 1990.

10. Zimmerli W, Seligmann B, Gallin JI: Exudation primes human and guinea pig neutrophils for subsequent responsiveness to the chemotactic peptide N-formylmethionylleucylphenylalanine and increases complement component C3bi receptor expression. *J Clin Invest* 1986;77:925–933.

11. Fyfe A, Holme ER, Zoma A, et al: C3b receptor (CR1) expression on the polymorphonuclear leukocytes from patients with systemic lupus erythematosus. *Clin Exp Immunol* 1987;67:300–308.

12. Mathes SJ, Feng LJ, Hunt TK: Coverage of the infected wound. *Ann Surg* 1983;198:420–429.

13. Altieri DC, Edgington TS: A monoclonal antibody reacting with distinct adhesion molecules defines a transition in the functional state of the receptor CD11b/CD18 (Mac-1). *J Immunol* 1988;141:2656–2660.

14. Moelleken BRW, Mathes SJ, Amerhauser A, et al: An adverse wound environment activates leukocytes prematurely. *Arch Surg*, 1991;126:225–231.

15. Davis LG, Dibner MD, Battey JF: *Basic Methods in Molecular Biology.* New York, Elsevier, 1986, pp 302–305.

16. Trezzini C, Jungi TW, Kuhnert P, et al: Fibrogen association with human monocytes: Evidence for constitutive expression of fibrinogen receptors and for involvement of Mac-1 (CD18, CR 3) in the binding. *Biochem Biophys Res Commun* 1988;156:477–484.

17. Jönsson K, Hunt TK, Mathes SJ: Oxygen as an isolated variable influences resistance to infection. *Ann Surg* 1988;208:783–787.

18. Gottrup F, Firmin R, Hunt TK, et al: The dynamic properties of tissue oxygen in healing flaps. *Surgery* 1984;95:527–536.

19. Mathes SJ, Alpert BS, Chang N: Use of the muscle flap in chronic osteomyelitis: Experimental and clinical correlation. *Plast Reconstr Surg* 1982;69:815–829.

20. Hunt TK, Twomey P, Zederfeldt B, et al: Respiratory gas tensions and pH in healing wounds. *Am J Surg* 1967;114:302–307.

21. Calderon W, Chang N, Mathes SJ: Comparison of the effect of bacterial inoculation in musculocutaneous and fasciocutaneous flaps. *Plast Reconstr Surg* 1986;77:785–794.

22. Jonsson K, Hunt TK, Brennan SS, et al: Tissue oxygen measurements in delayed skin flaps: A reconsideration of the mechanisms of the delay phenomenon. *Plast Reconstr Surg* 1988;82:328–336.

23. Loeffler DA, Keng PC, Baggs RB, et al: Lymphocytic infiltration and cytotoxicity under hypoxic conditions in the EMT6 mouse mammary tumor. *Int J Cancer* 1990;45:462–467.

24. Gillespie MN, Kojima S, Owasoyo JO, et al: Hypoxia provokes leukotriene-dependent neutrophil sequestration in perfused rabbit hearts. *J Pharmacol Exp Ther* 1987;241:812–816.

25. Anderson DC, Springer TA: Leukocyte adhesion deficiency: An inherited defect in the Mac-1, LFA-1, and p150,95 glycoproteins. *Annu Rev Med* 1987;38:175–194.

26. Andersson T, Dahlgren C, Lew PD, et al: Cell surface expression of fMet-Leu-Phe receptors on human neutrophils: Correlation to changes in the cytosolic free Ca^{2+} level and action of phorbol myristate acetate. *J Clin Invest* 1987;79:1226–1233.

27. Davis WB, Husney RM, Wewers MD, et al: Effect of O_2 partial pressure on the myeloperoxidase pathway of neutrophils. *J Appl Physiol* 1988;65:1995–2003.

28. Grisham MB, Jefferson MM, Melton DF, et al: Chlorination of endogenous amines by isolated neutrophils: Ammonia-dependent bactericidal, cytotoxic, and cytolytic activities of the chloramines. *J Biol Chem* 1984;259:10404–10413.

29. Grisham MB, Jefferson MM, Thomas EL: Role of monochloramine in the oxidation of erythrocyte hemoglobin by stimulated neutrophils. *J Biol Chem* 1984;259:6757–6765.

30. Pytela R: Amino acid sequence of the murine Mac-1 alpha chain reveals homology with the integrin family and an additional domain related to von Willebrand factor. *EMBO J* 1988;7:1371–1378.

31. Altieri DC, Morrissey JH, Edgington TS: Adhesive receptor Mac-1 coordinates the activation of factor X on stimulated cells of monocytic and myeloid differentiation: An alternative initiation of the coagulation protease cascade. *Proc Natl Acad Sci USA* 1988;85:7462–7466.

32. Pytela R, Pierschbacher MD, Ruoslahti E: Identification and isolation of a 140 kd cell surface glycoprotein with properties expected of a fibronectin receptor. *Cell* 1985;40:191–198.

33. Altieri DC, Bader R, Mannucci PM, et al: Oligospecificity of the cellular adhesion receptor Mac-1 encompasses an inducible recognition specificity for fibrinogen. *J Cell Biol* 1988;107:1893–1900.

34. Petrequin PR, Todd RF III, Devall LJ, et al: Association between gelatinase release and increased plasma membrane expression of the Mo1 glycoprotein. *Blood* 1987;69:605–610.

35. O'Shea JJ, Brown EJ, Seligmann BE, et al: Evidence for distinct intracellular pools of receptors for C3b and C3bi in human neutrophils. *J Immunol* 1985;134:2580–2587.

36. Wright DG, Gallin JI: Secretory responses of human neutrophils: Exocytosis of specific (secondary) granules by human neutrophils during adherence in vitro and during exudation in vivo. *J Immunol* 1979;123:285–294.

37. Jack RM, Fearon DT: Selective synthesis of mRNA and proteins by human peripheral blood neutrophils. *J Immunol* 1988;140:4286–4293.

38. Hughes V, Humphreys JM, Edwards SW: Protein synthesis is activated in primed neutrophils: A possible role in inflammation. *Biosci Rep* 1987;7:881–890.

39. Paty PB, Graeff RW, Waldman FM, et al: Biologic priming of neutrophils in subcutaneous wounds. *Arch Surg* 1988;123:1509–1513.

40. Paty PB, Graeff RW, Mathes SJ, et al: Superoxide production by wound neutrophils: Evidence for increased activity of the NADPH oxidase. *Arch Surg* 1990;125:65–69.

41. Zimmerli W, Lew PD, Cohen HJ, et al: Comparative superoxide-generating system of granulocytes from blood and peritoneal exudates. *Infect Immun* 1984;46:625–630.

42. Iwai A, Itoh M, Yokoyama Y, et al: Role of PAF in ischemia-reperfusion injury in the rat stomach. *Scand J Gastroenterol* 1989;162(suppl):63–66.

43. Rotstein OD, Fiegel VD, Simmons RL, et al: The deleterious effect of reduced pH and hypoxia on neutrophil migration in vitro. *J Surg Res* 1988;45:298–303.

Chapter 26

Pathophysiology of Osteomyelitis and Pharmacokinetics of Antimicrobial Agents in Normal and Osteomyelitic Bone

Robert H. Fitzgerald, Jr., MD
Joseph L. Whalen, MD, PhD
Steve A. Petersen, MD

Overview

Musculoskeletal sepsis, whether acute hematogenous osteomyelitis, a posttraumatic infection, or a postoperative prosthetic infection, has proven to be one of the more difficult disease processes to treat. Until recently, failure to understand the pathophysiology has hampered the development of innovative medical and surgical therapy. In acute hematogenous osteomyelitis, the failure of tissue-based phagocytes appears to be critical to the development of a significant infection. Although previous investigators have suggested that antimicrobial agents could not achieve therapeutic concentrations in normal or infected osseous tissue, recent experimentation suggests otherwise. The efficacy of a local muscle flap in the treatment of musculoskeletal infections relates not only to its ability to obliterate dead space but also to its ability to enhance the local blood supply during the healing process.

Acute Hematogenous Osteomyelitis

The metaphyseal ends of diaphyseal bones are the most common site of acute hematogenous osteomyelitis. Various investigators have suggested possible mechanisms—both anatomic and physiologic—to explain why this disease process so often occurs in the growth plate.[1,2] The failure of numerous investigators to develop a representative animal model hampered the development of an understanding of the pathophysiology of the disease process. Morrissy and associates[3] have developed an animal model in the rabbit that closely resembles the human disease process. These investigators created microscopic fractures of the physis, which altered its susceptibility to the development of an infection. Whalen and associates,[4] using light microscopy and ultrastructural techniques further characterized this model. These investigators were able to confirm that vascular loops, with a hairpin curve connecting the capillary and venule, do not exist. Instead, the capillaries that extend into the growth plate have both a variable con-

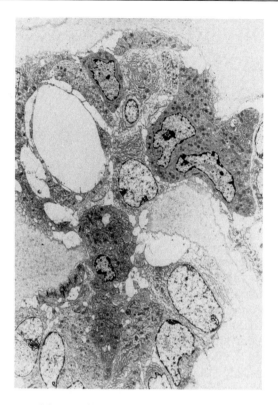

Fig. 1 *Cross-section of the vascular invasion of the cartilage columns. Macrophages associated with the endothelium of the invading capillary are removing a portion of the cartilage.*

tinuous and a discontinuous endothelium. Numerous tissue-based pericytes and cells that resemble macrophages were identified (Fig. 1). In the area of vascular invasion into the terminal cartilage cells of the physis, the capillary endothelium was invariably discontinuous, with extravasation of red blood cells into the extravascular space. Most notably these investigators described a consistent absence of circulating white blood cell granulocytes between the trabeculae of the primary spongiosa. This is in contrast to an abundance of neutrophils, eosinophils, basophils, and their precursors between the trabeculae of the secondary spongiosa in the lower portion of the metaphysis. Monocytes were observed in the loose connective tissue of the terminal vessels near the growth plate. In the primary spongiosa, therefore, protection from bacterial invasion rests with the tissue-based macrophages.

When a systemic bacteremia was created in the Morrissy rabbit model with a concomitant microscopic physical injury, osteomyelitis invariably occurred.[4] In physes not traumatized, bacteria were seen within the first 24 hours; but bacteria were not seen microscopically or recovered from tissue specimens incubated aerobically at any subsequent time period, and the animals did not develop any evidence of osteomyelitis. In contrast, in animals with a microscopic physeal injury, bacteria could be seen microscopically and isolated from clinical specimens from the proximal tibial physis beginning four hours following a bacteremia. The latter group of animals developed the characteristic clinical and roentgenographic findings consistent with osteomyelitis.

In the animals with a microscopic injury to the growth plate and a bacteremia the sequence of microscopic alterations exhibited a consistent pattern. Although an occasional neutrophil was observed in the terminal capillaries adjacent to the growth plate and extravasated red blood cells were present in the area of the microscopic injury to the physis, no free or phagocytosed bacteria were observed in the terminal capillaries, in the surrounding extravascular tissue, or in the void that was created by the injury (Fig. 2). The metaphyseal architecture revealed minor distortion and cellular debris where the injury had extended into the zone of vascular invasion, but was otherwise normal when examined four hours after injury and bacteremia. Again, no free or phagocytosed bacteria were observed in the metaphysis four hours after injury. In a few animals there was evidence of an inflammatory response within the metaphysis at 24 hours. However, by 48 hours following injury and a bacteremia, there was macroscopic and microscopic evidence of sepsis. With light microscopy, extensive necrosis of the primary spongiosa was observed, with numerous free bacteria between the bony trabeculae (Fig. 3). Inflammatory cells were distinctly absent. More distally, in the secondary spongiosa, an inflammatory reaction with neutrophil phagocytosis of bacteria was observed.

One week following injury and bacteremia, the inflammatory process extended from the diaphysis to the epiphysis. A monocytic infiltration resembling histocytes in a fibrovascular stroma replaced the normal cellular architecture of the metaphysis (Fig. 4). Isolated nests of neutrophils were also present. The primary and secondary spongiosa were replaced by granulation tissue, except for a few islands of calcified cartilage and osteoid that were being resorbed by osteoclasts. Phagocytosis of bacteria by mononuclear macrophages was evident. Neutrophils were present in large numbers in the area of the injury. Osteoclastic phagocytosis of cellular debris but not of bacteria was also observed.

These experiments document alteration of the host defense mechanisms in the proximal tibia by microscopic trauma to the physis.[4] The exact mechanisms have as yet to be defined. The cells responsible for phagocytosis of bacteria in the nontraumatized animal remain to be identified, because no evidence of bacteria or phagocytosis was identified during the first 24 hours even with ultrastructural techniques. The bacteria were most likely few in number and eluded detection in spite of a careful and tedious search. A new labeling technique has been developed that should help to determine whether tissue-based

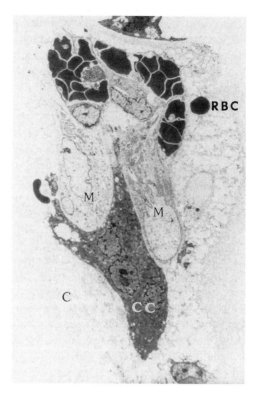

Fig. 2 *Electron micrograph of the proximal part of the tibia of a Group-IV rabbit, made four hours after physeal injury and bacterial seeding. The location is the terminal vascular zone, adjacent to the last transverse septum, distal to the lowermost hypertrophic chondrocyte (C). Red blood cells (RBC) can be seen extravascularly and packed within the terminal vessel. Two tissue-based macrophages (M) and a chondroclast (CC) are identified. No bacteria were observed after four hours (× 1500). (Reproduced with permission from Whalen JL, Fitzgerald RH Jr, Morrissy RT: A histological study of acute hematogenous osteomyelitis following physeal injuries in rabbits. J Bone Joint Surg 1988;70A:1386.)*

macrophages or other cells are responsible for the elimination of the invading bacteria.

Pharmacokinetics of Antimicrobial Agents in Normal and Osteomyelitic Bone

In the recent past, the ability to determine the distribution of antibiotics in various tissues—notably serum, urine, and spinal fluid—has been expanded by the development of bioassay techniques.[5] These techniques have not been applied to osseous tissue. Techniques used for assay of bone include: (1) assay of aliquots of a phosphate buffer in which fragments of bone have been agitated; (2) assay of a slurry

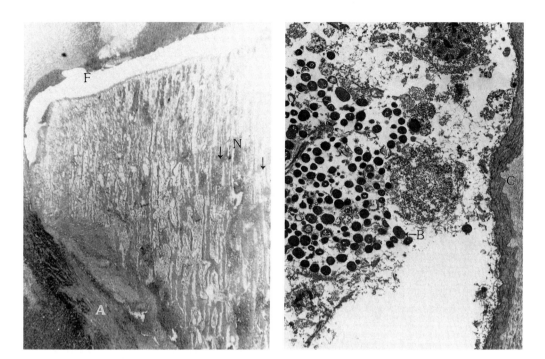

Fig. 3 *Micrographs of the proximal part of the tibia of a group-IV rabbit, made after 48 hours.* **Left,** *The arrows in this light micrograph indicate the advancing front of inflammatory cells. A zone of necrosis of tissue (N), which lacked inflammatory cells, is located below the injured area (F). A posterior subperiosteal abscess (A) can be seen in the lower left corner (× 16).* **Right,** *Electron micrograph of the upper part of the metaphysis in the zone of necrosis indicated in Figure 3,* **left.** *Free bacteria (B) occupy the spaces between cartilage columns (C). Note the loss of vessels and the cellular necrosis (× 3750). (Reproduced with permission from Whalen JL, Fitzgerald RH Jr, Morrissy RT: A histological study of acute hematogenous osteomyelitis following physeal injuries in rabbits.* J Bone Joint Surg *1988;70A:1388.)*

created by the mechanical crushing of bone, which is then added to a buffer solution; and (3) the assay of core specimens of cortical-cancellous bone placed on bacteria-laden plates.[6–8] Qualitative data have been obtained by using one or more of these techniques. Unfortunately, the data generated have not been consistent and have resulted in conflicting recommendations as to the application of various agents to the musculoskeletal system. Laboratory evaluation and in vivo animal experiments with several classes of agents have documented that antimicrobial agents can enter the interstitial fluid space of normal and osteomyelitic osseous tissue in concentrations equivalent to that obtained in serum under steady state conditions.[9–12]

Using triple tracer techniques it is possible to determine the quantity of a radioactive-labeled antibiotic entering normal or osteomyelitic bone (Fig. 5). These experiments document that, in the canine tibia,

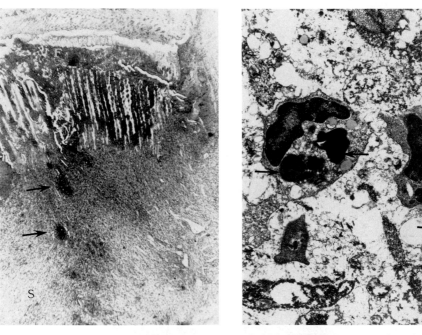

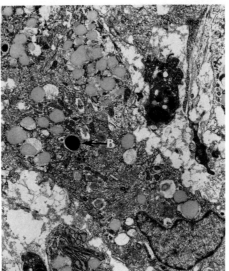

Fig. 4 *Micrographs of a group-IV rabbit made after seven days.* **Top left**, *Low-power light micrograph showing extensive destruction of tissue and subperiosteal reactive-bone formation. F = injured area. A fibrovascular stroma (S) occupies most of the metaphysis and epiphysis, and there are islands of inflammatory cells (arrows) and remnants of primary spongiosa (P) (× 16).* **Bottom**, *Electron micrograph of a macrophage containing a phagocytosed bacterium (B) in the fibrovascular tissue stroma in the metaphysis (× 5000).* **Top right**, *Electron micrograph of the injured area, showing phagocytosed bacteria (arrows) within neutrophils. Note the variable morphology, as seen in the control bacterial pellet. (Reproduced with permission from Whalen JL, Fitzgerald RH Jr, Morrissy RT: A histological study of acute hematogenous osteomyelitis following physeal injuries in rabbits.* J Bone Joint Surg *1988;70A:1389.)*

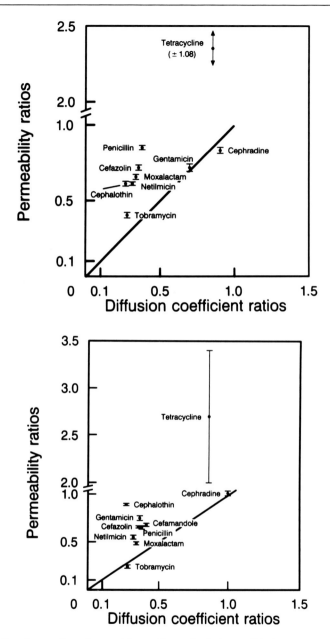

Fig. 5 *Top, Permeation of normal bone. For each of nine antibiotic agents, ratio of permeation by agent to permeation by sucrose (or strontium) is compared with ratio of diffusion coefficients of agent and of sucrose (or strontium). Each permeability ratio is essentially equal to or slightly greater than the corresponding diffusion-coefficient ratio, indicating that all agents studied are able to cross osseous capillary membrane. Each data point represents mean and standard deviation of at least five experiments. Bottom, Permeation of osteomyelitic tissue. Some ratios differ slightly from same-agent ratios in top figure. Data indicate that all agents studied are able to traverse the capillary membrane of osteomyelitic bone. Each data point represents mean and standard deviation of 4 to 11 experiments.*

the agents studied were able to leave the nutrient artery and its subsequent tributaries. Although these experiments did not address distribution in either normal or osteomyelitic tibias, they did define subtle differences in the passage of antibiotics from the capillary of bone. Five of the Beta-lactam agents studied—penicillin, cephalothin, cefazolin, cefamandole, and moxalactam—crossed the capillary membrane slightly more rapidly than could be explained by passive diffusion. The data suggest that the primary mode of transcapillary passage of these agents is through the intercellular pores. The lipophilic nature of these agents at physiologic pH may also allow them to pass through the proteinaceous material that lines the spaces and, possibly, through the intracytoplasmic vesicular system.

Cephradine exhibited an extraction pattern different from that of the other Beta-lactam agents. The permeability and diffusion coefficient ratio was unity, suggesting cephradine crossed the capillary membrane in a purely passive fashion. Cephradine is the only Beta-lactam agent which is a zwiterion (containing both an alkaline amino group and an acidic carboxy group) and exhibits lower protein binding (5% versus 80% or more for the other cephalosporins). These chemical and physiologic properties are most likely responsible for its altered capillary transport.

The three aminoglycosides studied—gentamicin, tobramycin, and netilmicin—varied in their ease of passage across the capillary membrane. Gentamicin crossed the capillary membrane of the osteomyelitic canine tibia in a passive fashion. In contrast, transcapillary passage of netilmicin and tobramycin in the canine tibia occurred more readily than could be explained by passive diffusion. These agents appeared to pass through the intercellular clefts and the intracytoplasmic vesicular system. In the normal canine tibia, gentamicin crossed the capillary membrane in a fashion similar to that of netilmicin. However, in osteomyelitic bone, its transcapillary passage was purely passive.

The variable behavior of gentamicin, which is composed of three molecules (C, C_{1a}, and C_2), probably reflects its molecular composition. All three molecules are heavily hydrated. The remaining two aminoglycosides are larger molecules than the Beta-lactam agents.

The extraction of tetracycline reflected the deposition of this agent into osteoid. It appeared to pass through the intercellular pores of the capillary membrane and intracytoplasmic vesicular system. There was no evidence of any impediment to the transcapillary passage of this agent.

The Beta-lactam agents and aminoglycosides are capable of traversing the capillary membrane of both normal and osteomyelitic bone without difficulty. Thus, in contrast to the bone-blood barrier proposed by Verwey and associates,[5] it can be concluded that there is no physiologic bone-blood barrier to the passage of antibiotics from the vascular system to interstitial fluid.[5]

Volume-of-distribution studies are used to analyze the distribution of substances within the various fluid spaces of normal and osteomyelitic bone. When studies testing the volume of distribution of Beta-

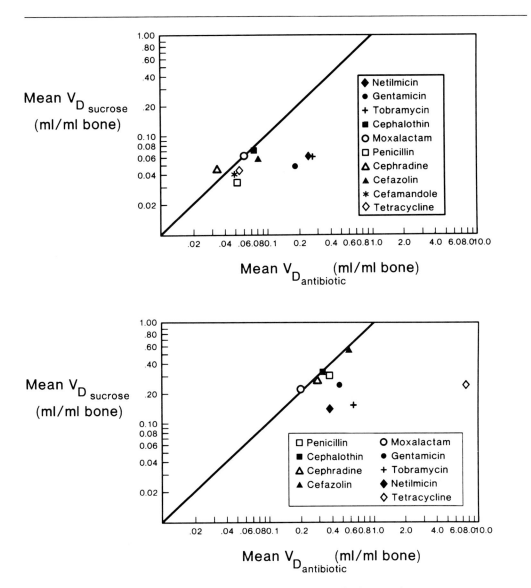

Fig. 6 *Top, Distribution in fluid spaces of normal cortical bone. Each of ten antibiotic agents is compared with sucrose.* **Bottom,** *Distribution in fluid spaces of osteomyelitic cortical bone. Each of nine antibiotic agents is compared with sucrose.*

lactam agents, aminoglycosides, and tetracyclines were performed, results showed the same variability (Fig. 6). In both normal and osteomyelitic bone, the Beta-lactam agents had a volume of distribution similar to that of sucrose. Because sucrose is limited to the extracellular fluid space of bone, the data imply that these agents are distributed within the extracellular fluid compartments of osseous tissue—the plasma and the interstitial fluid spaces.

The volume of distribution of the aminoglycoside agents exceeded that of sucrose. In normal cortical bone, these agents had a volume of distribution equivalent to the exchangeable water space of cortical bone (Fig. 6, *top*). In osteomyelitic cortical bone, gentamicin and netilmicin had volumes of distribution that were similar to the exchangeable water space (Fig. 6, *bottom*). Tobramycin had a volume of distribution one and one-half times the exchangeable water space of osteomyelitic bone, indicating that this agent was accumulating in one or more of the fluid spaces. These data suggested that the aminoglycosides were entering not only the extracellular fluid spaces but the cellular fluid spaces as well. Because the toxic side effects of these agents are created intracellularly, it is not surprising to find physiologic data supporting an intracellular distribution in normal and infected osseous tissue. In summary, the volume-of-distribution studies document that all of the agents studied are able to enter the interstitial fluid space of both normal and infected osseous tissue.

The use of an isotope assay makes it possible to calculate the concentration of antibiotics in the various fluid spaces of neuromonosteomyelytic bone. These concentrations were compared with serum concentrations determined at the same time by such readily available techniques as bioassay, high pressure liquid chromatographic assay, and immunoassay. The relationships between the interstitial fluid concentration and the simultaneous serum concentration showed a close correlation in most experiments (Fig. 7).

The interstitial fluid concentration of the Beta-lactam agents in normal osteomyelitic bone agreed with the serum concentration. The minor variations observed were within the limitations of the techniques. Except for tobramycin, the aminoglycoside agents had a similar relationship. For tobramycin, the variance related to the unusually large dose administered. In osteomyelitic bone, gentamicin seemed to concentrate in either interstitial fluid space, cellular fluid space, or both. The elevated serum and interstitial fluid levels of tobramycin reflect the high specificity and biologic activity of the labelled agent. The high concentrations of tetracycline in bone reflect its ability to be deposited in areas of new bone formation.

Under steady state conditions, the serum concentrations of antimicrobial agents reflect the interstitial fluid concentrations. Factors other than bone concentration should dictate the selection of an agent used to prevent and treat musculoskeletal infections. Other factors that should be evaluated include the potential for toxicity and activity against the causal organism, based on in vitro activity, susceptibility testing, and cost.

Physiologic Impact of a Local Muscle Flap on Osteomyelitic Bone

During the acute stages of the infectious process, the flow of blood through osteomyelitic bone increases. Subsequently, varying degrees

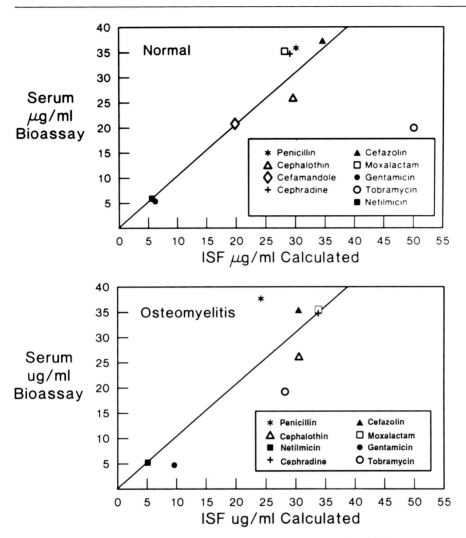

Fig. 7 *Top, Antibiotic concentrations in serum and in interstitial-space fluid (ISF) of normal bone (nine antibiotic agents: serum concentrations by bioassay, ISF concentrations calculated). Except for tobramycin, correlation is close. The dose of tobramycin was inordinately high and possibly led to concentrations in one or more of the fluid spaces. Each data point represents the mean of five experiments. Bottom, Antibiotic concentrations in serum and in interstitial-fluid space (ISF) of osteomyelitic tissue (eight antibiotic agents: serum concentrations by bioassay, ISF concentrations calculated). ISF concentrations match serum concentrations, except for penicillin. Each data point represents the mean of five experiments.*

of reduced blood flow have been reported. Although successful treatment of osteomyelitis with surgery and antimicrobial therapy restores the blood flow, it never returns to normal levels. The addition of a local muscle flap to the surgical therapy enhances a local bone-blood flow, which can improve the local host defense in the delivery of anti-microbial agents.

Treuta and Morgan[13] demonstrated that chronic osteomyelitis is more an ischemic disease of bone than an infectious problem of bone. Histologic examination of chronic osteomyelitis demonstrates a pre-dominance of fibrotic scar with minimal vascular tissue. Intermedul-lary oxygen tension measurements are markedly decreased in osseous sepsis, suggesting an unfavorable environment for healing. An is-chemic environment may be responsible for the chronicity of osseous infections, because the organisms responsible are known to survive in avascular and marginally vascularized tissues. The vascularity of bone appears to be a critical factor influencing the outcome of any therapy for osseous infections.

Twenty-seven adult mongrel dogs were studied following the crea-tion of osteomyelitis of the right proximal tibia. Twelve weeks after creation of the infection, the animals were randomly assigned to one of three groups. The first group of animals was treated with surgical debridement, a local muscle flap, and four weeks of parenteral gen-tamicin therapy. The second group was treated with debridement and four weeks of parenteral gentamicin therapy. The third group of ani-mals received no treatment and served as controls. Sixteen weeks after the initiation of treatment (28 weeks after creation of the infection), 85 strontium microspheres were administered, providing an accurate measurement of osseous blood flow. The animals were sacrificed im-mediately after microsphere measurement of blood flow, using pre-viously detailed techniques.[14] Ten of the eleven dogs treated with de-bridement, insertion of a local muscle flap, and four weeks of parenteral gentamicin therapy had no evidence of infection. Five of seven animals treated with debridement and four weeks of parenteral gentamicin therapy had eradication of their infectious process. All animals in the untreated control group had microbiologic, histologic, and roentgen-ographic evidence of osteomyelitis. Blood flow in the right tibias of those animals of group 1 was statistically greater ($P > 0.005$, paired Student's T-test) than in the unoperated left tibia. In contrast, the blood flow to the right proximal tibia in those animals successfully treated with surgical debridement without a local muscle flap (group 2) was no different from that measured in the unoperated left tibia ($P < 0.05$ paired Student's T-test).

Recent experience from multiple orthopaedic centers suggests a high incidence of eradication of osteomyelitis with the use of a local muscle flap.[15,16] Fitzgerald and associates[17] previously substantiated a high de-gree of success in the treatment of chronic osteomyelitis with the use of local muscle flap with two or more years of followup evaluation.[17]

The virtues of a local muscle flap in the treatment of osteomyelitis have been thought to be multifactorial. It has been suggested that a local muscle flap enhances healing through osseous revascularization as well as through obliteration of dead space. In this study, blood flow measurements with 85 strontium microspheres support the contention that a muscle flap improves local blood flow. Those dogs successfully treated with a local muscle flap had tibial blood flows that remained significantly higher than those of their contralateral unoperated tibias.

References

1. Trueta J: The three types of acute haematogenous osteomyelitis: A clinical and vascular study. *J Bone Joint Surg* 1959;41B:671–680.

2. Hobo T: Zur Pathogenese der akuten haematogenen Osteomyelitis, mit Berucksichtigung der Vitalfarbungslehre. *Acta Schol Med Univ Imper Kioto* 1921;4:1–29.

3. Morrissy RT, Haynes DW, Nelson CL: Acute hematogenous osteomyelitis: The role of trauma in a reproducible model. *Trans Orthop Res Soc* 1980;5:324.

4. Whalen JL, Fitzgerald RH Jr, Morrissy RT: A histological study of acute hematogenous osteomyelitis following physeal injuries in rabbits. *J Bone Joint Surg* 1988;70A:1383–1392.

5. Verwey WF, Willams HR Jr, Kalsow C: Penetration of chemotherapeutic agents into tissues. *Antimicrob Agents Chemother* 1965;5:1016–1024.

6. Smilack JD, Flittie WH, Wiliams TW Jr: Bone concentrations of antimicrobial agents after parenteral administration. *Antimicrob Agents Chemother* 1976;9:169–171.

7. Cunha BA, Gossling HR, Pasternak HS, et al: The penetration characteristics of cefazolin, cephalothin, and cephradine into bone in patients undergoing total hip replacement. *J Bone Joint Surg* 1977;59A:856–859.

8. Kolczun MC, Nelson CL, McHenry MC, et al: Antibiotic concentrations in human bone: A preliminary report. *J Bone Joint Surg* 1974;56A:305–310.

9. Bloom JD, Fitzgerald RH Jr, Washington JA II, et al: The transcapillary passage and interstitial fluid concentrations of penicillin in canine bone. *J Bone Joint Surg* 1980;62A:1168–1175.

10. Lunke RJ, Fitzgerald RH Jr, Washington JA II: Pharmacokinetics of cefamandole in osseous tissue. *Antimicrob Agents Chemother* 1981;19:851–858.

11. Fitzgerald RH: Antibiotic distribution in normal and osteomyelitic bone. *Orthop Clin North Am* 1984;15:537–546.

12. Daly RC, Fitzgerald RH Jr, Washington JA II: Penetration of cefazolin into normal and osteomyelitic canine cortical bone. *Antimicrob Agents Chemother* 1982;22:461–469.

13. Trueta J, Morgan JD: The vascular contribution to osteogenesis: I. Studies by the injection method. *J Bone Joint Surg* 1960;42B:97–109.

14. Heymann MA, Payne BD, Hoffman JIE, et al: Blood flow measurements with radionuclide-labeled particles. *Prog Cardiovasc Dis* 1977;20:55–79.

15. Ger R: Muscle transposition for treatment and prevention of chronic post-traumatic osteomyelitis of the tibia. *J Bone Joint Surg* 1977;59A:784–791.

16. Mathes SJ, Nahai F: *Clinical Atlas of Muscle and Musculocutaneous Flaps.* St. Louis, CV Mosby, 1979.

17. Fitzgerald RH Jr, Ruttle PE, Arnold PG, et al: Local muscle flaps in the treatment of chronic osteomyelitis. *J Bone Joint Surg* 1985;67A:175–185.

Chapter 27

Osteomyelitis: Lessons Learned From Animal Models and Clinical Application

Carl W. Norden, MD

In this chapter, important clinical issues in the treatment of osteo-myelitis will be discussed. Although osteomyelitis is an old disease, there have been relatively few advances in the understanding of certain aspects of therapy. The apparent failure of antimicrobial agents in chronic osteomyelitis is not easy to understand when compared with the success of these drugs in so many other infections. Clinical research has been difficult because of the marked variability of the disease and the important role of surgical treatment. In this chapter, certain aspects of research with animal models that have mimicked the human disease will be reviewed, which may offer insights into these problems.[1]

Before doing that, it is important to review information regarding osteomyelitis therapy. Excellent clinical studies[2] have established that a three-week course of antimicrobial therapy is effective in acute os-teomyelitis, and that this therapy may be either parenteral or oral as long as there are effective levels of antimicrobial agents in serum.[3] In contrast, the definition of "optimal therapy" for chronic osteomyelitis is unclear. The critical duration of therapy and the relative efficacy of various types of microbial agents are unknown. The significance of the penetration of agents into bone and "bone levels" is beyond the scope of this chapter, but further information is necessary in this area. The value of measuring serum bactericidal titers in chronic osteomyelitis is still uncertain. Perhaps most disturbing is the uncertainty about the prognosis of chronic osteomyelitis, which may be a lifelong disease.[4] How can "cure" be defined for such a disease?

Lessons Learned From Experimental Models

A brief review of the history of experimental osteomyelitis models is in order. The first experimental infection of bone was performed by Rodet,[5] who injected *Staphylococcus aureus* into rabbits and produced bone abscesses. These observations were extended by Lexer[6] who re-duced the amount of bacteria injected so that he could keep animals alive and allow bone changes to develop. An important observation subsequently made by Scheman and associates[7] was that in order to produce osteomyelitis it was necessary to injure the bone and then proceed with injection of bacteria; prior efforts that involved inoculation of bacteria directly or intravenously into uninjured bone failed to produce osteomyelitis and usually resulted in death of the animal.

A model was developed in 1970 that involved the intramedullary injection of sodium morrhuate, a sclerosing agent, and then *S aureus*.[8] This model has produced progressive osteomyelitis in all rabbits so infected and has also been used for the study of infection of bone with *Pseudomonas aeruginosa*.

This rabbit model of chronic osteomyelitis has been used to examine the effects of treatment with different antimicrobial agents. A series of observations has been made[1] and can be summarized as follows: (1) Penicillin or cephalosporin therapy, given for four weeks, has generally not been effective in treating experimental osteomyelitis caused by *S aureus*. (2) In single-agent therapy against *S aureus*, the most effective agent has been clindamycin. (3) Vancomycin has been ineffective in the treatment of experimental osteomyelitis caused by *S aureus*. (4) Rifampin, in conjunction with another agent active against *S aureus*, was highly effective when administered for either two weeks or four weeks. (5) The results of tests for synergism, where rifampin was one element of the combination, have not been predictive of the success of therapy in the experimental model. This is probably because the function of the second agent is to kill rifampin-resistant organisms and this action is not predicted as synergism by classic methods (checkerboard or time-kill curves). (6) Therapy with ciprofloxacin or ofloxacin has been extremely effective in the treatment of experimental osteomyelitis resulting from *P aeruginosa*; therapy with penicillins and aminoglycosides has not.

What characteristics might explain the success of clindamycin, rifampin, and quinolones in treating experimental osteomyelitis resulting from *S aureus* or *P aeruginosa*? One quality that all three drugs share is their ability to penetrate macrophages. I believe that this quality is of more than theoretical importance because *S aureus* can take up residence within macrophages and be protected from the action of antimicrobial agents that do not penetrate well into macrophages (such as penicillins and cephalosporins).

Can results from animal models be extrapolated and verified by clinical trials? In a multicenter trial that compared rifampin and nafcillin with nafcillin alone in the treatment of chronic staphylococcal osteomyelitis, the results (not statistically significant because of small sample size) suggest that the combination was more effective than single-drug therapy.[9] These results were predicted by the animal studies previously discussed. Also, the success of ciprofloxacin in the treatment of experimental osteomyelitis resulting from *P aeruginosa* has also been seen clinically with the same drug and the same infecting agent in man. The animal model provides a more difficult test for antimicrobial agents than most clinical trials because it requires complete sterilization of bone and this cannot be determined in patients. However, I believe that the animal model is a good predictor of potential success of agents in clinical trials and offers a uniform testing situation in which to compare different agents.

Clinical Issues in the Treatment of Osteomyelitis

Serum Bactericidal Levels

A general tenet of therapy for osteomyelitis has been the need to deliver high concentrations of antimicrobial agents in serum in order to achieve adequate levels in bone. One measure of serum levels is to determine the serum bactericidal titer (SBT), either peak or trough. In the pediatric literature, Tetzlaff and associates[10] and Prober and Yeager[11] have examined SBT in patients receiving oral therapy. Prober and Yeaker[11] suggested that a peak SBT of 1:16 or greater and a trough of 1:2 or greater would reflect adequate levels for the treatment of osteomyelitis. They basically used the SBT to assure that oral therapy was equivalent in intensity to parenteral therapy and that compliance was achieved with oral therapy.

Weinstein and associates[12] attempted to determine whether a standardized SBT would predict the outcome of treatment of osteomyelitis. They studied 30 episodes of acute osteomyelitis, and 18 chronic cases. They drew the following conclusions: (1) In patients with acute osteomyelitis, peak SBT was not predictive, whereas trough SBT of 1:2 or greater predicted cure. (2) In chronic osteomyelitis, a peak SBT of 1:16 or greater and a trough of 1:4 or greater predicted cure. (3) SBT "appears to be useful in the management of patients with osteomyelitis." (4) "It would seem prudent that patients with acute osteomyelitis have an SBT of 1:2 or greater at all times and that patients with chronic osteomyelitis have an SBT of 1:4 or greater at all times."

Several questions can be raised regarding these conclusions: (1) As the authors noted, it is possible that serum inhibitory activity would be equally predictive because there is no evidence to suggest that antimicrobial agents that are bactericidal are superior to agents that are only bacteriostatic in the treatment of osteomyelitis. (2) Regarding the conclusion that patients with acute osteomyelitis should have an SBT of 1:2 or greater at all times—of seven patients who had trough levels of less than 2, two were cured; treatment was unsuccessful in five. (3) The number of patients with chronic osteomyelitis is small (18) and the predictive value of a trough titer of less than 2 might change if more patients were studied.

What seems to be the most meaningful conclusion, at this time, about the use of the SBT in the management of osteomyelitis? I believe the test has value and that one should aim for trough values of 1:2 or greater whenever possible. However, one should not draw rigid lines such that potentially toxic concentrations of antimicrobial agents will be achieved in order to keep an SBT level of 1:2 or greater at all times. If a patient appears to be doing clinically well and the erythrocyte sedimentation rate is falling, and yet at the same time the SBT trough is not 1:2 or greater, I would not attempt to push the serum concentration higher, but would rather be guided by clinical parameters and the erythrocyte sedimentation rate.

Outpatient Management of Osteomyelitis

Patients receiving antimicrobial therapy for osteomyelitis are frequently ambulatory and are in otherwise good health. In such patients, home health care is a strong consideration if the patient, with assistance, can administer the antibiotics through a vascular access catheter. These catheters are surgically inserted while the patient is in the hospital and remain in place throughout the course of home therapy. The advantages of home care for the patient include a more normal life with family and a decreased risk of superinfection.

Outpatient therapy of osteomyelitis with intravenous antibiotics has been effective.[13-15] Although none of these studies compared home intravenous antimicrobial therapy with therapy in which the patient was kept in the hospital for the entire duration of treatment, the results with home intravenous antibiotic therapy seem entirely comparable in terms of efficacy to those previously reported in other controlled trials. One alternative to the use of home intravenous antimicrobial therapy is the use of intramuscular agents such as ceftriaxone, which can be given once daily. Russo and associates[16] treated 16 patients with osteomyelitis with this regimen and had excellent results. Intramuscular therapy was well tolerated and the use of lidocaine appeared to reduce pain from the injection. The advantage of the intramuscular route, used once daily, is the avoidance of an intravascular catheter and more frequent injection of antimicrobial agents. Outpatient therapy with orally administered agents is an alternative form of therapy that would be highly desirable, if effective, because it also would obviate the need for an intravascular access device.

Several studies[17-19] reviewed the economic advantages of outpatient intravenous antibiotic therapy in the management of osteomyelitis. Estimated savings per patient ranged from $500 to $2,200, which, according to Eisenberg and Kitz,[17] demonstrates a wide difference in savings if different sources of data for hospital costs are employed. These researchers point out that the large decreases in inpatient cost are often shifted to an increased outpatient cost. They also caution that because outpatient costs are more often borne by patients than are inpatient costs, outpatient therapy could be more expensive to the patient individually despite the savings to the hospital and to society as a whole.[17]

Oral Antimicrobial Therapy

As previously noted, the use of oral antimicrobial therapy for osteomyelitis is highly desirable, both from an economic point of view and from avoidance of intravascular catheterization. Administration of oral antimicrobial agents after initial intravenous therapy became widely accepted as a means of treating bone and joint infections in children.[10,20] Kolyvas and associates[21] extended these observations by comparing children with osteomyelitis or septic arthritis who were switched to oral antibiotics within 72 hours of intravenous therapy with another group continuing intravenous therapy for four weeks. They observed a similar clinical course and outcome in both groups and no treatment failures. They argued that antibiotic therapy could be safely changed to an oral route as soon as an organism was isolated and antimicrobial susceptibility determined.

In adults, the use of oral antimicrobial therapy for osteomyelitis has lagged behind that in children. Bell,[22] in Australia, reported excellent results, with periods of follow-up lasting as long as nine years, for treatment of adults with chronic staphylococcal osteomyelitis with oral doses of cloxacillin or phenoxymethylpenicillin. All patients received at least six months of therapy and for some patients, who were apparently well, therapy was maintained at a lower dose for periods as long as seven years. In all cases, probenecid was given in addition to the penicillin. These encouraging reports were not given wide credence because of the objections raised that the doses seemed extremely high and that continued maintenance therapy did not allow for determination of relapse or failure.

More recently, Black and associates[3] conducted a retrospective review of 21 adults with osteomyelitis or septic arthritis who received oral antimicrobial agents after an initial course of intravenous therapy. Oral therapy lasted a mean of 43 days and trough serum bactericidal titers were adjusted to be equal to or greater than 1:8. Eighteen of 21 patients had no clinical signs of recurrence; the follow-up period ranged from six to 66 months with a mean of 42 months. The oral agents used included cloxacillin, trimethoprim-sulfamethoxazole, and cephalexin. The authors noted that their preference for maintaining a trough serum bactericidal titer of 1:8 or greater was empirical and that there was no data to indicate that such measurements or adjustments of dosage improved efficacy. Gentry and Rodriguez[23] recently compared oral ciprofloxacin with parenteral therapy (a cephalosporin or nafcillin combined with an aminoglycoside) for the treatment of biopsy proven osteomyelitis. Mean durations of therapy were 56 days in the oral group and 47 in the intravenous group. The clinical success rates were 77% for the ciprofloxacin group and 79% for the parenteral therapy group. In each group, the majority of failures were the result of recurrence of the infection within one year of therapy. Of interest, and not totally explained, is the fact that infection with *P aeruginosa* as a single pathogen was successfully treated by both regimens, whereas polymicrobial infection, in which *P aeruginosa* was one pathogen, failed in almost every instance despite the regimen chosen. Resistance to ciprofloxacin did not occur except in a single strain of *P aeruginosa* that was resistant at the time of relapse. Superinfection with *S aureus* occurred in a few patients receiving ciprofloxacin despite in vitro susceptibility to ciprofloxacin of these strains. Gentry and Rodriguez[23] concluded that oral ciprofloxacin "is as safe and effective as parenteral antibiotics in cases of chronic osteomyelitis caused by susceptible organisms. For the vast majority of cases of chronic osteomyelitis, however, oral ciprofloxacin offers an attractive alternative to traditional parenteral therapies." Although these conclusions need to be verified in other studies, they seem plausible and support the approach and philosophy stated by Kolyvas and associates: "Given adequate absorption and distribution of active antibiotic, there is no fundamental reason why the oral route should be inferior to parenteral administration."[21]

Controlled Clinical Trials

It is difficult to perform well-controlled clinical trials of the treatment of chronic osteomyelitis. There is tremendous variability from patient to patient, and, in addition to the use of antimicrobial therapy, surgical debridement is an important part of management. Nonetheless, it appears that there are differences in the efficacy of different antimicrobial agents in the treatment of chronic osteomyelitis and, therefore, well conducted trials are necessary. Presently, through a contract between the Infectious Diseases Society of America and the Food and Drug Administration, guidelines are being written for controlled clinical trials. The following are important criteria in calling a trial "well conducted": (1) Precise inclusion and exclusion criteria; (2) Precise definitions of acute and chronic osteomyelitis; (3) Correct identification and sensitivity testing of infecting organisms; (4) Definition of the antimicrobial regimen and acceptable exceptions from that regimen; (5) Appropriate adjunctive surgical drainage for debridement; and (6) Definition of clinical and microbiologic responses.

References

1. Norden CW: Lessons learned from animal models of osteomyelitis. *Rev Infect Dis* 1988;10:103–110.
2. Dich VQ, Nelson JD, Haltalin KC: Osteomyelitis in infants and children: A review of 163 cases. *Am J Dis Child* 1975:129:1273–1278.
3. Black J, Hunt TL, Godley PJ, et al: Oral antimicrobial therapy for adults with osteomyelitis or septic arthritis. *J Infect Dis* 1987;155:968–972.
4. Waldovogel FA, Papageorgiou PS: Osteomyelitis: The past decade. *N Engl J Med* 1980;303:360–370.
5. Rodet A: Étude expérimentale sur l'ostéomyelíte infectieuse. *Compt Rend Acad Sci* 1884;99:569–571.
6. Lexer E: Zur experimentellen Erzeugung osteomyelitischer Herde. *Arch Klin Chir* 1894;48:181–200.
7. Scheman L, Janota M, Lewin P: The production of experimental osteomyelitis: Preliminary report. *JAMA* 1941;117:1525–1529.
8. Norden CW: Experimental osteomyelitis: I. A description of the model. *J Infect Dis* 1970;122:410–418.
9. Norden CW, Bryant R, Palmer D, et al: Chronic osteomyelitis caused by *Staphylococcus aureus*: Controlled clinical trial of nafcillin therapy and nafcillin-rifampin therapy. *South Med J* 1986;79:947–951.
10. Tetzlaff TR, McCracken GH Jr, Nelson JD: Oral antibiotic therapy for skeletal infections of children: II. Therapy of osteomyelitis and suppurative arthritis. *J Pediatr* 1978;92:485–490.

11. Prober CG, Yeager AS: Use of the serum bactericidal titer to assess the adequacy of oral antibiotic therapy in the treatment of acute hematogenous osteomyelitis. *J Pediatr* 1979;95:131–135.
12. Weinstein MP, Stratton CW, Hawley HB, et al: Multicenter collaborative evaluation of a standardized serum bactericidal test as a predictor of therapeutic efficacy in acute and chronic osteomyelitis. *Am J Med* 1987;83:218–222.
13. Wagner DK, Collier BD, Rytel MW: Long-term intravenous antibiotic therapy in chronic osteomyelitis. *Arch Intern Med* 1985;145:1073–1078.
14. Ingram C, Eron LJ, Goldenberg RI, et al: Antibiotic therapy of osteomyelitis in outpatients. *Med Clin North Am* 1988;72:723–738.
15. Menon J, Bown TM, Neri C: Long term outpatient intravenous antibiotic therapy for orthopedic patients. *Orthopedics* 1984;7:1280–1282.
16. Russo TA, Cook S, Gorbach SL: Intramuscular ceftriaxone in home parenteral therapy. *Antimicrob Agents Chemother* 1988;32:1439–1440.
17. Eisenberg JM, Kitz DS: Savings from outpatient antibiotic therapy for osteomyelitis: Economic analysis of a therapeutic strategy. *JAMA* 1986;255:1584–1588.
18. Balinsky W, Nesbitt S: Cost-effectiveness of outpatient parenteral antibiotics: A review of the literature. *Am J Med* 1989;87:301–305.
19. Chamberlain TM, Lehman ME, Groh MJ, et al: Cost analysis of a home intravenous antibiotic program. *Am J Hosp Pharm* 1988;45:2341–2345.
20. Bryson YJ, Connor JD, LeClerc M, et al: High-dose oral dicloxacillin treatment of acute staphylococcal osteomyelitis in children. *J Pediatr* 1979;94:673–675.
21. Kolyvas E, Ahronheim G, Marks MI, et al: Oral antibiotic therapy of skeletal infections in children. *Pediatrics* 1980;65:867–871.
22. Bell SM: Further observations on the value of oral penicillins in chronic staphylococcal osteomyelitis. *Med J Aust* 1976;2:591–593.
23. Gentry LO, Rodriguez GG: Oral ciprofloxacin compared with parenteral antibiotics in the treatment of osteomyelitis. *Antimicrob Agents Chemother* 1990;34:40–43.

Chapter 28

Adult Septic Arthritis

John L. Esterhai, Jr, MD
Vincent Ruggiero, BS

Introduction

Any patient with the acute onset of monoarticular arthritis should be approached as if the causative agent was a bacterial septic arthritis. The purpose of this chapter is to describe bacterial infectious arthritis, including its etiology, organisms, joint involvement, pathophysiology, differential diagnosis, treatment, prognosis, and areas for future research.

Septic arthritis continues to be a major health problem in urban medical centers. Incidence figures range from 0.034% to 0.13% for nongonococcal arthritis. The incidence may be increasing as a result of the advancing age of the population, particularly the longer life expectancy of patients at risk, such as diabetic patients, those with chronic illness, and other immunocompromised individuals.[1]

Etiology

Septic arthritis can result from: (1) Hematogenous seeding secondary to bacteremia from distant infection or intravenous drug abuse; (2) Direct inoculation secondary to penetrating trauma or joint aspiration; (3) The spread of contiguous soft tissue infection through the joint capsule from local cellulitis, abscess, septic bursitis, or tenosynovitis; and (4) Joint contamination from periarticular osteomyelitis. The major predisposing factors for developing septic arthritis include: (1) Preexisting joint disease, especially rheumatoid arthritis; (2) Closed trauma to the joint; (3) Direct penetration of the joint; (4) Intravenous drug abuse; and (5) Impaired host defense mechanisms, including malignancy, steroid and cytotoxic drug use, diabetes and other chronic debilitating diseases, and extreme old age.

Hematogenous Contamination Septic arthritis is most frequently caused by joint invasion during bacteremia. Because the synovial membrane of the joint is vascular and has no limiting basement membrane, it is a likely site for bacterial seeding during a bacteremia. The joint is protected from infection by local host factors in most cases. Histologic evidence of synovitis, with and without the demonstrated presence of bacteria, is common in bacteremic states and may correlate with the frequent arthralgias reported by patients.[2]

Direct Inoculation The incidence of septic arthritis increases in individuals with a history of trauma to the joint. The mechanism of injury with open trauma is obvious, because bacteria are introduced directly into the joint space. However, the mechanism whereby closed trauma leads to increased rates of infection is not clear. Possible explanations include hyperemia causing an increased exposure to microorganisms, damage to local anatomy allowing easier access to the joint, and hematoma formation providing a local culture medium.

At times, direct inoculation of the offending organism can be iatrogenic. Septic arthritis has been found to complicate arthroscopy in 0.004% to 3.4% of procedures.[3,4] A large study from Toronto documented an incidence of 0.23% and demonstrated the potential cost benefits of antibiotic prophylaxis.[3] Septic arthritis as a result of infection during open joint surgery is uncommon, occurring in less than 1% of patients.

There may be an increased rate of colonization with *Staphylococcus aureus* in patients receiving intra-articular steroid injections. It follows that there is a higher likelihood of infection with this organism in patients receiving such injections.[5] The actual risk of infection from such an injection is rare if strict aseptic technique is employed. Large series have demonstrated septic arthritis secondary to a corticosteroid injection to occur with an incidence of less than 0.008%. A recent study of nine rheumatoid arthritis patients with septic arthritis suggested that steroid injection made the patients more susceptible to septic arthritis, but that direct inoculation was a rare event.[6]

Contiguous Spread Soft-tissue infection from cellulitis, septic bursitis, infectious tenosynovitis, or local abscess formation can invade the joint capsule directly. After growth-plate closure, a vascular connection between the metaphysis and epiphysis allows intra-articular invasion of a metaphyseal osteomyelitis by chondral disruption into the joint space or by vascular extension via the synovial plexus.

Predisposing Factors Chronic inflammation and joint damage, such as that found in rheumatoid arthritis, is associated with increased incidence of joint infection, perhaps secondary to factors such as hyperemia and neovascularization, which can lead to increased exposure to infectious organisms, and abnormal joint structure, which can allow organisms to escape local defense mechanisms. Rheumatoid patients are also at increased risk secondary to systemic corticosteroid usage, intra-articular corticosteroid injections, a postulated lower resistance to infection in general, and a defect in granulocyte phagocytic function.[7] It has been shown that any increase in the extent of the patient's disease increases the susceptibility to septic arthritis. This is thought to be because of an increase in the number of injections received and an increase in the use of immunosuppressive agents.[6] In many large series, rheumatoid arthritis is the most common predisposing factor to joint infection. There is a reported prevalence of septic arthritis of 0.3% to 3% among rheumatoid arthritis patients.[6,7]

Additionally, in rheumatoid arthritis patients, infectious arthritis has a much worse prognosis than in other subgroups affected.[7] Complete recovery of joint function to preinfection level is achieved in 35% of rheumatoid arthritis patients versus 70% of others. A mortality rate of approximately 20% in rheumatoid arthritis patients compared with 5% to 10% for others demonstrates the seriousness of these infections. Polyarticular infection in association with rheumatoid arthritis is associated with a particularly poor prognosis.[8] Polyarticular septic arthritis alone is associated with an elevated mortality when compared to monoarticular arthritis. The mortality rate in a large series was 23% and 9%, respectively. When rheumatoid arthritis was an additional factor in the patient, the mortality rates were 56% and 8%, respectively.[8] The reasons for these statistics are not completely clear.

One contributing factor to the poor outcome in rheumatoid arthritis patients is the longer delay in diagnosis that often accompanies these infections. The difficulty arises in distinguishing a rheumatoid flare from an acute infection. The rheumatoid patient may even have polyarticular symptoms with only one septic joint. The infected joint may not be especially hot, and fever and leukocytosis may be absent. Pseudoseptic arthritis is well-described in rheumatoid patients and further complicates the picture. The patient has fever, monoarthritis, and a synovial fluid analysis that is compatible with infection, but will have negative culture and gram stains and will respond to intra-articular steroids. These factors make the diagnosis difficult, and they will often delay it.

Patients with systemic lupus erythematosus are another subgroup at high risk for developing septic arthritis.[9] The reasons for this susceptibility include depression of cell- and antibody-mediated immune responses, deficient opsonic capacity, and the use of immunosuppressive therapy. Patients with systemic lupus erythematosus have a high frequency of chronic Salmonella carriage as well as infection with this organism. Systemic lupus erythematosus is the most frequent predisposing factor for development of Salmonella septic arthritis. Thus, patients with systemic lupus erythematosus and signs and symptoms suggestive of infectious arthritis should be cultured for this organism and treated with appropriate antibiotics until culture results are obtained. Additionally, patients with active systemic lupus erythematosus and life-threatening complications requiring immunosuppressive therapy should be screened for carriage of Salmonella and treated appropriately.[9]

The elderly are more susceptible to infectious diseases. Immune function declines with age and the frequency and seriousness of infections increases with extreme age.[10] Although the reported incidence of septic arthritis in the elderly is lower than that for the rest of the population (estimated at 0.005%),[11] septic arthritis in individuals over the age of 60 may have a worse prognosis, with an increased risk of osteomyelitis and increased mortality. One study of 21 patients over the age of 60 with septic arthritis reported a mortality rate of 29% (20% died secondary to sepsis). There is a paucity of clinical findings on initial presentation, which may delay diagnosis.[11]

Organisms Involved in Adult Suppurative Arthritis

Although *Neisseria gonorrhea* has been reported to be the most common organism causing septic arthritis, recent studies have suggested that *Staphylococcus aureus* may actually be more common., A ten-year study from England found *S aureus* to be responsible for infection in 44% of the patients and *N gonorrhea* to account for only 11%.[12] However, this may have been secondary to the difficulty encountered when attempting to culture the gonococcus. *S aureus* is the most common cause of nongonococcal septic arthritis. In a recent study from Denmark it was shown that there is currently not a specific phage type of *S aureus* that is more likely to cause septic arthritis. A bacteriophage is a virus whose DNA can become incorporated into the bacterial genome. This will give the bacteria different properties (i.e. antibiotic resistance). The strains that were isolated from cases of septic arthritis were found less likely to be resistant to antibiotics and are, therefore, easier to treat than those strains that caused osteomyelitis.[13]

The other common organisms are streptococci and gram-negative organisms, including *Escherichia coli* and *Pseudomonas*. The gram-negative organisms have been implicated in intravenous drug abuse, but *S aureus* is probably more common even in this subset.[1,14] In a study of 28 patients with nongonococcal septic arthritis at Wayne County General Hospital, intravenous drug abuse was found to be the most common predisposing factor for developing septic arthritis.[1] *S aureus*, the most common organism identified, was present in 64% of patients. The authors found that the *S aureus* was methicillin resistant in 39% of patients.[1] *Streptococcus* species and gram-negative bacteria were also isolated.[1]

Anaerobic organisms account for approximately 1% of bacterial septic arthritis.[15] Clostridial infections are associated with significant morbidity. Aggressive treatment, including surgical debridement with complete synovectomy, has been recommended for these patients.[16]

There have been cases of fungal septic arthritis reported in AIDS patients. The infections were usually insidious in nature and associated with a contiguous osteomyelitis.[17] One case of an HIV positive, intravenous drug user with Candida septic arthritis of the sternoclavicular joint following a fungemia has been reported. This case did occur in the setting of a contiguous osteomyelitis.[18]

Lyme disease is caused by the spirochete *Borrelia burgdorferi*. Among its manifestations is its effect on the large joints, where it causes pain and swelling. It is reported that up to 60% of affected patients experience joint symptoms months to years after being infected. Arthritis can be the only manifestation in some cases. Beck and associates showed that Lyme disease spirochetes are a potent stimulator of interleukin-1 (IL-1) production. Their lipopolysaccharide (an endotoxin of the bacteria) causes stimulated cells to make IL-1. This protein (IL-1) can be found in the fluid of an inflamed joint. Antibodies against IL-1 inhibited the synovial fluid isolate from stimulating lymphocytes. *B burgdorferi* has been isolated from the synovial fluid of patients with chronic Lyme arthritis, which suggests that perhaps the arthritis is caused by persistent infection.[19] The role of IL-1 in septic arthritis is discussed in detail later in this chapter.

Joint Involvement The knee is the joint most commonly affected in infection (40%–50%). The hip (20%–25%) is more commonly involved than the shoulder (10%–15%), wrist (10%), ankle (10%–15%), elbow (10%–15%), or hand.

In intravenous drug abusers the sternoclavicular, sacroiliac[20] and manubriosternal[14] joints are the joints more commonly affected. The reason for this distribution is unexplained at present. Infection of the sacroiliac joint is often associated with diagnostic delay because the joint is relatively inaccessible, has limited range of motion, lacks the classic signs of infection, and is associated with symptoms easily confused with more common diagnoses.[21]

Septic arthritis of the shoulder usually causes pain and decreased range of motion. Infection of the glenohumeral joint is also associated with a poor outcome, in part attributed to the delay in diagnosis. In many patients, the initial diagnosis is either tendinitis or bursitis.[5]

Pathophysiology The pathophysiology of septic arthritis has been studied extensively using animal models. Signs of septic arthritis are pronounced by the second day after bacterial injection. Glycosaminoglycan depletion occurs by Day 5, with cartilage softening and fissuring by Day 7. Pannus overgrowth occurs by Day 11, with erosion of the joint capsule by Day 17. Fibrous ankylosis and complete destruction of the joint occurs by five weeks.[22]

The articular surface of a septic joint is affected both by direct interaction with the bacteria and by the host's own inflammatory system.[23] Interleukin-1 (IL-1) is produced by the body in response to infection. This protein causes further activation of the inflammatory process and is grouped into a class of molecules called cytokines for this reason. It is considered to be one of the most important cytokines contributing to the destruction of articular cartilage.[24] Exposure of the joint surface to IL-1 can cause cartilage degradation; proteoglycan release; increased secretion of collagenase; release of metalloproteases, which degrade cartilage; and activation of latent collagenases. IL-1 also inhibits the synthesis of glycosaminoglycan, which is an integral part of cartilage. There is evidence that levels of protease inhibitors are decreased in arthritic conditions. This decrease has been shown to occur in infections caused by *S aureus*. IL-1 levels are also found to be elevated in osteoarthritis. Osteoarthritis, like septic arthritis, causes inflammation in the joint, which is stimulated in part by IL-1 release.

Studies by Williams and associates[23] show that staphylococcal culture medium or an IL-1 injection into the joint space will result in elevated collagenase and caseinase activity compared with controls. This stimulation of enzymatic activity is thought to be a critical factor in the degradation of cartilage in a septic joint. It is postulated that the bacteria cause IL-1 to be released, which in turn stimulates the inflammatory cascade.[23] The signal transduction method by which the chondrocytes respond to the IL-1 is not known. It is thought that nitric oxide is the key. In in vitro studies, the levels of nitric oxide rose with injection of IL-1 or lipopolysaccharide. More work needs to be done to determine what is the definite signal.[25] Inflammatory cells must be induced to produce IL-1 in normal subjects. It is believed that polymorphonuclear leucocytes (i.e. neutrophils) of rheumatoid arthritis patients already have IL-1 and its precursor stored in their granules.[24]

As stated earlier, there are natural inhibitors to the destruction of the articular surface. These are present in lower than normal amounts in the inflamed joint. Piroxicam, a nonsteroidal anti-inflammatory used to treat rheumatoid arthritis and osteoarthritis, can enhance the production of these inhibitors and induce the formation of new inhibitors. The work being done is very new, and further research is needed to determine its full significance.[26]

There may be specific characteristics and interactions between the infecting organisms and the host in septic arthritis. Most patients with bacteremia do not develop septic joints. Specific joints are affected preferentially. Septic arthritis occurs much more frequently in patients with underlying disease. There is a predominance of specific organisms causing septic arthritis that is out of proportion to the incidence of bacteremia with those specific bacteria. One important bacterial property for the initiation of infection is adherence to the substrate. This has been demonstrated for many of the organisms that infect the respiratory and gastrointestinal tracts. Studies have documented specific binding of *S aureus* to articular cartilage and collagen and have shown that the specific binding of *S aureus* to cartilage is important for the hematogenous seeding of joints.[27,28] More specifically, scanning and transmission electron microscopic studies of rabbit and human material have demonstrated specific binding of *S aureus* to collagen, and further studies have provided strong evidence of a specific collagen receptor on the surface membrane on certain strains of *S aureus*. Although this receptor has not yet been isolated, enzymatic degradation studies demonstrate that it contains protein components.[27-29]

A comparison of *S aureus* and *E coli* infections in the rabbit knee model showed that by 48 hours knees infected with *S aureus* had lost 42% of their glycosaminoglycan whereas knees infected with *E coli* had lost only 20%. Thus, the extent of damage varies, depending on the organism involved.[30]

Treatment

The goals of treatment include: sterilization of the joint; decompression; removal of the inflammatory cells, enzymes, debris, or foreign body; elimination of destructive pannus; and return to full functional recovery.[31]

Antibiotic therapy is fundamental to the treatment of septic arthritis.[32] The initial choice of antibiotics, made before culture results are received, is based on the following data: patient age; risk factors such as IV drug abuse, rheumatoid arthritis, chronic illness, and extra-articular sites of infection; and gram stain. In adults, treatment may be initiated with a penicillinase-resistant antistaphylococcal antibiotic. The choice of treatment is modified if there is a high likelihood of gram-negative or methicillin-resistant organisms. When culture and sensitivity information become available, the regimen should be modified to maximize efficiency and decrease risk to the patient. Patients suspected of gonococcal infection may receive 10 million units per day of intravenous penicillin-G until there is clinical improvement, followed by 2g per day of amoxicillin or ampicillin to complete a seven-day course.

The route of antibiotic treatment is controversial. The use of local infusion versus systemic administration has been in question for years. Human studies of intra-articular antibiotic concentrations through systemic administration have been conducted with many different antibiotics. These include penicillin-G, phenoxymethyl penicillin, nafcillin, cephaloridine, cloxacillin, tetracycline, erythromycin, lincomycin, ampicillin, cephalothin, and kanamycin. All except erythromycin achieved intra-articular concentrations that exceeded the level necessary to inhibit or kill infecting organisms.[33] Direct injection of antibiotics into the joint, which can cause a chemical synovitis, should be avoided.[34]

A more controversial issue related to antibiotic therapy is the use of oral versus intravenous medications. Oral therapy should be adequate in the setting of normal absorption and distribution of the antibiotic.[35] A number of studies have supported this statement, reporting successful use of oral antibiotics to treat septic arthritis. The advantages of oral administration over parenteral administration include cost savings, convenience, comfort, and decreased length of hospitalization.[35] Maintenance of adequate serum levels is the only real concern. Patients must be instructed to take their medications in proper dosage with the necessary timing relative to meals, and they must be followed appropriately to ensure that adequate serum levels are achieved.

Another issue in antibiotic therapy is the duration of treatment. Generally, it is recommended that antibiotics be given for a total of four to six weeks for nongonococcal infections and for two weeks for gonococcal arthritis. However, animal studies have shown that the joint actually may be sterilized within days of the initiation of treatment. Drainage and lavage of the joint also aid in elimination of bacteria. There are no controlled studies that document the optimal length of treatment. The ultimate length of antibiotic treatment is influenced by the specific microorganism, the patient's underlying condition, and the complementary surgery or medical treatment. Antibiotics alone cannot prevent ongoing cartilage destruction caused by a sterile and progressive postinfectious arthritis secondary to lysosomal enzymes and antigenic bacterial debris.

In light of research, which has shown IL-1 to be a major factor in the pathogenesis of septic arthritis or any inflammatory arthritis, new methods of treatment are being devised. In a study by Smith, it was shown that an IL-1 receptor antagonist protein (IRAP) inhibited IL-1-induced matrix erosion and normalized glycosaminoglycan production. This IRAP also inhibits collagenase, gelatinase, and stromelysin, which all play a part in the destruction of cartilage via IL-1 stimulation. IRAP is produced in a variety of cells in the body. These findings suggest that in the future IRAP may have a role in antiarthritis therapy.[36] Other research has shown that glucocorticoids suppress the production of the metalloproteases. Metalloproteases are enzymes that are known to destroy cartilage after being stimulated by the normal inflammatory response. Administration of glucocorticoids has been shown to make the chondrocytes refractory to cytokine stimulation.[37] It has been found that steroids are protective to the joint. Osteophyte formation is decreased and chondrocyte proteoglycan synthesis is normalized.[38] These latest findings are found to be true in osteoarthritis. The degree to which they will be effective in terms of treatment of septic arthritis is not known.

The effects of nonsteroidal anti-inflammatory drugs used adjunctively with antibiotic treatment is being explored in animal models.[39] Naproxen treatment was begun two days before infection of the knee with S aureus. Quantitation of glycosaminoglycan and collagen losses showed that, while animals treated with the combination of naproxen and antibiotic therapy lost 38% of their glycosaminoglycans, animals treated only with antibiotic lost 51%. Collagen losses were 19% and 30% respectively. These data suggest that supplementing early antibiotic treatment with nonsteroidal anti-inflammatory medication can reduce the destruction of articular cartilage during S aureus infection. However, the use of nonsteroidal anti-inflammatory drugs in patients in whom a firm bacteriologic diagnosis has not been reached may cause confusion. In such patients, response to therapy is one of the criteria by which adequacy of antibiotic coverage is assessed. Improvement secondary to nonsteroidal anti-inflammatory use may delay realization of inadequate antibiotic coverage.[39]

The controversy over continuous passive motion of a septic joint has not been resolved. During the acute phase of infection and before treatment, motion is painful. Thus, external splinting often provides some initial relief. However, prolonged immobilization of a injured joint carries with it the risks of degenerative arthritis, disuse osteoporosis, muscle atrophy, pain, and stiffness. Salter[40] had demonstrated prevention of progressive cartilage damage in septic joints treated with continuous passive motion compared with joints subjected to either immobilization or intermittent active motion. Proposed mechanisms have included improvement of cartilage nutrition via increased diffusion of synovial fluid, better clearance of the enzymes present in the purulent exudate, prevention of adhesions and pannus formation, and stimulation of chondrocyte synthetic processes.

Ongoing research is needed to further outline the new and redefine the old methods of treatment. Optimal route and duration of antibiotic therapy must be further worked out. The mechanism by which the organisms cause destruction of the articular cartilage is being sought in hopes that it can be exploited. How bacteria adhere and how they initiate infection is also being explored. Once more information is known perhaps a method of treatment can be devised that will spare the cartilage and allow the joint to return to full function without any compromise.

References

1. Ang-Font GZ, Rozboril MB, Thompson GR: Changes in nongonococcal septic arthritis: Drug abuse and methicillin-resistant *Staphylococcus aureus*. *Arthritis Rheum* 1985;28:210–213.
2. Steigbigel NH: Diagnosis and management of septic arthritis. *Curr Clin Top Infect Dis* 1983, pp 1–29.
3. D'Angelo GL, Ogilvie-Harris DJ: Septic arthritis following arthroscopy with cost/benefit analysis of antibiotic prophylaxis. *Arthroscopy* 1988;4:10–14.
4. Toye B, Thomson J, Karsh J: Case report: *Staphylococcus epidermidis* septic arthritis postarthroscopy. *Clin Exp Rheumatol* 1987;5:165–166.
5. Lesile BM, Harris JM III, Driscoll D: Septic arthritis of the shoulder in adults. *J Bone Joint Surg* 1989;71A:1516–1522.
6. Östensson A, Geborek P: Septic arthritis as a non-surgical complication in Rheumatoid Arthritis: Relation to disease severity and therapy. *Br J Rheumatol* 1991;30:35–38.
7. Goldenberg DL: Infectious arthritis complicating rheumatoid arthritis and other chronic rheumatic disorders. *Arthritis Rheum* 1989;32:496–502.
8. Epstein JH, Zimmerman B III, Ho G Jr: Polyarticular septic arthritis. *J Rheumatol* 1986;13:1105–1107.
9. Medina F, Fraga A, Lavalle C: Salmonella septic arthritis in Systemic Lupus Erythematosus: The importance of the chronic carrier state. *J Rheumatol* 1989;16:203–208.
10. Yoshikawa TT: Geriatric infectious diseases: An emerging problem. *J Am Geriatr Soc* 1983;31:34–39.
11. Vincent GM, Amirault JD: Septic arthritis in the elderly. *Clin Orthop* 1990;251:241–245.
12. Cooper C, Cawley MID: Bacterial arthritis in an English health district: A 10 year review. *Ann Rheum Dis* 1986;45:458–463.
13. Espersen F, Frimodt-Møller N, Thamdrup Rosdahl V, et al: Changing pattern of bone and joint infections due to *Staphylococcus aureus*: Study of cases of bacteremia in Denmark, 1959–1988. *Rev Infect Dis* 1991;13:347–358.
14. López-Longo FJ, Monteagudo I, Vaquero FJ, et al: Primary septic arthritis of the manubriosternal joint in a heroin user. *Clin Orthop* 1986;202:230–231.
15. Clarke HJ, Allum R: Anaerobic septic arthritis due to bacteroides: Brief report. *J Bone Joint Surg* 1988;70B:847–848.
16. Fauser DJ, Zuckerman JD: Clostridal septic arthritis: Case report and review of the literature. *Arthritis Rheum* 1988;31:295–298.

17. Zimmerman B III, Erickson AD, Mikolich DJ: Septic acromioclavicular arthritis and osteomyelitis in a patient with acquired immunodeficiency syndrome. *Arthritis Rheum* 1989;32:1175–1178.

18. Edelstein H, McCabe R: *Candida albicans* septic arthritis and osteomyelitis of the sternoclavicular joint in a patient with HIV. *J Rheumatol* 1991:18:110–111.

19. Beck G, Benach JL, Habicht GS: Isolation of interleukin 1 from joint fluids of patients with Lyme disease. *J Rheumatol* 1989;16:800–806.

20. Hodgson BF: Pyogenic sacroiliac joint infection. *Clin Orthop* 1989;246:146–149.

21. Shanahan MDG, Ackroyd CE: Pyogenic infection of the sacroiliac joint: A report of 11 cases. *J Bone Joint Surg* 1985;67B:605–608.

22. Riegels-Nielsen P, Frimodt-Møller N, Jensen JS: Rabbit model of septic arthritis. *Acta Orthop Scand* 1987;58:14–19.

23. Williams RJ III, Smith RL, Schurman DJ: Purified Staphylococcal culture medium stimulates neutral metalloprotease secretion from human articular cartilage. *J Orthop Res* 1991;9:258–265.

24. Watanabe S, Horimoto T, Matsumoto T, et al: IL-1 from human PMN leucocytes. *Trans Orthop Res Soc* 1991;16:383.

25. Stadler J, Billiar TR, Curran RD, et al: Interleukin-1 induces nitric oxide synthesis in articular chondrocytes. *Trans Orthop Res Soc* 1991;16:322.

26. Herman JH, Sowder WG, Donaldson JB, et al: NSAID modulation of catabolin production reflects induction of interleukin-1 inhibitory activity. *Trans Orthop Res Soc* 1991;16:200.

27. Nade S, Speers DJ: Staphylococcal adherence to chicken cartilage. *Acta Orthop Scand* 1987;58:351–353.

28. Speziale P, Raucci G, Visai L, et al: Binding of collagen to *Staphylococcus aureus* Cowan 1. *J Bacteriol* 1986;167:77–81.

29. Naylor PT, Myrvik QN, Webb LS, et al: Adhesion and antibiotic resistance of slime producing and nonslime producing coagulase-negative staphylococcus. *Trans Orthop Res Soc* 1990;15:292.

30. Riegels-Nielsen P, Frimodt-Møller N, Sorensen M, et al: Antibiotic treatment insufficient for established septic arthritis: *Staphylococcus aureus* experiments in rabbits. *Acta Orthop Scand* 1989;60:113–115.

31. Goldenberg DL, Cohen AS: Acute infectious agent arthritis: A review of patients with nongonococcal joint infections (with emphasis on therapy and prognosis). *Am J Med* 1976;60:369–377.

32. Cawston TE, Weaver L, Coughlan RJ, et al: Synovial fluids from infected joints contain active metalloproteinases and no inhibitory activity. *Br J Rheumatol* 1989;28:386–392.

33. Frimodt-Møller N, Riegels-Nielson P: Antibiotic penetration into the infected knee. *Acta Orthop Scand* 1987;58:256–259.

34. Sáez-Llorens X, Jafari HS, Olsen KD, et al: Induction of suppurative arthritis in rabbits by *Haemophilus* endotoxin, tumor necrosis factor α and interleukin-1β. *J Infect Dis* 1991;163:1267–1272.

35. Black J, Hunt TL, Godley PJ, et al: Oral antimicrobial therapy for adults with osteomyelitis or septic arthritis. *J Infect Dis* 1987;155:968–972.

36. Smith RJ, Chin JE, Sam LM, et al: Biologic effects of an interleukin-1 receptor antagonist protein on interleukin-1--stimulated cartilage erosion and chondrocyte responsiveness. *Arthritis Rheum* 1991;34:78–83.

37. DiBattista JA, Martel-Pelletier J, Wosu LO, et al: Glucocorticoid receptor mediated inhibition of Interleukin-1 stimulated neutral metalloprotease synthesis in normal human chondrocytes. *J Clin Endocrinol Metab* 1991;72:316–326.

38. Van den Berg WB: Impact of NSAID and steroids on cartilage destruction in murine antigen induced arthritis. *J Rheumatol* 1991;27(suppl):122–123.

39. Smith RL, Schurman DJ, Kajiyama G, et al: Effect of NSAID and antibiotic treatment in a rabbit model of staphylococcal infectious arthritis. *Trans Orthop Res Soc* 1990;15:296.
40. Salter RB: The biologic concept of continuous passive motion of synovial joints. *Clin Orthop* 1989;242:12–25.

Chapter 29

Antibiotic Therapy for Osteomyelitis

Layne O. Gentry, MD

Introduction

Osteomyelitis is an infection that involves native bone or orthopaedic prostheses. Despite occasional reports to the contrary, there is no credible evidence that these deep-seated infections can be cured without complete surgical debridement of necrotic bone and soft tissue and replacement of an infected prosthesis, followed by systemic antimicrobial therapy for at least four to six weeks. Surgical management alone cannot eradicate pathogenic bacteria that may have been disseminated, and reliance upon chemotherapy alone fails in the presence of devascularized material, which serves as a continued focus for bacterial growth.

Review

The antibiotic therapy for osteomyelitis and its changing etiology and the role of biopsy in confirming the disease have been reviewed.[1] While osteomyelitis is primarily associated with trauma and is caused by strains of *Staphylococcus aureus* susceptible to penicillinase-resistant penicillins such as nafcillin, this classic presentation is diminishing in relative importance. Hospital-acquired infections are now more prevalent. The incidence of pure *S aureus* osteomyelitis diminished from 45% to 27% between 1970 and 1988, and the incidence of pure gram-negative infection increased from 13% to 35% over the same period.[1]

Undoubtedly, improved diagnostic procedures have contributed to these apparent epidemiologic changes. Before a definitive study in 1978 established the lack of correlation of sinus tract cultures with bone biopsies,[2] many gram-negative organisms present in aspirated specimens were not considered to be pathogens in the infected bone, but rather to reflect nosocomial colonization. The pathogenicity of gram-negative organisms in bone was confirmed by a series of patients with mixed osteomyelitis who were treated with nafcillin and gentamicin. Nafcillin monotherapy invariably failed when the gentamicin was discontinued because of nephrotoxicity associated with prolonged regimens.

Modern Therapy

Many of the newer antimicrobial agents are appropriate in treating osteomyelitis because of the recent emphasis upon the development of drugs that are active against unusual and resistant pathogens, can be absorbed extravascularly, and can be administered safely for prolonged regimens. Pharmacokinetic considerations are important in osteomyelitis, especially drug penetration into bone, yet there is little standardization in the methods by which these drug levels are measured in bone. Serum bactericidal titers may be useful in predicting the outcome of therapy; trough titers with a ratio of 1:4 or greater are associated with a favorable prognosis when parenteral therapy is used.[3]

Toxicity may be the primary consideration in selecting therapy among equally effective agents. Indeed, in many cases of recurrent osteomyelitis or infected prostheses in elderly patients for whom surgical replacement is not advised, chronic or lifelong antibiotic suppression may be required. I rarely use aminoglycosides to treat nonenterococcal osteomyelitis; newer, less toxic agents that are active against resistant gram-negative organisms are preferred.

Economics relevant to the care of osteomyelitis patients have been studied. Most cases of osteomyelitis are diagnosed in the hospital because bone biopsy, which is usually done following a radiograph or computed tomography, magnetic resonance imaging, or radionuclide scan, is required to confirm the etiology of the infection. Unlike many nosocomial infections, prevalent symptoms of osteomyelitis are often subacute, and the condition is rarely life-threatening. Outpatient or home care, when compared with four to six weeks of hospitalization, is economically advantageous and convenient for the patient.

Literature Review

During the past ten years, the third-generation cephalosporins, monobactams, beta-lactam/beta-lactamase inhibitor combinations, carbapenems, and the oral fluoroquinolones have been extensively evaluated in osteomyelitis. A review of the published clinical trials, including osteomyelitis cases treated with these agents and excluding duplicate data, case reports, or open series where data specific to osteomyelitis cannot be discerned, has been attempted. Although there are several third-generation cephalosporins in use, I have focused on cefotaxime, which was the first such agent developed, ceftazidime, which is currently popular, and ceftriaxone, which has the most favorable pharmacokinetic profile (feasibility of once-daily administration). Osteomyelitis results have been published for ciprofloxacin, ofloxacin, and pefloxacin among the oral fluoroquinolones.

Diagnostic criteria include identification of a known pathogen from biopsy or surgical specimen, or positive blood culture. Deep-swab culture of an aspirate was not considered a diagnostic procedure, except

Table 1 Pharmacodynamics of antimicrobial agents*

Agent	Dosage	Cmax(bone)† (μg/g)	Minimal Inhibitory Concentration 90%	
			S aureus	P aeruginosa
Cefotaxime	2 g every 12 hrs	12.4	<8	Total resistance
Ceftazidime	2 g every 12 hrs	31.1	<16	<16
Ceftriaxone	2 g every 24 hrs	25.6	<8	<64
Aztreonam	2 g every 8 hrs	16.0	Total resistance	<4
Timentin(r)‡	3.1 g every 6 hrs	34.2	<1	<64
Imipenem	1 g every 8 hrs	4.3	<1	<2
Ciprofloxacin	750 mg every 12 hrs	5.7	<1	<1
Ofloxacin	400 mg every 12 hrs	2.2	<1	<2
Pefloxacin	400 mg every 12 hrs	18.5	<1	<2
Teicoplanin	400 mg every 24 hrs	5.8	<1	Total resistance

*Data are representative values taken from a compilation of the literature.
†Data are taken from small, noncomparative studies and, thus, should not be used to draw inferences as to the relative pharmacokinetic profiles of two different antibiotics, but, rather, to demonstrate activity in bone for each of the agents (Cmax=maximum concentration).
‡Ticarcillin/clavulanic acid

in cases where pathologic fracture might have resulted from biopsy. Antimicrobial therapy is considered successful when signs and symptoms of infection disappear and no further antimicrobial therapy is necessary. Most importantly, while the clinical symptoms of osteomyelitis may abate with therapy, long-term follow-up is required to assess the true efficacy of such therapy, and priority is given to series of patients for which follow-up data are available. Bacteriologic results are compiled, where available, for *S aureus* and *Pseudomonas aeruginosa*, the two most common causes of osteomyelitis. Unfortunately, insufficient data are published for a similar breakdown for the Enterobacteriaceae.

In this review, there is no attempt to validate statistically a compilation of the results from separate clinical trials. Arithmetic tabulations only are made, which may uncover large-scale trends that might not be apparent from the numerous small series that have been published.

Antibiotics

Third-Generation Cephalosporins

Cefotaxime, ceftazidime, and ceftriaxone are typically administered in doses of 2 g every six, 12, and 24 hours, respectively. Each of these agents achieves drug levels in bone exceeding 90% of the minimal inhibitory concentration (MIC90) for *S aureus*, the most common cause of osteomyelitis (Table 1). Against *P aeruginosa*, the most common gram-negative pathogen in bone, cefotaxime is not routinely active, ceftazidime is present in bone levels greater than the inhibitory concentration for this pathogen, and ceftriaxone is not predictably active in bone.

Cefotaxime

Six published clinical trials involving cefotaxime have provided osteomyelitis data.[4-9] A total of 148 patients received cefotaxime, typically 2.0 g every six hours, and 146 (99%) of these patients were able to complete a regimen of therapy, which averaged 29 days, without experiencing an adverse reaction that required cefotaxime discontinuation. Cefotaxime therapy produced a resolution of the clinical symptoms of infection at the end of therapy ("remission") in 89% of the patients. The two largest series[4,7] provided six-month follow-up data, and cefotaxime had long-term success in 88% of these subjects.

S aureus was eradicated—or was assumed to be eradicated in those cases where clinical resolution precluded follow-up microbiologic evaluation—in 81% of the infected subjects, while only three of seven (43%) cases of *P aeruginosa* osteomyelitis were successfully treated with cefotaxime. Not surprisingly, *Enterococcus faecalis* was responsible for each of the adverse microbiologic events, namely, five clinically significant colonizations or superinfections. Enterococci are routinely unresponsive to the cephalosporins and have emerged as a troublesome cause of infection nationwide.[10]

Ceftazidime

At least eight clinical trials involving ceftazidime in osteomyelitis have been reported, involving at least 155 subjects.[11-18] Ceftazidime, 2 g every 12 hours for an average of 39 days, was successful in resolving the clinical symptoms of infection in 92% of these subjects, and the incidence of adverse effects precluding completion of ceftazidime therapy was only 3%. Dutoy and Wauters[17] reported 86% success with an average of nine months' follow-up, Bach and Cocchetto[12] and Gentry[14] had success rates of 68% and 92%, respectively, after 12 months. Sheftel and Mader's[13] smaller series had a mean of 21 months of follow-up with a 67% long-term success rate.

Bacteriologic eradication rates were high with ceftazidime for both *S aureus* (92%) and *P aeruginosa* (86%), with follow-up on most of these cases. While ceftazidime is noted for its activity against *P aeruginosa*, the excellent results in eradicating *S aureus* may be considered surprising. Adverse microbiologic events associated with ceftazidime included two cases of resistance in *P aeruginosa* and one in *Enterobacter cloacae*, as well as two recurrences of *E cloacae* infection. Enterobacter species are typically highly resistant to the cephalosporins, especially those agents used frequently. Significantly, there is no evidence of superinfections or resistance with gram-positive organisms and ceftazidime in osteomyelitis.

Ceftriaxone

Ceftriaxone has been evaluated in treating osteomyelitis in four trials; however, few follow-up data are available.[5,19-21] At dosages of 2 g daily or 1 g every 12 hours, end-of-therapy assessment was a success for 166 (89%) of 186 patients, with none needing to stop therapy because of an adverse effect. Three patients for whom some follow-up data are available (average follow-up time is three months) were all successfully treated. In Eron and associates'[20] study, which is the largest, bacteriologic data are available, with eradication rates of 95% for *S aureus* and 71% for *P aeruginosa*. The long-term efficacy in *P aeruginosa* will probably be significantly less than 71% because of the lack of in vitro activity for ceftriaxone against most strains of this organism. Despite these otherwise impressive data, and current interest in ceftriaxone for treatment of osteomyelitis because of its convenient, once daily administration, more comprehensive follow-up data are necessary before ceftriaxone can be accepted for osteomyelitis therapy.

Newer Beta-Lactams

Aztreonam, ticarcillin/clavulanic acid, and imipenem/cilastatin are representative of the newer classes of beta-lactams; namely, the monobactams, beta-lactam/beta-lactamase inhibitor combinations, and carbapenems, respectively (Table 1). Aztreonam (typical dosage is 2 g every eight hours) is active against most gram-negative bacteria in bone, including Enterobacteriaceae and *P aeruginosa*, yet most gram-positive organisms, including *S aureus*, are resistant. Aztreonam has only limited potential as monotherapy for osteomyelitis, as gram-positive cocci must be carefully excluded from the diagnosis. Ticarcillin/clavulanic acid is very effective extravascularly, achieving concentrations greater than the inhibitory concentration for *S aureus*, and in lesser concentrations with *P aeruginosa*. Imipenem/cilastatin, a potent and important mode of therapy, is active in bone against *S aureus*, Enterobacteriaceae, and *P aeruginosa*.

Aztreonam

The first of the class of monobactams to become widely available, aztreonam is characterized by activity against Enterobacteriaceae and *P aeruginosa*, excellent tissue penetration, and a lack of significant toxicity. While aztreonam is not active against gram-positive cocci, interest in its potential for fighting osteomyelitis has coincided with the disease's increasing gram-negative etiology. A total of 64 cases of aztreonam monotherapy for gram-negative osteomyelitis have been reported in eight small series,[22-29] with therapy discontinued only once because of an adverse effect. The average length of therapy was 25 days. For most of the patients, follow-up data were obtained for at least three months, with long-term success averaging 71%. *P aeruginosa* was eradicated in 22 (65%) of 34 cases. As might be predicted, adverse microbiologic events associated with aztreonam in osteomyelitis include emergence of gram-positive organisms, (one strain of *E faecalis* and three strains of *S aureus*) acquired resistance in one strain of *P aeruginosa*, and reinfection in one strain each of *Serratia marcescens* and *E cloacae*.

Ticarcillin/Clavulanic Acid

The ureidopenicillin/beta-lactamase inhibitor combination of ticarcillin/clavulanic acid has been evaluated in at least five trials involving 84 subjects.[30-34] Of these, 77 (92%) were able to tolerate a complete regimen of therapy, which averaged 28 days. The success rate at the end of therapy for ticarcillin/clavulanic acid appears to be 90%. Long-term follow-up data are available for at least half of these reported subjects, with a "cure" rate averaging 74%; these data include seven (78%) of nine subjects cured in one series with an average of 21 months of follow-up data obtained.[34]

Eradication of *S aureus* by ticarcillin/clavulanic acid was only 72%, with follow-up data available for almost all of these cases, and *P aeruginosa* eradication was 75%, with follow-up data provided for all. One strain each of *E cloacae* and *S marcescens* were resistant to therapy. These results in vivo are not completely consistent with the in vitro profile for ticarcillin/clavulanic acid of high activity against *S aureus* and lesser activity against *P aeruginosa*. For osteomyelitis, theoretical considerations may not always correspond to clinical experience.

The every-six-hours dosage regimen of ticarcillin/clavulanic acid is a significant impediment to its routine use in osteomyelitis patients.

Imipenem/Cilastatin

One of the newest and most important antimicrobial agents for the treatment of nosocomial infections is imipenem/cilastatin, which is highly active against most pathogenic bacteria. The high cost of the drug and its relatively short half-life (dose needed every six hours) substantially limit its usefulness in osteomyelitis. Nonetheless, osteomyelitis results are available from three trials,[9,35,36] including one series of 34 patients,[9] 33 of whom completed therapy, with sustained cure one year after therapy in 24 (73%). Bacteriologic eradication was 88% for *S aureus* and 75% for *P aeruginosa*, with two of the three persisting strains of *P aeruginosa* acquiring resistance to imipenem/cilastatin during therapy.

Oral Fluoroquinolones

Perhaps no class of antimicrobials is of as much interest in osteomyelitis as the oral fluoroquinolones. Ciprofloxacin and ofloxacin are approved for use in this country, and approval for enoxacin is pending. The quinolones penetrate bone at sufficient levels to inhibit *S aureus* and *P aeruginosa*, and are highly active against the Enterobacteriaceae (Table 1). Although the quinolones are similar in many regards, some comparisons can be made. Ciprofloxacin is more active in vitro and in vivo against *P aeruginosa* than is ofloxacin, while ofloxacin is more active in vivo against *S aureus* than is ciprofloxacin because of the higher serum levels of ofloxacin. As previously noted,[1] oral quinolone monotherapy may cost considerably less than parenteral alternatives, with added benefits of safety and convenience for the patient.

Ciprofloxacin

Ciprofloxacin has been the most extensively studied drug in osteomyelitis, with at least 23 trials published involving at least 368 subjects.[15,37-58] The percentage of patients able to complete the regimen, typically 750 mg every 12 hours for an average of 74 days, appears to be over 98%. With such extended regimens, long-term success rates and adverse microbiologic events must be carefully investigated in subjects with poor wound healing associated with diabetes mellitus or peripheral vascular disease. From those 14 studies that have provided follow-up data,[37-39,41,44,46,47,51,52,54-58] the long-term success rate of oral ciprofloxacin monotherapy is predicted at 75%. Included among these data are 29 subjects in one series with a 12–month cure rate of 66%, all of whom had underlying diabetes mellitus and/or peripheral vascular disease.

Microbiologic response has been equally consistent, with eradication rates for *S aureus* of 78% and of *P aeruginosa* 79%, the latter being an extensive data set of 95 cases for whom long-term follow-up data are available. Despite numerous Enterobacteriaceae cases treated, adverse microbiologic events, namely superinfections or acquired resistance during therapy, are concentrated among *S aureus* and *P aeruginosa*. Twelve (11%) of 107 isolates of *P aeruginosa* and six *S aureus* strains acquired resistance to treatment or caused superinfection.

Ofloxacin

Data from ofloxacin and osteomyelitis are available for at least 44 subjects in three trials,[52,59,60] all of whom were able to safely complete a regimen of 400 mg every 12 hours averaging over 100 days. Long-term follow-up data predict efficacy in 73% of patients.[52,59] Bacteriologic eradication rates were 74% for *S aureus* and 67% for *P aeruginosa*, with one strain of this organism acquiring resistance to ofloxacin. *S aureus* has not shown the ability to acquire resistance to ofloxacin in osteomyelitis.

Also presented in Table 1 are corresponding data for pefloxacin, a quinolone approved for use in Europe, yet whose status in the United States remains unclear. Twenty-eight cases have been published, remarkable for the ability of each to tolerate a pefloxacin regimen averaging 163 days.

Historical Review-Oral Penicillins

It is worthwhile to review earlier attempts to treat chronic staphylococcal osteomyelitis with oral penicillins, especially cloxacillin/dicloxacillin. In 1964, Borchardt and Hoffmeister[61] reported disappointing results for cloxacillin therapy (1 g/day), in chronic osteomyelitis; treatment was unsuccessful in four of six patients. Bell[62] in 1968 reported results with a higher dose (5 g/day) of cloxacillin in chronic *S aureus* osteomyelitis; 15 (94%) of 16 patients completed a regimen that averaged 200 days, with complete resolution of symptoms in 13 patients (87%). Remarkably, in a follow-up publication eight years later,

Bell[63] reported that one of the two patients with persistent drainage had since been cured by continued chronic cloxacillin suppression (1 g/day), and there had been no additional relapses, for a long-term success rate of 93%. Hedstrom[64] in 1974, using similar high-dose regimens of cloxacillin and dicloxacillin, successfully treated 29 (88%) of 33 patients with six months of therapy. Finally, in 1975, Hodgin[65] reported the results of oral penicillins in treating chronic *S aureus* osteomyelitis, with a successful outcome 18 months after therapy for nine (64%) of 14 patients.

These historical results represent carefully conducted trials that acknowledged the need for careful surgical management prior to drug therapy, as well as long-term patient follow-up. Obviously, these results compare favorably with other antistaphylococcal therapies, and support a hypothesis that effective, tolerable antibiotics can resolve osteomyelitis when close attention is paid to complete surgical debridement followed by reliance upon an extended regimen of antimicrobial therapy.

Parenteral Versus Oral Therapy

Prospective, randomized comparisons have been conducted of ciprofloxacin and ofloxacin with standard parenteral therapies, for cases of chronic osteomyelitis resulting from susceptible organisms. Parenteral therapies included nafcillin or cefazolin for treating osteomyelitis resulting from *S aureus*, and ceftazidime for treating gram-negative osteomyelitis.

In the ciprofloxacin trial,[38] 24 (77%) of 31 subjects evaluated remained cured 12 months after a therapeutic regimen that averaged 56 days, while in the intravenous group, 22 (79%) of 28 remained symptom-free 12 months after a regimen averaging 47 days. Diabetic subjects fared equally well in both groups, and polymicrobial osteomyelitis resulting from *P aeruginosa* was equally troublesome for the two approaches. There were two *S aureus* superinfections in the ciprofloxacin group. In an identical protocol for ofloxacin versus parenteral therapy,[59] ofloxacin was successful for 14 (74%) of 19 subjects with 18–months follow-up, with a successful outcome for 12 (86%) of 14 in the parenteral group. Again, diabetic subjects were not adversely affected by ofloxacin therapy, which in this trial averaged 56 days as compared with only 28 days for parenteral therapy.

Resistant Organisms

P aeruginosa

High levels of success in eradicating *P aeruginosa* from bone have been reported for parenteral ceftazidime and oral ciprofloxacin therapy, which have become the treatments of choice for this condition.

Ticarcillin/clavulanic acid and imipenem/cilastatin are not first-line agents for treating osteomyelitis, and the long-term efficacy for ceftriaxone in *P aeruginosa* osteomyelitis is related to its diminished in vitro activity. Although extensive data are not available for diabetic subjects, in whom *P aeruginosa* infection often spreads from contiguous soft tissue, and for whom wound healing may be delayed, a recent comprehensive review of the combined literature for infections of the skin and skin structure[66] showed no evidence to suggest that the extended therapeutic regimens associated with oral therapy as compared with parenteral therapy are associated with a higher degree of failure in diabetic patients.

P aeruginosa may be resistant to ceftazidime and ciprofloxacin therapy. Adverse effects are somewhat more likely with ciprofloxacin than with ceftazidime, despite theoretical considerations that predict lower instances of resistance to ciprofloxacin because of the mutational nature of such occurrences.[67] Microbiologic surveillance is necessary in either case, so oral ciprofloxacin therapy is the treatment of choice for osteomyelitis resulting from susceptible strains of *P aeruginosa*, in patients able to tolerate an extended regimen of oral therapy.

E faecalis

With the increasing use of broad-spectrum agents active against gram-negative enteric flora, enterococci have emerged as important nosocomial pathogens. *E faecalis* are routinely unresponsive to the cephalosporins and many of the newer beta-lactams, and the antibiotics of choice for enterococcal infection include vancomycin and synergistic combinations of penicillinase-resistant penicillins and aminoglycosides (e.g., nafcillin plus amikacin). Vancomycin suffers from poor kinetics in bone,[68] ototoxicity, and nephrotoxicity, and osteomyelitis patients in whom vancomycin therapy is attempted will often experience severe adverse effects of the medication prior to bacteriologic cure. As for combination therapy involving aminoglycosides, nephrotoxicity remains an important concern, although the clinical response is usually much more rapid. Literature reports of isolation of gentamicin-resistant enterococci are disturbing,[69] yet have not been substantiated in clinical practice in our center.

Methicillin-Resistant *S aureus* and Teicoplanin

A newer glycopeptide, teicoplanin, is under investigation as an alternative to vancomycin for infection resulting from methicillin-resistant staphylococci, and possibly enterococci. Preliminary safety results have been encouraging, with lower toxicity associated with teicoplanin, when compared with vancomycin. Six open, noncomparative trials have provided results for teicoplanin in osteomyelitis (Table 2),[70–75] with long-term success rates averaging 75%, and 92% eradication of *S aureus*. Seven of eight subjects with infection associated with foreign material were cured in one series. The most recent data, with more complete follow-up, confirm a 73% success rate of six

429

Table 2 Clinical Trials: Teicoplanin

Study	Daily Dosage	Total No. of Patients (Completed Therapy)	Mean Length of Treatment (days)	Remission (%)	Mean Follow-up (months)	No. of Patients Cured (%)	No. with Pathogen/Total* S aureus	Adverse Effects
Greenberg[70]	6–15 mg/kg	20(15)	53	—	6	11(73)	10/12	—
de Latta[71]	200–400 mg	8(8)	—	—	3	7(88)	—	1**
Van Laethem[72]	400 mg	1(1)	42	—	3	0(0)	0/1**	—
Galanakis[73]	200 mg	3(3)	36	—	2	1(33)	—	—
Bibler[74]	200–600 mg	1(1)	42	100	—	—	1/1†	—
Glupczynski[75]	200 mg	14(14)	28	—	1	11(79)	13/14	1‡

*Number of patients with *P aeruginosa* = 0 for all studies.
**Methicillin resistant *S aureus*
†Methicillin resistant *S epidermidis*
‡*S marcescens* superinfection

months, although the dosage now used is much higher (6 to 15 mg/kg versus 400 mg) because of dose-effect studies in methicillin-resistant *S aureus* bacteremia.[74,75] At these higher dosages, five of 20 osteomyelitis patients could not tolerate teicoplanin, developing a severe, macropapular rash distant to the infusion site. It remains to be seen whether osteomyelitis patients can tolerate teicoplanin at doses adequate to eradicate methicillin-resistant staphylococci from bone.

Conclusion

Many of the newer antimicrobial agents developed over the past ten years are appropriate in osteomyelitis caused by particular organisms. The various antibiotics active against gram-negative organisms complement the emerging pathogenesis of infections involving bone, and more recent attention has been paid to agents active against the resistant gram-positive bacteria that are increasingly troublesome. Economic considerations and patient comfort contribute to a full investigation of the role of oral antimicrobials, from traditional agents to the newer quinolones. Historical and recent results suggest that, with careful and complete surgical debridement of necrotic bone and soft tissue, oral therapy remains a viable alternative to intravenous care.

References

1. Gentry LO: Antibiotic therapy for osteomyelitis. *Infect Dis Clin North Am* 1990;4:485–499.
2. Mackowiak PA, Jones SR, Smith JW: Diagnostic value of sinus-tract cultures in chronic osteomyelitis. *JAMA* 1978;239:2772–2775.
3. Weinstein MP, Stratton CW, Hawley HB, et al: Multicenter collaborative evaluation of a standardized serum bactericidal test as a predictor of therapeutic efficacy in acute and chronic osteomyelitis. *Am J Med* 1987;83:218–222.
4. Gomis M, Herranz A, Aparicio P, et al: Cefotaxime in the treatment of chronic osteomyelitis caused by gram-negative bacilli. *J Antimicrob Chemother* 1990;26(suppl A):45–52.

5. Mandell LA, Bergeron MG, Ronald AR, et al: Once-daily therapy with ceftriaxone compared with daily multiple-dose therapy with cefotaxime for serious bacterial infections: A randomized, double-blind study. *J Infect Dis* 1989;160:433–441.

6. LeFrock JL, Carr BB: Clinical experience with cefotaxime in the treatment of serious bone and joint infections. *Rev Infect Dis* 1982;4(suppl):S465–S471.

7. Mader JT, LeFrock JL, Hyams KC, et al: Cefotaxime therapy for patients with osteomyelitis and septic arthritis. *Rev Infect Dis* 1982;4(suppl):S472–S480.

8. Löffler L, Bauernfeind A, Keyl W, et al: An open, comparative study of sulbactam plus ampicillin vs. cefotaxime as initial therapy for serious soft tissue and bone and joint infections. *Rev Infect Dis* 1986;8(suppl 5):S593–S598.

9. Stamboulian D, Argüello EA, Jasovich A, et al: Comparative clinical evaluation of imipenem/cilastatin vs. cefotaxime in treatment of severe bacterial infections. *Rev Infect Dis* 1985;7(suppl 3):S458–S462.

10. Horan TC, White JW, Jarvis WR, et al: Nosocomial infection surveillance, 1984. *MMWE CDC Surveill Sum* 1986;35:5517–5529.

11. Bragman S, Sage R, Booth L, et al: Ceftazidime in the treatment of serious Pseudomonas aeruginosa sepsis. *Scand J Infect Dis* 1986;18:425–429.

12. Bach MC, Cocchetto DM: Ceftazidime as single-agent therapy for gram-negative aerobic bacillary osteomyelitis. *Antimicrob Agents Chemother* 1987;31:1605–1608.

13. Sheftel TG, Mader JT: Randomized evaluation of ceftazidime or ticarcillin and tobramycin for the treatment of osteomyelitis caused by gram-negative bacilli. *Antimicrob Agents Chemother* 1986;29:112–115.

14. Gentry LO: Treatment of skin, skin structure, bone, and joint infections with ceftazidime. *Am J Med* 1985;79(suppl 2A):67–74.

15. Peacock JE Jr, Pegram PS, Weber SF, et al: Prospective, randomized comparison of sequential intravenous followed by oral ciprofloxacin with intravenous ceftazidime in the treatment of serious infections. *Am J Med* 1989;87(suppl 5A):185S–190S.

16. Gaut PL, Carron WC, Ching WTW, et al: Intravenous/oral ciprofloxacin therapy versus intravenous ceftazidime therapy for selected bacterial infections. *Am J Med* 1989;87(suppl 5A):169S–175S.

17. Dutoy JP, Wauters G: The treatment of bone infections with ceftazidime. *J Antimicrob Chemother* 1983;12(suppl A):229–233.

18. Giamarellou H, Perdikaris G, Galanakis N, et al: Pefloxacin versus ceftazidime in the treatment of a variety of gram-negative-bacterial infections. *Antimicrob Agents Chemother* 1989;33:1362–1367.

19. McCloskey RV: Clinical and bacteriologic efficacy of ceftriaxone in the United States. *Am J Med* 1984;77(suppl 4C):97–103.

20. Eron LJ, Goldenberg RI, Poretz DM: Combined ceftriaxone and surgical therapy for osteomyelitis in hospital and outpatient settings. *Am J Surg* 1984;148(suppl 4A):1–4.

21. Scully BE, Neu HC: Ceftriaxone in the treatment of serious infections, particularly after surgery. *Am J Surg* 1984;148(suppl 4A):35–40.

22. Pribyl C, Salzer R, Beskin J, et al: Aztreonam in the treatment of serious orthopedic infections. *Am J Med* 1985;78(suppl 2A):51–56.

23. Scully BE, Neu HC: Use of aztreonam in the treatment of serious infections due to multiresistant gram-negative organisms, including *Pseudomonas aeruginosa. Am J Med* 1985;78:251–261.

24. Romero-Vivas J, Rodríguez-Créixems M, Bouza E, et al: Evaluation of aztreonam in the treatment of severe bacterial infections. *Antimicrob Agents Chemother* 1985;28:222–226.

25. Giamarellou H, Galanakis N, Douzinas E, et al: Evaluation of aztreonam in difficult-to-treat infections with prolonged posttreatment follow-up. *Antimicrob Agents Chemother* 1984;26:245–249.

26. LeFrock JL, Smith BR, Chandrasekar P, et al: Efficacy and safety of aztreonam in the treatment of serious gram-negative bacterial infections. *Arch Intern Med* 1987;147:325–328.

27. Greenberg RN, Reilly PM, Luppen KL, et al: Treatment of serious gram-negative infections with aztreonam. *J Infect Dis* 1984;150:623–630.

28. McKellar PP: Clinical evaluation of aztreonam therapy for serious infections due to gram-negative bacteria. *Rev Infect Dis* 1985;7(suppl 4):S803–S809.

29. Simons WJ, Lee TJ: Aztreonam in the treatment of bone and joint infections caused by gram-negative bacilli. *Rev Infect Dis* 1985;7(suppl 4):S783–S788.

30. Meylan PR, Calandra T, Casey PA, et al: Clinical experience with Timentin in severe hospital infections. *J Antimicrob Chemother* 1985;17(suppl C):127–139.

31. Roselle GA, Bode R, Hamilton B, et al: Clinical trial of the efficacy and safety of ticarcillin and clavulanic acid. *Antimicrob Agents Chemother* 1985;27:291–296.

32. Gentry LO, Macko V, Lind R, et al: Ticarcillin plus clavulanic acid (Timentin) therapy for osteomyelitis. *Am J Med* 1985;79(suppl 5B):116–121.

33. Johnson CC, Reinhardt JF, Wallace SL, et al: Safety and efficacy of ticarcillin plus clavulanic acid in the treatment of infections of soft tissue, bone, and joint. *Am J Med* 1985;79(suppl 5B):136–140.

34. Siebert WT, Kopp PE: Ticarcillin plus clavulanic acid versus moxalactam therapy of osteomyelitis, septic arthritis, and skin and soft tissue infections. *Am J Med* 1985;79(suppl 5B):141–145.

35. Iannini PB, Kunkel MJ, Hilton E, et al: Imipenem/cilastatin: General experience in a community hospital. *Am J Med* 1985;78(suppl 6A):122–126.

36. MacGregor RR, Gentry LO: Imipenem/cilastatin in the treatment of osteomyelitis. *Am J Med* 1985;78(suppl 6A):100–103.

37. Dan M, Siegman-Igra Y, Pitlik S, et al: Oral ciprofloxacin treatment of *Pseudomonas aeruginosa* osteomyelitis. *Antimicrob Agents Chemother* 1990;34:849–852.

38. Gentry LO, Rodriquez GG: Oral ciprofloxacin compared with parenteral antibiotics in the treatment of osteomyelitis. *Antimicrob Agents Chemother* 1990;34:40–43.

39. Mader JT, Cantrell JS, Calhoun J: Oral ciprofloxacin compared with standard parenteral antibiotic therapy for chronic osteomyelitis in adults. *J Bone Joint Surg* 1990;72A:104–110.

40. Ramirez CA, Bran JL, Mejia CR, et al: Open, prospective study of the clinical efficacy of ciprofloxacin. *Antimicrob Agents Chemother* 1985;28:128–132.

41. Peterson LR, Lissack LM, Canter KI, et al: Therapy of lower extremity infections with ciprofloxacin in patients with diabetes mellitus, peripheral vascular disease, or both. *Am J Med* 1989;86:801–808.

42. Modai J: Treatment of serious infections with intravenous ciprofloxacin: French Multicenter Study Group. *Am J Med* 1989;87(suppl 5A):243S–247S.

43. Greenberg RN, Wilson KM, Brusca PA: Intravenous and oral ciprofloxacin treatment of 52 infections. *Am J Med* 1989;87(suppl 5A):238S–239S.

44. Gudiol F, Cabellos C, Pallares R, et al: Intravenous ciprofloxacin therapy in severe infections. *Am J Med* 1989;87(suppl 5A):221S–224S.

45. Abadie-Kemmerly S, Pankey GA: Safety and efficacy of intravenous ciprofloxacin in the treatment of selected infections. *Am J Med* 1989;87(suppl 5A):213S–220S.

46. Neu HC, Davidson S, Briones F: Intravenous/oral ciprofloxacin therapy of infections caused by multiresistant bacteria. *Am J Med* 1989;87(suppl 5A):209S–212S.

47. Report from a Swedish study group: Therapy of acute and chronic gram-negative osteomyelitis with ciprofloxacin. *J Antimicrob Chemother* 1988;22:221–228.

48. Notari MA, Mittler BE: Ciprofloxacin: A study of usage in pedal infections with case reports. *J Foot Surg* 1989;28:521–523.

49. Follath F, Bindschedler M, Wenk M, et al: Use of ciprofloxacin in the treatment of *Pseudomonas aeruginosa* infections. *Eur J Clin Microbiol* 1986;5:236–240.

50. Giamarellou H, Galanakis N, Dendrinos C, et al: Evaluation of ciprofloxacin in the treatment of *Pseudomonas aeruginosa* infections. *Eur J Clin Microbiol* 1986;5:232–235.

51. Dellamonica P, Bernard E, Etesse H, et al: Evaluation of pefloxacin, ofloxacin and ciprofloxacin in the treatment of thirty-nine cases of chronic osteomyelitis. *Eur J Clin Microbiol Infect Dis* 1989;8:1024–1030.

52. Greenberg RN, Tice AD, Marsh PK, et al: Randomized trial of ciprofloxacin compared with other antimicrobial therapy in the treatment of osteomyelitis. *Am J Med* 1987;82(suppl 4A):266–269.

53. Scully BE, Neu HC, Parry MF, et al: Oral ciprofloxacin therapy of infections due to Pseudomonas aeruginosa. *Lancet* 1986;1:819–822.

54. Daly JS, Worthington MG, Razvi SA, et al: Intravenous and sequential intravenous and oral ciprofloxacin in the treatment of severe infections. *Am J Med* 1989;87(suppl 5A):232S–234S.

55. Lesse AJ, Freer C, Salata RA, et al: Oral ciprofloxacin therapy for gram-negative bacillary osteomyelitis. *Am J Med* 1987;82(suppl 4A):247–253.

56. Gilbert DN, Tice AD, Marsh PK, et al: Oral ciprofloxacin therapy for chronic contiguous osteomyelitis caused by aerobic gram-negative bacilli. *Am J Med* 1987;82(suppl 4A):254–258.

57. Slama TG, Misinski J, Sklar S: Oral ciprofloxacin therapy for osteomyelitis caused by aerobic gram-negative bacilli. *Am J Med* 1987;82(suppl 4A):259–261.

58. Hessen MT, Ingerman MJ, Kaufman DH, et al: Clinical efficacy of ciprofloxacin therapy for gram-negative bacillary osteomyelitis. *Am J Med* 1987;82(suppl 4A):262–265.

59. Gentry LO, Rodriguez-Gomez G: Ofloxacin versus parenteral therapy for chronic osteomyelitis. *Antimicrob Agents Chemother* 1991;35:538–541.

60. Regamey C, Steinbach-Lebbin C: Severe infections treated with intravenous ofloxacin: A prospective clinical multicentre Swiss study. *J Antimicrob Chemother* 1990;26(suppl D):107–114.

61. Borchardt KA, Hoffmeister RA: Peroral oxacillin in chronic osteomyelitis: Preliminary evaluation. *NY State J Med* 1964;64:2414–2417.

62. Bell SM: Oral penicillins in the treatment of chronic staphylococcal osteomyelitis. *Lancet* 1968;2:295–297.

63. Bell SM: Further observations on the value of oral penicillins in chronic staphylococcal osteomyelitis. *Med J Aust* 1976;2:591–593.

64. Hedström SA: The prognosis of chronic staphylococcal osteomyelitis after long-term antibiotic treatment. *Scand J Infect Dis* 1974;6:33–38.

65. Hodgin UG Jr: Antibiotics in the treatment of chronic staphylococcal osteomyelitis. *South Med J* 1975;68:817–823.

66. Black J, Hunt TL, Godley PJ, et al: Oral antimicrobial therapy for adults with osteomyelitis or septic arthritis. *J Infect Dis* 1987;155:968–972.

67. Hooper DC, Wolfson JS, Ng EY, et al: Mechanisms of action of and resistance to ciprofloxacin. *Am J Med* 1987;82(suppl 4A):12–20.

68. Wilson KJ, Mader JT: Concentrations of vancomycin in bone and serum of normal rabbits and those with osteomyelitis. *Antimicrob Agents Chemother* 1984;25:140–141.

69. Rhinehart E, Smith NE, Wennersten C, et al: Rapid dissemination of beta-lactamase-producing aminoglycoside-resistant *Enterococcus faecalis* among patients and staff on an infant-toddler surgical ward. *N Engl J Med* 1990;323:1814–1818.

70. Greenberg RN: Treatment of bone, joint, and vascular-access-associated gram-positive bacterial infections with teicoplanin. *Antimicrob Agents Chemother* 1990;34:2392–2397.

71. De Lalla F, Santoro D, Rinaldi E, et al: Teicoplanin in the treatment of infections by staphylococci, *Clostridium difficile* and other gram-positive bacteria. *J Antimicrob Chemother* 1989;23:131–142.

72. Van Laethem Y, Hermans P, De Witt S, et al: Teicoplanin compared with vancomycin in methicillin-resistant *Staphylococcus aureus* infections: Preliminary results. *J Antimicrob Chemother* 1988;21(suppl A):81–87.

73. Galanakis N, Giamarellou H, Vlachogiannis N, et al: Poor efficacy of teicoplanin in treatment of deep-seated staphylococcal infections. *Eur J Clin Microbiol Infect Dis* 1988;7:130–134.

74. Bibler MR, Frame PT, Hagler DN, et al: Clinical evaluation of efficacy, pharmacokinetics, and safety of teicoplanin for serious gram-positive infections. *Antimicrob Agents Chemother* 1987;31:207–212.

75. Glupczynski Y, Lagast H, Van der Auwera P, et al: Clinical evaluation of teicoplanin for therapy of severe infections caused by gram-positive bacteria. *Antimicrob Agents Chemother* 1986;29:52–57.

Chapter 30

Antiseptics

Jon T. Mader, MD
Hans Hager, MD
Jose Cobos, MD
Jason H. Calhoun, MD

Introduction

Antiseptics are substances used on or in living tissue to inhibit or destroy microorganisms; they are used for hand washing, surgical preparation, on wounds, or in body cavities. Commonly used classes of antiseptics include phenols, alcohols, acids, halogens, oxidizing agents, chlorhexidine, heavy metals and their salts, quaternary ammonium compounds, anti-adherence compounds, organic acids, and soaps. Important properties of antiseptics include germicidal potency, rapidity of action, length of activity, surface tension, potency in presence of inflammatory exudates and soaps, and effect on the mechanisms of healing and tissue repair.

Often, no distinction is made between antiseptics, disinfectants, and germicides. Germicide is a general term for any agent that destroys microorganisms; both antiseptics and disinfectants are germicides. A disinfectant is a chemical germicide that is used solely for destroying microorganisms on inanimate objects. Germicides may be categorized according to their antimicrobial action as bactericides, fungicides, protozoacides, virucides, or a combination thereof. Some chemicals, such as the iodophors, are used as active agents in chemical germicides formulated for use both as disinfectants and as antiseptics. However, precise formulations are usually significantly different depending on the intended use, and germicidal efficacy often varies substantially from antiseptics to disinfectants. In general, disinfectants should never be used as antiseptics and vice versa. Disinfectants harshly denature proteins and are not approved for use on wounds or in body cavities.

The clinical use of topical antimicrobial agents to cleanse contaminated and chronic wounds is common. Honey and resins were used by the ancient Egyptians.[1] In the 1800s, Lister developed the premise that the reduction of superficial bacterial contamination would promote wound healing. Although the antibacterial efficacy of topical antimicrobials is well documented, their effect on living tissue and on the process of wound healing is poorly understood. Antiseptics are also used for hand washing (Fig. 1) and surgical preparation.

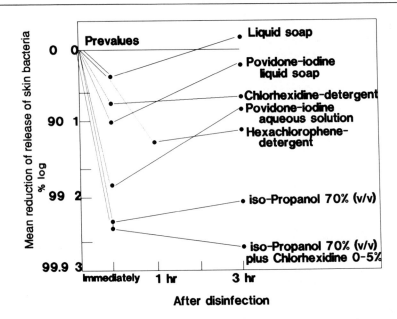

Fig. 1 *Examples of the efficacy of various antiseptics for surgical hand disinfection. All solutions used for five minutes apart from chlorhexidine detergent (three minutes). (Adapted with permission from Rotter M: Are models useful for testing hand antiseptics?* J Hosp Infect *1988;11(suppl A):236–243.)*

Antiseptics are a heterogeneous group of compounds with respect to chemical structure, mechanism of action, and therapeutic use. Most authors classify antiseptics loosely using a chemical classification. The commonly used classes of antiseptics (Table 1) include: phenolics, alcohols, acids, halogens, oxidizing agents, chlorhexidine, metallic ions, quaternary ammonium compounds, anti-adherence compounds, organic acids, and soaps.

Classes of Antiseptics

Phenols and Phenol Derivatives

Phenol   Phenol (carbolic acid) was first used by Lister in 1867. Phenol causes protein denaturation, leakage of essential intracellular metabolites through the cell wall, and inactivation of many intracellular enzymes. The phenol coefficient test, developed by Rideal in 1903, compares the bactericidal activities of various germicides with that of standard phenol.[2] Because of its toxicity, phenol is rarely used today. Even unabraded skin may be deeply penetrated and necrosed.[3,4] Currently, less toxic and more bactericidal derivatives of phenol are used.

Table 1 Standard antiseptic chemical classes and agents

Group	Effective Against	Effect on Spores	Speed	Nature of Activity
Phenolics	Gram +, gram −, mycobacteria	Moderate	Good	Bactericidal
Alcohols	Gram +, gram −, and acid fast	Poor Bacteriostatic	Rapid	Bactericidal Fungistatic
Acids	± gram +, gram −		Moderate	Bactericidal
Halogens	Gram +, gram −, mycobacteria	Moderate	Rapid	Bactericidal
Oxidizing agents	Gram +, gram −	Poor	Rapid	Bactericidal
Chlorhexidine	Gram +, ± gram −, fungi	Moderate	Moderate	Bactericidal
Metallic ions	Gram +, gram −	Poor	Moderate	Bactericidal Fungicidal
Quaternary ammonium compounds	Gram +, gram −	Poor	Moderate	Bactericidal or bacteriostatic
Anti-adherence compounds	Gram +, gram −	Unknown	Unknown	Anti-adherence

Hexachlorophene   Hexachlorophene (chlorine-substituted bis-phenol) is the most commonly used phenol derivative. When used in high concentrations, it disrupts microbial cell walls and precipitates cell proteins. In lower concentrations, it is thought to act by inactivation of oxidative and other essential enzyme systems within the microorganism.[5] Although it is active against gram-positive bacteria, it is relatively inactive against gram-negative bacteria, the tubercle bacillus, fungi, and viruses. Occasional outbreaks of gram-negative nosocomial infections have been traced to this antiseptic.[5,6,7] Although hexachlorophene is highly bacteriostatic, prolonged contact is required to kill microorganisms.

Organic matter, such as serum and pus, reduces the efficacy of hexachlorophene, but it does not lose potency in the presence of soap. Three percent hexachlorophene is a synthetic detergent vehicle. Hexachlorophene liquid soap and other hexachlorophene preparations are frequently used as operative scrubs and/or germicidal soaps for hand washing. However, maximal reduction of skin flora is attained only after several successive days of hand washing because the chemical must gradually accumulate on the skin surface before it reaches optimal concentrations. Washing the hands with hexachlorophene exclusively and frequently deposits a film of hexachlorophene on the skin, where it then performs a continuous degerming action.[8] An approximate 40% reduction in skin flora is noted with the first hand washing using a hexachlorophene detergent combination. This extends to approximately 93% after one hour, and then the bacterial counts begin to return toward baseline.[9] Hexachlorophene is absorbed through the skin and tissues where it can produce both transient and permanent neurologic symptoms, especially after repeated use in high concentrations.[10] Additionally, this agent is teratogenic.[3] For these reasons, the Food and Drug Administration (FDA) has banned nonprescription sales of products that contain more than 0.1% hexachlorophene. Its use for total body bathing, on denuded skin, mucous membranes, or newborn infants is contraindicated. Approved FDA uses of hexachlorophene are now limited to surgical scrubbing and hand washing.

Alcohols

Alcohols evaporate readily and are bactericidal and inexpensive. These substances have excellent antibacterial activity against most gram-positive and gram-negative organisms, as well as the tubercle bacillus, but are minimally sporicidal. Alcohols are believed to exert their antibacterial action by denaturing proteins. Proteins are not as easily denaturized in the absence of water as they are in the presence of water; therefore absolute ethyl alcohol is less bactericidal than mixtures of alcohol and water. The bactericidal activity of alcohols increases with molecular weight. Currently, ethyl and isopropyl alcohol are the ones used extensively in clinical practice.

The rapidly volatile nature of alcohol prevents it from leaving a lasting antiseptic effect on the skin or wound, but because of its continued lethal effect on damaged organisms, bacterial counts continue to decrease for several hours after use.[4]

Ethyl Alcohol   Ethyl alcohol is widely used as an antiseptic before venipuncture, needle injection, and finger pricks. For skin antisepsis, alcohol concentrations between 70% and 92% by weight are equally effective.[11] In addition to its effect on bacteria, ethyl alcohol also exerts substantial fungicidal and virucidal activity.

Isopropyl Alcohol   Isopropyl alcohol is the most commonly used alcohol clinically. It is the highest molecular weight alcohol miscible with water in all proportions. Because isopropyl alcohol is not potable, it is not subject to the legal restrictions and taxation imposed on ethyl alcohol. It is more bactericidal than ethyl alcohol and also has no effect on spores. Isopropyl alcohol is not harmful to human skin, although its vapors can be absorbed through the lungs and produce toxic side effects, usually narcosis in children. For skin antisepsis, solutions of 70% or more recommended. The bactericidal action of isopropyl alcohol increases with its concentration. Seventy percent isopropyl alcohol immediately eradicates 99.3% of the skin flora with a subsequent gradual return toward baseline bacterial counts. When isopropyl alcohol is combined with chlorhexidine, bacterial reduction continues for more than three hours.[9]

Acids

Several acids are used as antiseptics. The germicidal action of most acids is caused by hydrogen ions, but others have a more selective type of action.

Acetic Acid   Acetic acid in a 5% concentration is bactericidal to many types of microorganisms and is bacteriostatic at lower concentration. Gram-negative organisms, especially *Pseudomonas aeruginosa*, are particularly susceptible to acetic acid. However, recent studies imply that 0.25% acetic acid is harmful to fibroblasts.[12]

Halogens and Halogen-Containing Compounds

Iodine Iodine is one of the oldest antiseptics. Elemental iodine is bactericidal and sporicidal over a wide pH range against bacteria, fungi, viruses, and protozoa; however, acid solutions markedly increase its germicidal efficiency. A 1:20,000 solution of iodine kills almost all bacteria within one minute, but takes 15 minutes to kill spores.

Because toxicity of iodine is extremely low in relation to its germicidal capacity, it is a safe antiseptic agent. However, strong iodine solutions (> 5% iodine) can cause chemical burns if placed on large areas of the skin, and systemic absorption of iodine has resulted in hyperthyroidism.[3]

Iodine Preparations Containing Free Iodine Two percent iodine tincture, USP, contains 2% iodine and 2% sodium iodide in 44% to 55% ethyl alcohol. The solution spreads evenly, dries slowly, does not burn the skin, and rarely causes any patient discomfort. Aqueous iodine is also an effective antiseptic, although an iodide salt must be added to solubilize the iodine.

Iodophors An iodophor is iodine combined with a solubilizing agent or carrier that liberates free iodine in solution. Iodophors act by penetrating the bacterial cell wall, oxidizing, and substituting free iodine for the microbial cell contents. The iodophors have a wide range of antibacterial actions against gram-positive and gram-negative bacteria, mycobacteria, fungi, and viruses. The antimicrobial action of iodophors declines rapidly as they dry because of the unavailability of free iodine.[13] Iodophors require about two minutes of contact time to allow sufficient release of free iodine.[14] They are nonirritating to the eyes, skin, nose, mouth, and vaginal mucosa and produce minimal discomfort when applied to abrasions and wounds. Moreover, no allergic response to iodine occurs, even in sensitive individuals, when it is applied in the form of an iodophor. In low dilutions, they do not permanently stain skin or natural fabrics. Their stability permits easy storage.

Povidone-iodine is a complex of iodine and polyvinylpyrrolidone. The compound slowly releases free iodine when dissolved in water. It is claimed that povidone-iodine is more effective and less toxic than aqueous or alcohol solutions. Blatt and Maloney[15] found that the germicidal properties of three different iodophors were similar to those of iodine solutions of equivalent iodine content. The 98% immediate reduction of skin flora noted with aqueous povidone-iodine is followed by gradual return of the normal skin flora. Povidone-iodine detergents reduce skin flora by 90% but lack continuous action.[9]

Chlorine Chlorine appears to exert its antibacterial action in the form of undissociated hypochlorous acid (HOCl). Chlorine combines with water to form HOCl and dissociated hydrochloric acid (HCl). HOCl is undissociated in neutral or acid solutions and exerts a strong bactericidal effect. It dissociates in alkaline solution, and the hypochlorite ion is much less effective. Dakin's solution, a buffered solution of sodium hypochlorite introduced in World War I as an antiseptic irrigant for wounds, is injurious to tissues. Modified Dakin's solution contains 0.5% sodium hypochlorite, instead of 5.0% sodium hypochlorite, and is much less toxic to tissues. Unfortunately, even with a 0.1% solution of modified Dakin's, an inflammatory response has been noted in normal skin within 14 days. This solution, however, is a good antiseptic with an immediate two log reduction (99%) in *Staphylococcus aureus*, *Candida albicans*, and *P aeruginosa*.[16]

Oxidizing Agents

Hydrogen Peroxide   Hydrogen peroxide is frequently used in granulating and other open wounds to reduce bacterial contamination. Low concentrations of unstable preparations are rapidly inactivated by catalase in the tissues. Consequently, numerous bubbles of oxygen gas, which signify rapid inactivation of the hydrogen peroxide, are formed when it is placed into open tissues. Unstable preparations of hydrogen peroxide are almost totally ineffective as an antiseptic and have been generally abandoned. Recently, however, hydrogen peroxide has become available in pure stabilized preparations with a long shelf life. Even though it is not commonly used, tests have shown stabilized hydrogen peroxide to be an effective germicide.[4]

Chlorhexidine

Chlorhexidine is a cationic bisbiguanide that kills bacterial cells by disrupting their cell membranes and precipitating the cell contents. Although its spectrum of activity is broad, it is somewhat more effective against gram-positive than gram-negative organisms. *Proteus* species, *Providencia* species, and *Serratia* species are particularly resistant. Most bacterial organisms are inhibited by concentrations below 50 µg/ml; however, the lowest concentration recommended is 200 µg/ml. Although chlorhexidine is a good fungicide, its action is fair against the tubercle bacillus and poor against the viruses.[17,18] Chlorhexidine retains its antibacterial activity in the presence of blood and other organic material. However, because its activity is pH dependent, it may be neutralized by hard tap water, natural soaps, and certain pharmaceuticals containing nonionic surfactants or inorganic anions.

Chlorhexidine is used extensively for skin antisepsis before operative procedures. There is no absorption through intact skin, and it has a low potential for causing skin reactions.[19] Chlorhexidine can be used many times for hand antisepsis without causing dryness, irritation, or discomfort. Chlorhexidine 0.005% is not reported to cause additional tissue injury or delayed healing when used for cleaning superficial wounds. Chlorhexidine is recommended for topical use only.

Chlorhexidine's long duration of action is a major advantage when used for hand washing. Although it produces only a 70% immediate reduction in skin flora, a residual remains because of its strong affinity for skin, which sustains chlorhexidine's activity for several hours.[9,20,21] When it is combined with alcohol there is a synergistic effect producing 99% immediate and long-term reduction of the skin flora. Its duration of action with alcohol is somewhat less than with soap combinations. With greater than three washings per day, 98% continuous reduction in skin flora can be anticipated after five days of use. However, skin overgrowth has occurred with gram-positive bacteria and *Candida* species.[3] Concentrations greater than 2% chlorhexidine seem to provide little increased bactericidal advantage.[22]

Heavy Metals and Their Salts

Mercurials   Inorganic mercury compounds were among the earliest antiseptics used. Organic and inorganic mercurials are bacteriostatic compounds that combine with sulfhydryl groups on cytoplasmic or cell wall enzymes. The sulfhydryl inibition is reversible and bacteria may regain their virulence when exposure to the agent has ended. Numerous sulfhydryl groups are readily available in the body. In addition to bacteria, mercury also inactivates enzymes in tissues. Thus, mercurials are toxic and have a low therapeutic index.

Organic mercurial compounds are more bacteriostatic, less irritating, and less toxic than the inorganic mercurial salts. However, they are slow acting and are inactivated by blood and other organic material.[23] Merbromin (mercurochrome) has minimal bacteriostatic activity and is relatively inactive at the pH of body fluids. Thimerosal (merthiolate) is commonly applied to cuts and abrasions. Tinctures of organic mercurials are more effective than aqueous solutions but not as effective as 70% ethyl alcohol.

Silver   Silver exerts its antimicrobial activity by inhibiting cellular enzymes and by blocking DNA replication. Silver compounds are bactericidal in high concentrations ($\geq$ 10%) but only bacteriostatic in lower concentrations. Silver nitrate solutions are applied as antiseptics to mucous membranes. One percent silver nitrate is used as eye drops at birth to prevent ophthalmia neonatorum.

Currently, silver sulfadiazine cream is applied to burns to prevent bacterial infections. It penetrates the eschar particularly well. Silver sulfadiazine is bactericidal and is easier to work with than silver nitrate; however, it is painful when applied to burn injuries. Furthermore, silver sulfadiazine is a carbonic anhydrase inhibitor and can cause metabolic acidosis.

Other silver salts of acetate, citrate, and lactate are used for eye lotions and treatment of burn wounds or wound surfaces. Silver proteinates are colloidal preparations of silver used for eye drops, urethral irrigations, throat and nose sprays, and vaginal and rectal suppositories. Recently, silver-impregnated devices, such as Foley catheters and central line cuffs, have become available. Their efficacy is being evaluated.

Quaternary Ammonium Compounds

For many years, quaternary ammonium compounds were popular disinfectants because of their inertness and low cost. These are cationic surface-active agents that can precipitate or denature protein, thereby destroying the microorganisms. Unfortunately, quaternary ammonium compounds are relatively inactive against gram-negative bacteria. They form a thin film on the skin under which bacteria can remain viable. In addition, they are rapidly inactivated by any trace of soap left on the skin after regular washing. If allowed to stand, the solutions may become contaminated by *Pseudomonas* species and have been the source of some hospital-acquired infections.[24]

Commonly used commercial preparations include benzalkonium chloride and cetylpyridinium chloride. Tincture of benzalkonium chloride is more effective than an aqueous solution. A considerable portion of the benefit is attributed to the alcohol-acetone solvent.

Anti-adherence Compounds

Taurolidine (Taurolin) Taurolidine—Taurolin, bis-(1,1-dioxoperhydro-1,2,4 methylene thadiazinyl-4) methane—is a novel antimicrobial for local and parenteral use. It is active against gram-positive organisms, gram-negative organisms, and fungi. Recent reports have shown that taurolidine and the related compound noxythiolin blocked the in vitro adherence of bacteria to tissues, including epithelial and fibroblast cells.[25] The clinical significance of these observations remains uncertain. However, the potential ability to block the adherence of pathogenic organisms to wound surfaces may have a significant effect in preventing bacterial colonization and infection.[26]

Other Antiseptics and Detergents

Organic Agents Organic agents, such as ether, acetone, chloroform, and xylene, have also been used for skin antisepsis but are drying agents and are somewhat injurious to tissue. In addition, ether and acetone are extremely flammable.

Soaps Soap is a poor antiseptic. While a bar of soap will quickly sterilize itself after it has been used, it is relatively ineffective as a skin antiseptic. Its value lies in its ability to remove gross dirt, grease, oils, and other surface debris that might contain microorganisms. A 30% immediate reduction in skin flora has been noted after hand washing with soap.[9] However, bacteriologic rebound is almost immediate. Because detergents tend to cause significant damage when applied to denuded tissue, these agents should be reserved for intact skin.[3]

Discussion

One of the most important properties of antiseptics is their germicidal potency. An agent that is lethal to microorganisms is superior to one that merely inhibits growth. A broad antimicrobial spectrum is essential, especially for microorganisms that inhabit the skin or wounds. Bactericidal and fungicidal properties are much more important than virucidal or protozoacidal actions. Other important properties of antiseptic agents include low surface tension, because they must spread over skin or wound surfaces, and retention of potency in the presence of inflammatory exudates. Antiseptics should be rapid acting so that bacteria and fungi are killed during routine hand-washing or skin preparation times. Sustained activity of the antiseptic is an additional advantage. Antiseptics should not be systemically absorbed or cause hypersensitivity reactions. They should not be inactivated by soaps used for cleansing the skin. Antiseptic agents should not cause irritation of skin or tissues and should not interfere with the mechanisms of healing and tissue repair.

The germicidal potency of antiseptics has been best tested in vivo by hand-washing experiments (Fig. 1). These studies are relatively easy to perform, contribute information on skin antisepsis, and allow the formulation of products that cause minimal irritation to the skin. Most of the work has been done with gram-positive organisms and with normal skin flora.[27] Complete sterilization of the skin is impossible; however, various formulations of chlorhexidine, hexachlorophene, alcohols, and iodines have been shown to be adequate for hand antisepsis. In most cases, reducing the skin flora to a bacterial concentration range of 10^4 to 10^5 appears to be adequate for antisepsis. The gram-negative efficacy of some of these antiseptics has been questioned. Epidemics have been traced to surgical scrubs contaminated with *Pseudomonas* species. However, it has been difficult to blame the antiseptics used in hand washing as the cause of nosocomial infections caused by gram-negative organisms. Except for *Acinetobacter* species and *Klebsiella* species, most common gram-negative pathogens will not colonize normal skin for longer than 90 minutes.[28]

Given the variety of nonstandardized data, absolute conclusions about antiseptics and hand washing are impossible; however, the following data exist. After physical cleansing, alcohols and organic iodines appear to provide the best and broadest immediate antiseptic action on intact skin. Chlorhexidine, especially in combination with alcohol, has the advantage of broad antiseptic action and continuous action when used regularly. With the exception of hexachlorophene, the combination of soap with an antiseptic seldom works as well as the antiseptic alone.[9]

In 1919, Alexander Fleming stated that antiseptics will exercise a beneficial effect in a septic wound only if they possess the property of stimulating or conserving the natural defense mechanism of the body against infection.[29] The efficacy of topical antiseptic agents must be considered in relation to their potential detrimental effects on wound

443

healing. However, the evidence that antiseptics are toxic to healing tissue is scanty and confusing. Many commonly used antiseptics have a toxic effect on fibroblasts grown in tissue culture. Lineaweaver and associates[12] tested four antiseptics on human fibroblast cultures: 1% povidone-iodine, 0.5% sodium hypochlorite, 0.25% acetic acid, and 3% hydrogen peroxide. All four antiseptics were found to be cytotoxic, and all of the cytotoxic agents except hydrogen peroxide were found to adversely affect wound healing. Comparison of bactericidal and cytotoxic effects of serial dilutions of these four topical agents indicated the cellular toxicity of hydrogen peroxide and acetic acid exceeded their bactericidal potency. Bactericidal noncytotoxic dilutions of povidone-iodine (0.001%) and sodium hypochlorite (0.005%) were identified. Blenkharn[30] found 0.05% chlorhexidine but not noxythiolin to be cytotoxic to three lines of fibroblasts. Silver sulfadiazine has likewise been shown to have in vitro toxicity to human fibroblasts.[31]

In the rabbit ear chamber model, Brennan and Leaper[32] studied 1.0% and 5.0% povidone-iodine, chlorhexidine, hypochlorite (Euson, Chloramine T), hydrogen peroxide, and saline. All the antiseptics caused some adverse effects but the two hypochlorite antiseptics caused irreversible damage to capillary circulation of the granulation tissue, leading to a delay in wound healing. Aqueous chlorhexidine was found to be innocuous in this model.

Adverse effects on the host defense system may also counteract any benefit afforded by the reduction in numbers of viable bacteria. Aqueous povidone iodine is toxic to phagocytic cells at very low concentrations.[33] Sodium hypochlorite (Dakin's solution) has been found to inhibit neutrophil chemotaxis at low concentrations.[34]

Almost all agents are injurious to open wound tissues to varying degrees. Soaps increase tissue injury. Possibly, chlorhexidine or dilute solutions of sodium hypochlorite or povidone-iodine will offer some bactericidal ability without significantly damaging tissue. However, further studies are necessary to definitely prove efficacy and lack of tissue toxicity of these agents. Given the available toxicity data, continuous irrigation with any of the antiseptics cannot be recommended. Silver-based agents and their relationship to burns should be considered separately. The anti-adherence agents taurolidine and noxythiolin need to be further explored.

A great deal is known about the antiseptics including chemistry, mode of action, antimicrobial activity, duration of effect, and toxicity. Further studies documenting the interactions between antiseptics, bacteria, skin surfaces, wounds, and the immune system are needed to identify those clinical situations where antiseptic use is beneficial or harmful to the patient.

References

1. Efem SE: Clinical observations on the wound healing properties of honey. *Br J Surg* 1988;75:679–681.
2. Rideal S, Walker JTA: Standardisation of disinfectants. *J Sanit Inst* 1903;24:424.

3. Harvey SC: Antiseptics and disinfectants; fungicides; ecotparasiticides, in Gilman AG, Goodman LS, Rall TW, et al (eds): *Goodman and Gillman's The Pharmacological Basis of Therapeutics*, ed 7. New York, Macmillan, 1985, pp 959–979.

4. Laufman H: Current use of skin and wound cleansers and antiseptics. *Am J Surg* 1989;157:359–365.

5. Miller JM, Jackson DA, Collier CS: The microbicidal property of Phisohex. *Milit Med* 1962;127:576–578.

6. Chisholm TC, Duncan TL, Hufnagel CA, et al: Disinfecting action of phisoderm containing 3 percent hexachlorophene on the skin of hands. *Surgery* 1950;28:812–818.

7. Smith CR: Disinfection for tuberculous hygiene. *Soap Sanit Chem* 1951;2–6.

8. Price PB: Fallacy of a current surgical fad: The 3–minute preoperative scrub with hexachlorophene soap. *Ann Surg* 1951;134:476–485.

9. Rotter M: Are models useful for testing hand antiseptics? *J Hosp Infect* 1988;11(suppl A):236–243.

10. Hargiss C, Larson E: The epidemiology of *Staphylococcus aureus* in a newborn nursery from 1970 through 1976. *Pediatrics* 1978;61:348–353.

11. Price PB: Ethyl alcohol as a germicide. *Arch Surg* 1939;38:528–542.

12. Lineaweaver W, Howard R, Soucy D, et al: Topical antimicrobial toxicity. *Arch Surg* 1985;120:267–270.

13. Altemeier WA: Surgical antiseptics, in Block SS (ed): *Disinfection, Sterilization, and Preservation*, ed 3. Philadelphia, Lea & Febiger, 1983, pp 493–504.

14. Lavelle KJ, Doedens DJ, Kleit SA, et al: Iodine absorption in burn patients treated topically with povidone-iodine. *Clin Pharmacol Ther* 1975;17:355–362.

15. Blatt R, Maloney JV Jr: An evaluation of the iodophor compounds as surgical germicides. *Surg Gynecol Obstet* 1961;113:699–704.

16. Cotter JL, Fader RC, Lilley C, et al: Chemical parameters, antimicrobial activities, and tissue toxicity of 0.1 and 0.5% sodium hypochlorite solutions. *Antimicrob Agents Chemother* 1985;28:118–122.

17. Ayliffe GA, Noy MF, Babb JR, et al: A comparison of pre-operative bathing with chlorhexidine-detergent and non-medicated soap in the prevention of wound infection. *J Hosp Infect* 1983;4:237–244.

18. Gardner JF, Gray KG: Chlorhexidine, in Block SS (ed): *Disinfection, Sterilization, and Preservation*, ed 3. Philadelphia, Lea & Febiger, 1983, pp 251–270.

19. O'Neill J, Horner M, Challop RM, et al: Percutaneous absorption potential of chlorhexidine in neonates. *Curr Ther* 1982;31:435–437.

20. Ayliffe GAJ: Surgical scrub and skin disinfection. *Infect Control* 1984;5:23–27.

21. Ojajärvi J: An evaluation of antiseptics used for hand disinfection in wards. *J Hyg* 1976;76:75–82.

22. Larson EL, Laughon BE: Comparison of four antiseptic products containing chlorhexidine gluconate. *Antimicrob Agents Chemother* 1987;31:1572–1574.

23. Morton HE, North LL Jr, Engley FB Jr: The bacteriostatic and bactericidal actions of some mercurial compounds on hemolytic streptococci: In vivo and in vitro studies. Council on Pharmacy & Chemistry. *JAMA* 1948;136:37–41.

24. Sanford JP: Disinfectants that don't. *Ann Intern Med* 1970;72:282–283.

25. Blenkharn JI: Sustained anti-adherence activity of taurolidine (Taurolin) and noxythiolin (Noxyflex S) solutions. *J Pharm Pharmacol* 1988;40:509–511.

26. Gorman SP, McCafferty DF, Woolfson AD, et al: A comparative study of the microbial antiadherence capacities of three antimicrobial agents. *J Clin Pharm Ther* 1987;12:393–399.

27. Isenberg HD, D'Amato RF: Indigenous and pathogenic microorganisms of humans, in Lennette EH, Balows A, Hausler WJ Jr, et al (eds): *Manual of Clinical Microbiology*, ed 4. Washington, DC, American Society for Microbiology, 1985, pp 24–35.

28. Ayliffe GAJ, Babb JR, Davies JG, et al: Hand disinfection: A comparison of various agents in laboratory and ward studies. *J Hosp Infect* 1988;11:226–243.

29. Fleming A: The action of chemical and physiological antiseptics in a septic wound. *Br J Surg* 1919;7:99–129.

30. Blenkharn JI: The differential cytotoxicity of antiseptic agents. *J Pharm Pharmacol* 1987;39:477–479.

31. McCauley RL, Poole B, Heggers JP, et al: Differential in-vitro toxicity of topical antimicrobial agents to human keratinocytes, in *Proceedings of the 22nd Annual Meeting of the American Burn Association*. 1990, vol 22, p 2.

32. Brennan SS, Leaper DJ: The effect of antiseptics on the healing wound: A study using the rabbit ear chamber. *Br J Surg* 1985;72:780–782.

33. Van den Broek PJ, Buys LFM, Van Furth R: Interaction of povidone-iodine compounds, phagocytic cells, and microorganisms. *Antimicrob Agents Chemother* 1982;22:593–597.

34. Kozol RA, Gillies CD, Elgebaly SA: Effects of sodium hypochlorite (Dakin's solution) on cells of the wound module. *Arch Surg* 1988;123:420–423.

Future Directions

Role of Growth Factors

Although it is generally recognized that growth factors are involved in initiating or mediating many aspects of wound healing, the biological interrelationships of growth factors remain poorly understood. Continued experimental and clinical studies are suggested to broaden our understanding of how growth factors interact with each other and their target cells. The interrelationship of growth factors and their target cells in vivo is complex. A systematic investigation into the actions of growth factors in isolated environments is also warranted. The mechanism of action of growth factors such as Fibroblast Growth Factor remains unknown. Defining these mechanisms will be an important step if we are to use these agents therapeutically to augment normal wound healing and to aid in the prevention of musculoskeletal infection. Furthermore, local delivery systems for growth factors will have to be developed and evaluated.

Role of Oxygen

Although considerable data exist linking wound healing and resistance to infection with local tissue oxygen tension in general surgery populations, specific studies in the orthopaedic population are necessary. It will be interesting to see if orthopaedic patients receive similar benefits from techniques, such as sympathetic blockade, epidural analgesia, and temperature maintenance, that have proved to be promising in the general surgical population.

Studies are needed to determine the role of subcutaneous wound tissue oxygen tension ($Psqo_2$) monitoring in improving outcome in different subpopulations of orthopaedic patients. Measurement of $Psqo_2$ may provide valuable information on the adequacy of oxygen supply to the injured bone. The value of hyperbaric oxygen as an adjuvant in the treatment of osteomyelitis has been limited in part by the difficulty in defining which patients can be expected to benefit from such care. Measurement of $Psqo_2$ may make it possible to assess the probability of benefit to each individual patient and to guide interventions aimed at improving perfusion. Techniques to measure bone tissue oxygen tension should also be developed. This can likely be done by some adaptation of the current technology.

Increasing blood flow to infected bone could be of value in increasing the oxygen supply and aiding the healing process. The identification of agents with vasodilator actions on the microcirculation of bone would prove valuable.

Role of Nutrition

While it is clear that appropriate nutritional support will benefit the malnourished, it is not clear what is the ideal treatment for malnutrition in the surgical setting. While literature-supported protocols are being sought by general surgeons, studies are needed to define the unique problems and ideal approaches in orthopaedic populations. Elucidation of the roles of vitamin D, calcium, and phosphorus in normal metabolism requires further study, given the enormous role of these factors in bone healing. Further investigation into the optimal replacement of these factors during trauma, sepsis, and surgery is needed.

Our knowledge of nutritional status and outcome in orthopaedic patients remains limited. The development of techniques that will rapidly, accurately, and inexpensively assess nutritional status is crucial for providing guidelines for therapy. The following questions need to be answered: Are certain orthopaedic surgery populations at higher risk of being malnourished at the time of admission as well as following surgery? Can patient groups at increased risk of postoperative morbidity and mortality be identified? Can nutritional intervention, before and/or after surgery have a positive impact on patient outcome? Can we identify those patients who will benefit from nutritional supplementation? What is the true financial cost of malnutrition in orthopaedic patients? Studies to answer these questions should use research designs analogous to those used in epidemiological studies. They should be prospective and randomized. Special attention should be given to the nutritional indicators used to evaluate patients.

Role of Antibiotics and Antiseptics

There are still gains to be made in the antibiotic treatment of osteomyelitis. More studies are needed to clarify whether bactericidal agents are more effective than bacteriostatic ones. Are antibiotics with a postantibiotic effect more successful (Beta-lactam drugs for gram-positive cocci, aminoglycosides and quinolones for gram-negative bacilli)? Ideal dosing remains unclear. Are shorter intervals or constant infusions more effective than standard intermittent therapy? Preliminary studies suggest that oral fluoroquinoline therapy is as safe and effective as parenteral therapy in the treatment of chronic osteomyelitis. These conclusions need to be verified in other studies. Recently, parenteral ciprofloxacin has been made available. Does this become our parenteral therapy of choice in the treatment of osteomyelitis?

The emphasis on preventive medicine will increase in the upcoming years. Thus, defining optimal prophylaxis for orthopaedic procedures is of utmost importance. We do not know the ideal drug, dose, or duration of treatment for any prophylactic regimen. A review of the bacteriology of postoperative infections is warranted to see if any conclusions can be drawn about the antibiotic sensitivity of the responsible pathogens. A randomized, double-blind study would be the best way to define optimal prophylaxis. However, such a study would require an extremely high number of patients because of the low rates of perioperative wound infection after orthopaedic procedures. The priorities in such a study should include the numbers of perioperative doses of antibiotics required. A single preoperative dose makes the most sense, although some case reports have shown that postoperative wound infection can occur via the incision after the incision is closed. Any study of prophylaxis should look particularly at coagulase negative staphylococci, the most important perioperative pathogens in orthopaedic surgery. The efficacy of perioperative antibiotics in preventing infections in other sites, such as urinary catheters and in the lungs, also needs to be addressed. It is now known that patients become transiently bacteremic during dental procedures. The increased risk of musculoskeletal infection and optimal prophylaxis for particular orthopaedic patients (for example, those who have undergone total hip replacement or total knee arthroplasty) undergoing dental procedures needs to be defined.

The relationship between serum antibiotic concentrations and concentrations reaching the wound site remains inconsistent. We need better ways to achieve locally high concentrations of antibiotic in the wound tissue or ischemic bone. The evaluation of antibiotic release systems, such as pumps, biodegradable carriers, polymethylmethacrylate beads, and antibiotic cement combinations, is an area of great interest. Although in vitro and in vivo studies offer data to support their use, there are virtually no valuable data concerning the efficacy of these systems. Carefully designed controlled trials among comparable groups of patients need to be carried out.

In the future, a great deal of our energy should be directed toward the discovery of adjuvant treatments that might improve therapeutic success. Immobilization, electric fields, and stimulation of vascular growth are some examples of known technology that may improve our treatment results. The effectiveness of treating musculoskeletal infection with both nonsteroidal inflammatory medications and antibiotics needs to be evaluated.

A great deal is known about antiseptics, including chemistry, mode of action, antimicrobial activity, duration of effect, and toxicity. Further studies should examine the interactions between antiseptics, bacteria, skin surfaces, wounds, and the immune system. Clinical situations where antiseptic use is beneficial or harmful should be identified. An extensive review of the literature is warranted to determine more precisely the role of antiseptics in protecting the surgeon, in protecting the skin, and in wound treatment. Information concerning cost, side effects, immunosuppression, spectrum, and route of administration needs to be readily available. Other clinical uses for antiseptics, for example, in the treatment of Lyme disease and syphilis, should be sought.

Role of Analogs

Understanding the basic mechanisms of foreign body infection permits us to develop novel strategies for prevention and treatment. Now that we are beginning to understand the adhesin-ligand interaction as it pertains to the interaction between bacterial and host tissue, our efforts should be devoted to establishing a clinical role for analogs and analog-derived vaccines as antibacterial agents. We must pursue the discovery of new receptors to deal with problematic organisms such as *Staphylococcus epidermidis*. Short-term goals would be to establish the role for induction/expression of receptors and to explore differential affinity for tissue type (bone, cartilage, soft tissue). The potential efficacy of monoclonal antibodies in blocking the attachment of bacteria to biomaterials needs to be determined. An unexplored topic that merits interest is why some bacteria, for example, staphylococci, are common infectors of foreign bodies whereas others (streptococci) are less common and more easily eradicated.

Role of Advances in Surgical Technique

Despite advances in the treatment of musculoskeletal infection, the outcome of treatment of chronic osteomyelitis remains intimately linked with the adequacy of surgical debridement. If necrotic or infected tissue remains following surgical debridement, it is unlikely that antibiotic therapy will eradicate the infection. We need to develop better means of establishing clean margins both preoperatively and intraoperatively. Currently, preoperative imaging techniques, as well as intraoperative inspection of bone, are inadequate for determining the limits of the infectious process. A means of defining soft-tissue and bone viability needs to be developed. Current tools, such as magnetic resonance imaging and laser doppler flowmetry, need to be perfected. We also must determine how devitalized tissue and foreign material complicate wound healing. Guidelines for the appropriate type and timing of soft-tissue transfer procedures should be sought and established. The role of bone replacement techniques, such as bone grafting and Ilizarov technique, needs to be defined.

Role of the Operating Room Environment

A reevaluation of current operating room air-handling standards is warranted. Furthermore, there are no well-controlled studies that clearly support or refute the absolute need for laminar clean airflow rooms. According to the American College of Surgeons, a clean wound infection rate of less than 1% to 2% should be achievable with standard operating room air handling. They point out that it is not

449

reasonable to consider adding the capital cost, maintenance expense, noise, and communication problems of laminar clean airflow rooms until less expensive infection control measures are rigorously applied in daily practice.[1] Large-scale, well-controlled studies are needed to determine more precisely the risk of airborne particulate contamination in orthopaedic procedures, and the benefits of laminar clean

airflow systems in reducing contamination need to be quantified. Finally, our energies should be devoted to the discovery of newer, less expensive air-handling systems that are as effective as laminar flow.[1]

References

1. McQuarrie DG, Glover JL: Laminar airflow systems: A 1991 update. *Am Coll Surg Bul* 1991;76:18–23.

Index